Carbohydrate Intake in Non-Communicable Disease Prevention and Treatment

Carbohydrate Intake in Non-Communicable Disease Prevention and Treatment

Special Issue Editor

Bernard Venn

MDPI • Basel • Beijing • Wuhan • Barcelona • Belgrade

MDPI

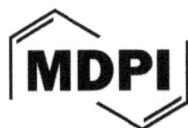

Special Issue Editor
Bernard Venn
University of Otago
New Zealand

Editorial Office
MDPI
St. Alban-Anlage 66
4052 Basel, Switzerland

This is a reprint of articles from the Special Issue published online in the open access journal *Nutrients* (ISSN 2072-6643) in 2018 (available at: https://www.mdpi.com/journal/nutrients/special_issues/carbohydrate_non-communicable)

For citation purposes, cite each article independently as indicated on the article page online and as indicated below:

LastName, A.A.; LastName, B.B.; LastName, C.C. Article Title. *Journal Name* **Year**, *Article Number, Page Range.*

ISBN 978-3-03897-818-3 (Pbk)
ISBN 978-3-03897-819-0 (PDF)

Contents

About the Special Issue Editor

Bernard Venn is a Senior Lecturer in the Department of Human Nutrition at the University of Otago, New Zealand. He teaches at undergraduate and postgraduate level to students of human nutrition and dietetics and supervises Masters (MSc and MDiet) and PhD candidates. Dr Venn has a longstanding interest in carbohydrate foods and in the food's carbohydrate components (sugars, starch, and fibre). His research has ranged from observational, laboratory benchtop through to human intervention trials. Collaboration with scientists at Plant and Food Research (Palmerston North, New Zealand) has enabled cross-discipline research to be undertaken between academia and a Crown Research Institute. Dr Venn participated in the Food and Agriculture Organization/World Health Organization's scientific update on carbohydrates in human nutrition, 2007. Dr Venn is research-active and enjoys his involvement in contemporary human nutrition through teaching and participating on editorial boards.

Preface to "Carbohydrate Intake in Non-Communicable Prevention and Treatment"

Carbohydrates contribute to the majority of dietary energy intake for most of the world's population. Humans' reliance on carbohydrate as an energy source dates back millennia and in more recent history, all large civilizations have depended on carbohydrate-rich food sources. Traditional diets of healthy populations have been based on starchy staple foods, for example: Corn in Mexico; rice in India and South-East Asia; wheat in the Middle East; Cassava and potatoes in South America; and soybeans in East Asia. Moves away from these traditional diets and lifestyles, enabled by an expanded range of foods, more refined products, a broader wealth base, and less active urban living are temporally associated with a greater burden of noncommunicable disease.In this Special Issue, carbohydrate foods were examined from a microbiota perspective, through to controlled trials on glycaemic and satiety outcomes, the impact of activity on glycaemia, assessing people's knowledge of carbohydrate, an intervention of a low carbohydrate diet, a review of potato in a healthy diet, and a review of the association between glycaemic index/load and non-communicable disease. Undoubtedly, carbohydrate-rich staple foods will continue to be major dietary components contributing both to the good health of people and to the sustainability of the Earth's resources. Given the importance of carbohydrate-rich foods, this is an area of research that will continue to flourish. I would like to acknowledge all of the contributing authors and the peer reviewers for their expertise and the staff at MDPI for their professionalism, enthusiasm, and efficiency.

Bernard Venn
Special Issue Editor

nutrients

MDPI

Article

Efficacy of a Moderately Low Carbohydrate Diet in a 36-Month Observational Study of Japanese Patients with Type 2 Diabetes

Mariko Sanada [1], Chinatsu Kabe [1], Hisa Hata [1], Junichi Uchida [1], Gaku Inoue [1], Yoko Tsukamoto [1], Yoshifumi Yamada [2], Junichiro Irie [3], Shogo Tabata [1], Mitsuhisa Tabata [1] and Satoru Yamada [1,*]

[1] Kitasato Institute Hospital, Diabetes Center, 5-9-1 Shirokane, Minato-ku, Tokyo 108-0072, Japan;
      mrksmd@insti.kitasato-u.ac.jp (M.S.); kabe@insti.kitasato-u.ac.jp (C.K.);
      h-izumi@insti.kitasato-u.ac.jp (H.H.); uchida-j@insti.kitasato-u.ac.jp (J.U.);
      inoueg@pharm.kitasato-u.ac.jp (G.I.); tsuka-y@insti.kitasato-u.ac.jp (Y.T.);
      sky_walker_718@a6.keio.jp (S.T.); mitsutabata@gmail.com (M.T.)
[2] Boei Ika Daigakko Boei Igagku Kenkyu Center, 3-2 Namiki, Tokorozawa, Saitama 359-0042, Japan;
      yamayoshi0718@yahoo.co.jp
[3] School of Medicine, Keio University, Internal Medicine, 35 Shinanomachi, Shinjuku, Tokyo 160-8582, Japan;
      j-irie@z8.keio.jp
*   Correspondence: yamada-s@insti.kitasato-u.ac.jp; Tel.: +81-3-3444-6161

Received: 27 March 2018; Accepted: 18 April 2018; Published: 24 April 2018

✓ check for updates

Abstract: We previously showed that a non-calorie-restricted, moderately low-carbohydrate diet (mLCD) is more effective than caloric restriction for glycemic and lipid profile control in patients with type 2 diabetes. To determine whether mLCD intervention is sustainable, effective, and safe over a long period, we performed a 36-month observational study. We sequentially enrolled 200 patients with type 2 diabetes and taught them how to follow the mLCD. We compared the following parameters pre- and post-dietary intervention in an outpatient setting: glycated hemoglobin (HbA1c), body weight, lipid profile (total cholesterol, low and high-density lipoprotein cholesterol, triglycerides), systolic and diastolic blood pressure, liver enzymes (aspartate aminotransferase, alanine aminotransferase), and renal function (urea nitrogen, creatinine, estimated glomerular filtration rate). Data from 157 participants were analyzed (43 were lost to follow-up). The following parameters decreased over the period of study: HbA1c (from $8.0 \pm 1.5\%$ to $7.5 \pm 1.3\%$, $p < 0.0001$) and alanine aminotransferase (from 29.9 ± 23.6 to 26.2 ± 18.4 IL/L, $p = 0.009$). Parameters that increased were high-density lipoprotein cholesterol (from 58.9 ± 15.9 to 61.2 ± 17.4 mg/dL, $p = 0.001$) and urea nitrogen (from 15.9 ± 5.2 to 17.0 ± 5.4 mg/dL, $p = 0.003$). Over 36 months, the mLCD intervention showed sustained effectiveness (without safety concerns) in improving HbA1c, lipid profile, and liver enzymes in Japanese patients with type 2 diabetes.

Keywords: low-carbohydrate diet; type 2 diabetes mellitus; observational study

1. Introduction

The most recent dietary guidelines of the American Diabetes Association (ADA) emphasize that no single diet is suitable for all people with diabetes, and likewise there is no ideal macronutrient balance [1]. Several dietary approaches have been proposed in Western countries for people with diabetes [1,2], with guidelines recommending that individuals discuss with health professionals (physicians and dietitians) which approach would be preferable, most effective, and sustainable for them.

Recently, the Japanese Diabetes Society relaxed their dietary approach, recommending a caloric restriction of 25–35 kcal/kg ideal body weight with carbohydrates composing 50–60% of total energy consumption. No other dietary approach is currently approved by the Japanese Diabetes Society guidelines [3]. In an endeavor to make dietary approaches more flexible and sustainable for diabetes patients in Japan, in August 2009 we adopted a non-calorie restricted, moderately low-carbohydrate diet (mLCD) with the approval of the Institutional Ethical Review Board of our hospital in Tokyo, Japan. In a randomized clinical trial, we found this mLCD to be more effective than caloric restriction for glycemic and lipid profile control in patients with type 2 diabetes [4]. However, this trial was limited to six months in duration. To evaluate the long-term efficacy and safety of mLCD as a sustainable dietary therapy and to check for rebound effects (which are common in dietary studies [5]), we conducted a 36-month observational study of patients with diabetes following our mLCD.

2. Materials and Methods

We retrospectively enrolled 200 patients with type 2 diabetes who received outpatient treatment in Kitasato Institute Hospital, Tokyo, Japan between August 2009 and October 2016. Participants were instructed to restrict their carbohydrate intake to 20–40 g per meal and 70–130 g per day, with 10 g of carbohydrates consumed as a snack or drink at least once daily. Although we did not recommend any percentage of carbohydrate, fat, and protein to total caloric intake, it was 30:45:20 in our previous study [4]. A dietary salt restriction intervention was also performed on patients for whom it was deemed appropriate. Patients who injected insulin were recommended to monitor their capillary glucose levels frequently after mLCD was initiated.

At the first nutritional intervention and at six-month intervals thereafter, we measured the following: glycated hemoglobin (HbA1c), body weight, lipid profile (total cholesterol (TC), low-density lipoprotein cholesterol (LDL-C), high-density lipoprotein cholesterol (HDL-C), triglyceride (TG)), blood pressure (systolic blood pressure (SBP), diastolic blood pressure (DBP)), liver enzymes (aspartate aminotransferase (AST), alanine aminotransferase (ALT)), and renal function (urea nitrogen (UN), uric acid (UA), creatinine (Cr), estimated glomerular filtration rate (eGFR)). We also recorded the incidence of hypoglycemia (defined as self-monitored blood glucose levels less than 70 mg/dL, with or without hypoglycemic symptoms) for 2 months before the first intervention and for 2-month intervals during the intervention, and calculated the corresponding before/after ratios. Missing values were replaced with values obtained during the previous or following two months.

To investigate the interactions between response to the mLCD and participant baseline HbA1c level or body mass index (BMI, kg/m^2), we conducted post hoc analyses. In one analysis, we classified participants according to their change in HbA1c during the 36 months of dietary intervention as follows: responder (decrease in HbA1c), unchanged (no change in HbA1c), or worsened (increase in HbA1c). In other analyses, we classified participants according to their baseline HbA1c (HbA1c < 7%, 7% ≤ HbA1c < 8%, 8% ≤ HbA1c < 9%, or 9% ≤ HbA1c) or BMI (BMI < 25, 25 ≤ BMI < 30, or 30 ≤ BMI).

Values are presented as the mean ± standard deviation (SD). Statistical analyses were performed using IBM SPSS 19 software (IBM Japan, Tokyo, Japan). We compared baseline and 36-month parameter values using the Wilcoxon signed-rank test. Multiple comparisons were made as appropriate using two-way analysis of variance (ANOVA).

This study was approved by the institutional review board of Kitasato Institution Hospital and performed in accordance with the Declaration of Helsinki. Informed consent was obtained in the form of an opt-out, by posting notices requesting that diabetes patients who had received guidance about low carbohydrate diets inform us if they did not want their records to be used for research purposes. This consent process was approved by the ethical review board at Kitasato Institution Hospital. All participants' anonymity is preserved. This study was registered as clinical trial ID UMIN000022910.

3. Results

The characteristics of the 200 patients enrolled are shown in Table 1. Of these, 43 participants were lost to follow-up during the 36-month study period. The most common reasons for drop-out were a discontinuation of visits to our hospital (n = 24) and referral to general physicians (n = 15). The other four participants lost to follow-up died (two from myocardial infarction, one from cardiac arrest, and one from a head injury). There were no differences in the baseline characteristics between the 43 patients who dropped out and the remaining 157.

Table 1. Baseline characteristics of the study participants

	All Participants	Retained	Lost to Follow-Up
n	200	157	43
Female/Male	71/129	51/106	20/23
Age	59.7 ± 12.9	59.5 ± 12.4	60.5 ± 13.9
BMI (kg/m^2)	26.4 ± 4.9	26.6 ± 4.7	25.4 ± 5.1
FPG (mg/dL)	151 ± 57	153 ± 58	145 ± 50
HbA1c (%)	8.0 ± 1.5	8.0 ± 1.5	8.0 ± 1.5
TG (mg/dL)	147 ± 120	147 ± 121	144 ± 106
LDL-C (mg/dL)	116 ± 33	116 ± 33	121 ± 45
HDL-C (mg/dL)	60 ± 17	59 ± 16	62 ± 21
BP (mmHg)	128 ± 15/76 ± 12	128 ± 15/77 ± 12	127 ± 16/72 ± 12

Values are the mean ± standard deviation. BMI, body mass index; FPG, fasting plasma glucose; HbA1c, glycated hemoglobin; TG, triglyceride; LDL-C, low-density lipoprotein cholesterol; HDL-C, high-density lipoprotein cholesterol; BP, blood pressure.

Among the 157 patients, HbA1c levels had improved (decreased) in 104 participants (i.e., the responder rate was 66.2%), remained unchanged in 10 participants, and worsened (increased) in 43 patients at 36 months after first mLCD intervention. From baseline to 36 months, there were statistically significant improvements in HbA1c (decrease), DBP (decrease), TC (decrease), LDL-C (increase), and ALT (decrease) (Table 2). For HbA1c levels, the improvement occurred during the first 6 months and was maintained through 36 months (Figures 1 and 2). The UN level increased significantly over 36 months, while Cr and eGFR showed no change. No significant changes were observed during the study period for body weight, HDL-C, TG, SBP, AST, or UA (Table 2). The record of hypoglycemic agents showed that the number of participants taking insulin injections and/or sulfonylureas did not change during the study period. As for dosage, the mean total daily dose of insulin per person decreased from 29.9 units at the start of the intervention to 23.6 units at 36 months post-intervention. The mean dose of glimepiride (which all sulfonylurea users were prescribed) per person also decreased, from 1.39 mg at the start of the intervention to 1.11 mg at 36 months. Participants who reduced their insulin and/or glimepiride dosage started taking metformin and/or dipeptidyl peptidase-4 inhibitors instead. Thus, the number of participants taking metformin and dipeptidyl peptidase-4 inhibitors increased during the 36 months (from 71 to 89 and 48 to 93, respectively).

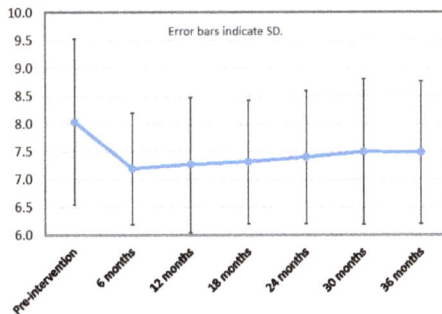

Figure 1. HbA1c level (%). Error bars indicate standard deviation (n = 157).

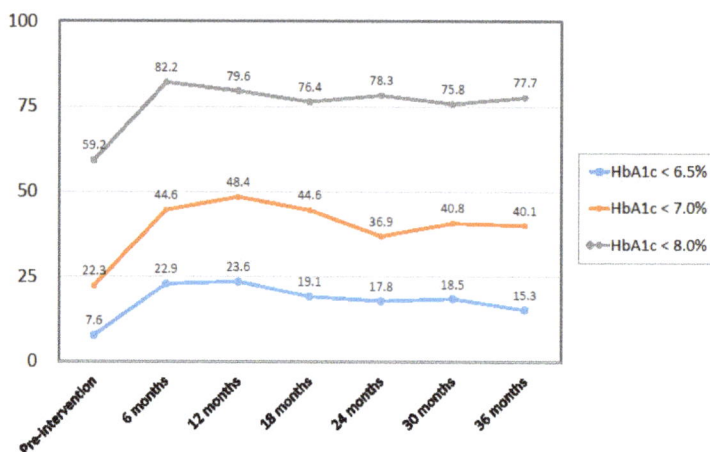

Figure 2. Percentage of patients who reached target HbA1c levels (%).

During the 36 months, there was also an increase in the prescription of anti-hyperlipidemic agents. Thus, we performed a last-observation carried forward (LOCF) analysis on lipid profiles using the values when anti-hyperlipidemic agents were started or when their dosages increased. This analysis showed that LOCF TC improved, and LOCF TG worsened (Table 2).

Table 2. Changes in the outcome measures of study participants on a moderately low-carbohydrate diet over 36 months.

	Pre-Intervention	12 Months	24 Months	36 Months	*p* Value
Body weight (kg)	72.5 ± 15.2	71.6 ± 14.9	72.0 ± 15.0	71.9 ± 15.1	n.s.
FBS (mg)	153.1 ± 58.0	143.3 ± 47.2	144.4 ± 48.6	140.6 ± 43.5	n.s.
SBP (mmHg)	127.7 ± 15.4	125.8 ± 13.3	127.1 ± 13.1	125.0 ± 13.1	n.s.
DBP (mmHg)	76.8 ± 11.8	74.8 ± 10.9	75.4 ± 9.5	74.5 ± 10.6	0.029
HbA1c (%)	8.0 ± 1.5	7.3 ± 1.2	7.4 ± 1.2	7.5 ± 1.3	<0.0001
TC (mg/dL)	200.7 ± 44.1	194.0 ± 39.0	192.8 ± 32.9	189.9 ± 33.3	0.003
LDL-C (mg/dL)	116.1 ± 33.0	107.2 ± 28.2	108.1 ± 26.7	106.7 ± 26.9	<0.0001
HDL-C (mg/dL)	59.0 ± 15.9	61.7 ± 16.7	61.2 ± 16.9	59.8 ± 18.3	n.s.
TG (mg/dL)	146.6 ± 120.7	142.7 ± 137.4	141.2 ± 102.9	152.5 ± 122.2	n.s.
LOCF TC (mg/dL)	200.8 ± 44.1	196.2 ± 40.3	196.2 ± 35.9	189.9 ± 33.3	0.0007
LOCF LDL-C (mg/dL)	116.1 ± 33.0	109.0 ± 29.7	110.6 ± 29.7	106.7 ± 26.9	n.s.
LOCF HDL-C (mg/dL)	59.1 ± 15.9	61.4 ± 16.4	61.3 ± 16.7	59.8 ± 18.3	n.s.
LOCF TG (mg/dL)	146.5 ± 120.7	147.7 ± 139.6	144.7 ± 113.6	152.5 ± 122.2	0.02
AST (IU/L)	26.6 ± 13.3	24.2 ± 10.8	25.1 ± 11.7	26.4 ± 13.6	n.s.
ALT (IU/L)	29.9 ± 23.6	23.4 ± 15.3	25.1 ± 18.5	26.2 ± 18.4	0.009
Cr (mg/dL)	0.8 ± 0.2	0.8 ± 0.2	0.8 ± 0.2	0.8 ± 0.2	0.046
eGFR (mL/(min·1.73 m^2))	74.4 ± 18.8	73.6 ± 19.2	73.1 ± 19.0	72.1 ± 20.8	0.007
UA (mg/dL)	5.8 ± 1.4	5.9 ± 1.4	5.9 ± 1.4	6.0 ± 1.7	n.s.
UN (mg/dL)	15.8 ± 5.0	17.5 ± 6.2	16.8 ± 5.0	17.0 ± 5.5	0.002
ACR (mg/g Cr)	196.6 ± 828.0	123.6 ± 517.1	166.4 ± 515.1	123.3 ± 287.4	n.s.
Urinary protein	(−)* 91 (58%) (+/−)* 38 (24%) (1+) * 20 (13%) (2+) * 8 (5%)	102 (65%) 38 (24%) 14 (9%) 3 (2%)	92 (59%) 40 (25%) 17 (11%) 8 (5%)	99 (63%) 31 (20%) 23 (15%) 4 (2%)	n.s. †

† Result of a chi-square test. Values are the mean ± standard deviation or number (percentage) of participants. * Although urinary protein test is qualitative, these content were similar with below; (−) 10 mg/dL, (+/−) 10–20 mg/dL, (1+) 100 mg/dL, (2+) 300 mg/dL. FBS, fasting blood sugar; SBP, systolic blood pressure; DBP, diastolic blood pressure; HbA1c, glycated hemoglobin; TC, total cholesterol; LDL-C, low-density lipoprotein cholesterol; HDL-C, high-density lipoprotein cholesterol; TG, triglyceride; LOCF, last-observation carried forward; AST, aspartate aminotransferase; ALT, alanine aminotransferase; Cr, creatinine; eGFR, estimated glomerular filtration rate; UA, uric acid; UN, urea nitrogen; ACR, albumin to creatinine ratio (from random spot urine sampling); n.s., not significant.

Of the 43 participants receiving insulin, 31 maintained blood glucose self-monitoring records. Among these 31 participants, the incidence of hypoglycemia was 1.46% before the introduction of mLCD, which then increased to a maximum of 2.43% for 1–2 months after the first intervention. Several months later, the incidence of hypoglycemia stabilized at approximately 1.0% (Table 3).

Table 3. Incidence of hypoglycemia in the 31 participants who received insulin and maintained blood glucose self-monitoring records while on a moderately low-carbohydrate diet for 36 months.

2-Month Pre-Intervention Period	1 to 2 Months	3 to 4 Months	5 to 6 Months	7 to 8 Months	9 to 10 Months	11 to 12 Months
31/2121 (1.46%)	73/3010 (2.43%)	60/2887 (2.08%)	39/2387 (1.63%)	49/2709 (1.81%)	53/2367 (2.24%)	17/2098 (0.81%)
	13 to 14 months	15 to 16 months	17 to 18 months	19 to 20 months	21 to 22 months	23 to 24 months
	44/2698 (1.63%)	26/2634 (0.99%)	26/2544 (1.02%)	12/2347 (0.51%)	30/2430 (1.23%)	20/2562 (0.78%)
	25 to 26 months	27 to 28 months	29 to 30 months	31 to 32 months	33 to 34 months	35 to 36 months
	19/2361 (0.80%)	26/2657 (0.98%)	23/2609 (0.88%)	33/2711 (1.22%)	44/2748 (1.60%)	31/3066 (1.01%)

Values are the number of hypoglycemic readings/total number of readings (percent incidence of hypoglycemia).

To identify characteristics of participants who responded to the mLCD, we classified the 157 participants according to their change in HbA1c levels from baseline to 36 months as either responders, unchanged non-responders, or worsened non-responders. At baseline, the responders were younger and had higher HbA1c levels than the other two groups (Table 4). We also classified participants according to their baseline HbA1c levels and found that the HbA1c ≥ 9% group had the greatest improvement in HbA1c (Figure 3). On the other hand, the ALT ≥ 9% group had the greatest improvement in ALT. Change in body weight was independent of baseline HbA1c.

Table 4. Baseline characteristics of participants classified as responders or non-responders according to their change in HbA1c levels over the 36-month study period.

Characteristic	All (n = 157)	Responders (n = 109)	Non-Responders	
			Worsened (n = 41)	Unchanged (n = 7)
Age (years)	59.5	57.7	63.8	62.6
BMI (kg/m^2)	26.6	26.9	26.2	25.3
FPG (mg/dL)	153	159	144	116
HbA1c (%)	8.0	8.3	7.4	7.0
TG (mg/dL)	147	159	119	112
LDL-C (mg/dL)	116	118	112	115
HDL-C (mg/dL)	59.0	56.9	61.8	76.6
BP (mmHg)	128/77	128/78	128/74	122/72
Dietary education sessions	2.2	2.3	2.2	2.1
Disease duration (years)	10.0	9.7	10.6	11.3

Values are the means. BMI, body mass index; FPG, fasting plasma glucose; HbA1c, glycated hemoglobin; TG, triglyceride; LDL-C, low-density lipoprotein cholesterol; HDL-C, high-density lipoprotein cholesterol; BP, blood pressure.

We then classified the participants according to baseline BMI. While HbA1c decreased independently of baseline BMI level, the change in body weight across the study period differed between BMI groups. While participants with a baseline BMI < 25 showed sustained body weight, and those with BMI ≥ 25 showed a decrease in body weight (Figure 4).

Although two participants experienced myocardial infarction and died, there was no incidence of stroke, peripheral artery disease, renal dysfunction, or liver dysfunction among the participants in this study. The two patients who died from myocardial infarction had a 10+ year history of diabetes and presented multiple risk factors including hypertension, type IIb dyslipidemia, obesity, and a history of smoking.

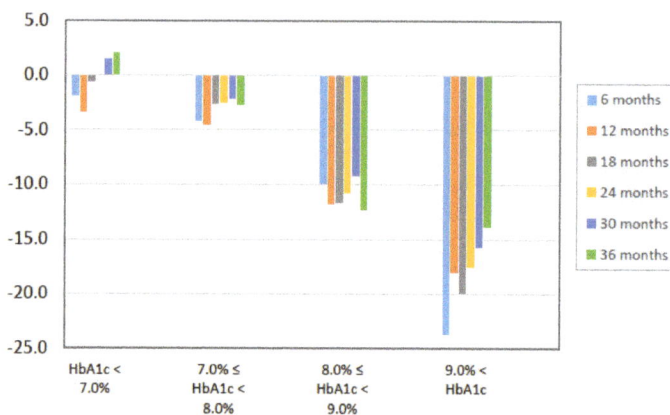

Figure 3. Percent changes in HbA1c stratified by baseline HbA1c (%).

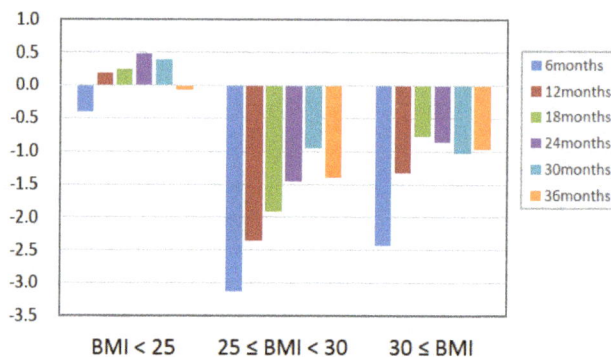

Figure 4. Absolute changes in body weight stratified by baseline BMI (kg).

4. Discussion

This study has three noteworthy aspects. First, this study is a long-term (36 months) observational study on a dietary approach for diabetes. To the best of our knowledge, this is the first long-term observational study on such a diet in East Asians. This moderately low-carbohydrate diet improved HbA1c levels within the first 6 months and then maintained that improvement for 36 months. According to the recently published ADA Standards of Medical Care [6], the effects of low-carbohydrate diets remain unclear because any improvements by such a diet tend to occur on a short-term basis and are not maintained. As described by the ADA, the wide range of definitions for a low-carbohydrate diet have created confusion. According to our current data, the improvements caused by a moderately low-carbohydrate diet can be maintained. Furthermore, the fact that East Asians have traditionally consumed a high-carbohydrate diet may explain the finding that a moderately low-carbohydrate diet is effective in reducing HbA1c in this population.

Second, we found that a moderately low-carbohydrate diet improved HbA1c levels without causing undernutrition in non-obese patients with diabetes. Previous dietary approaches for diabetes have been considered successful if they result in weight loss. While this may be acceptable for white and black patients with type 2 diabetes, almost all of whom are obese [7,8], such diets might cause undernutrition in East Asians who develop diabetes in the absence of obesity [9]. In fact, there have been almost no studies of East Asians consuming a Mediterranean diet or the DASH diet. The CALERIE trial indicated that caloric restrictions cause loss of muscle and bone mineral density in non-obese individuals [10,11]. Thus, a moderately low-carbohydrate diet might be a safe dietary approach for East Asians or diabetics who are not obese.

Third, our findings indicate the safety of a moderately low-carbohydrate diet. Diminished kidney function and a worse lipid profile are common concerns with a restricted carbohydrate diet [12]. In the current study, there were statistically significant changes in kidney function (eGFR; from 74.4 ± 18.8 to 72.1 ± 20.8 (mL/(min·1.73 m^2)) during 36 months) and lipid profiles, but those changes were either not clinically significant. As for kidney function it may represent improvements compared with previous data, which have shown an annual eGFR decline of 0.7–2.0 mL/(min·1.73 m^2) in diabetic patients [13,14]. In addition, the frequency of hypoglycemia increased in our patients using a sulfonylurea or insulin, but those patients recovered once the dose of that medication was adjusted. We therefore conclude that a moderately low-carbohydrate diet is a highly safe diet.

As for low-carbohydrate diets, there is a controversy whether high fat or high protein is more beneficial. Most of previous studies of low-carbohydrate diets were high fat and Feinman et al. described high fat as being recommended in general [15]. However, meta-analysis of Clifton et al. showed the importance of protein [16]. Our current study did not provide any information to this controversy.

This study has several limitations. Because this was an observational study and it did not compare subjects to a control group, bias, and confounding factors cannot be ruled out. In addition, the sample size of 200 patients precluded any examination of the effects of the low-carbohydrate diet on cancer or dementia.

In conclusion, we have shown that a moderately low-carbohydrate diet is highly effective, safe, and sustainable. To address the study's limitations, large-scale long-term randomized controlled trials should be conducted in the future.

Acknowledgments: This study was funded by a Kitasato Institute Hospital Research Grant (Grant No. 8125).

Author Contributions: M.S. analyzed the data and wrote the manuscript. J.U., H.H. and C.K. conceived and designed the experiments. Y.Y., J.I., S.T. and M.T. performed the experiments. G.I. and Y.T. analyzed the data. S.Y. conceived and designed the experiments, performed the experiments, and analyzed the data.

Conflicts of Interest: The authors report no conflicts of interest related to this work.

References

1. Evert, A.B.; Boucher, J.L.; Cypress, M.; Dunbar, S.A.; Franz, M.J.; Mayer-Davis, E.J.; Neumiller, J.J.; Nwankwo, R.; Verdi, C.L.; Urbanski, P.; et al. Nutrition therapy recommendations for the management of adults with diabetes. *Diabetes Care* **2013**, *36*, 3821–3842. [CrossRef] [PubMed]
2. Ley, S.H.; Hamdy, O.; Mohan, V.; Hu, F.B. Prevention and management of type 2 diabetes: Dietary components and nutritional strategies. *Lancet* **2014**, *383*, 1999–2007. [CrossRef]
3. Tajima, N.; Noda, M.; Origasa, H.; Noto, H.; Yabe, D.; Fujita, Y.; Goto, A.; Fujimoto, K.; Sakamoto, M.; Haneda, M. Evidence-based practice guideline for the treatment for diabetes in Japan 2013. *Diabetol. Int.* **2015**, *6*, 151–187. [CrossRef]
4. Yamada, Y.; Uchida, J.; Izumi, H.; Tsukamoto, Y.; Inoue, G.; Watanabe, Y.; Irie, J.; Yamada, S. A non-calorie-restricted low-carbohydrate diet is effective as an alternative therapy for patients with type 2 diabetes. *Intern. Med.* **2014**, *53*, 13–19. [CrossRef] [PubMed]
5. Banasik, J.L.; Walker, M.K.; Randall, J.M.; Netjes, R.B.; Foutz, M.S. Low-calorie diet induced weight loss may alter regulatory hormones and contribute to rebound visceral adiposity in obese persons with a family history of type-2 diabetes. *J. Am. Assoc. Nurse Pract.* **2013**, *25*, 440–448. [CrossRef] [PubMed]
6. American Diabetes Association. Lifestyle management: Standards of medical care in diabetes-2018. *Diabetes Care* **2018**, *41*, S38–S50. [CrossRef]
7. Looker, H.C.; Knowler, W.C.; Hanson, R.L. Changes in BMI and weight before and after the development of type 2 diabetes. *Diabetes Care* **2001**, *24*, 1917–1922. [CrossRef] [PubMed]
8. De Fine Olivarius, N.; Richelsen, B.; Siersma, V.; Andreasen, A.H.; Beck-Nielsen, H. Weight history of patients with newly diagnosed Type 2 diabetes. *Diabet. Med.* **2008**, *25*, 933–941. [CrossRef] [PubMed]

9. Heianza, Y.; Arase, Y.; Kodama, S.; Tsuji, H.; Saito, K.; Hara, S.; Sone, H. Trajectory of body mass index before the development of type 2 diabetes in Japanese men: Toranomon Hospital Health Management Center Study 15. *J. Diabetes Investig.* **2015**, *6*, 289–294. [CrossRef] [PubMed]
10. Villareal, D.T.; Fontana, L.; Das, S.K.; Redman, L.; Smith, S.R.; Saltzman, E.; Bales, C.; Rochon, J.; Pieper, C.; Huang, M.; et al. Effect of two-year caloric restriction on bone metabolism and bone mineral density in non-obese younger adults: A randomized clinical trial. *J. Bone Miner. Res.* **2016**, *31*, 40–51. [CrossRef] [PubMed]
11. Das, S.K.; Roberts, S.B.; Bhapkar, M.V.; Villareal, D.T.; Fontana, L.; Martin, C.K.; Racette, S.B.; Fuss, P.J.; Kraus, W.E.; Wong, W.W.; et al. Body-composition changes in the Comprehensive Assessment of Long-term Effects of Reducing Intake of Energy (CALERIE)-2 study: A 2-y randomized controlled trial of calorie restriction in nonobese humans. *Am. J. Clin. Nutr.* **2017**, *105*, 913–927. [CrossRef] [PubMed]
12. American Diabetes Association; Bantle, J.P.; Wylie-Rosett, J.; Albright, A.L.; Apovian, C.M.; Clark, N.G.; Franz, M.J.; Hoogwerf, B.J.; Lichtenstein, A.H.; Mayer-Davis, E.; et al. Nutrition recommendations and interventions for diabetes: A position statement of the American Diabetes Association. *Diabetes Care* **2008**, *31*, S61–S78. [CrossRef] [PubMed]
13. Araki, S.; Haneda, M.; Koya, D.; Isshiki, K.; Kume, S.; Sugimoto, T.; Kawai, H.; Nishio, Y.; Kashiwagi, A.; Uzu, T. Association between urinary type IV collagen level and deterioration of renal function in type 2 diabetic patients without overt proteinuria. *Diabetes Care* **2010**, *33*, 1805–1810. [CrossRef] [PubMed]
14. Araki, S.; Haneda, M.; Koya, D.; Sugaya, T.; Isshiki, K.; Kume, S.; Kashiwagi, A.; Uzu, T.; Maegawa, H. Predictive effects of urinary liver-type fatty acid-binding protein for deteriorating renal function and incidence of cardiovascular disease in type 2 diabetic patients without advanced nephropathy. *Diabetes Care* **2013**, *36*, 1248–1253. [CrossRef] [PubMed]
15. Feinman, R.D.; Pogozelski, W.K.; Astrup, A.; Bernstein, R.K.; Fine, E.J.; Westman, E.C.; Accurso, A.; Frassetto, L.; Gower, B.A.; McFarlane, S.I.; et al. Dietary carbohydrate restriction as the first approach in diabetes management. *Nutrition* **2015**, *31*, 1–13. [CrossRef] [PubMed]
16. Clifton, P.M.; Condo, D.; Keogh, J.B. Long term weight maintenance after advice to consume low carbohydrate, higher protein diets. *Nutr. Metab. Cardiovasc. Dis.* **2014**, *24*, 224–235. [CrossRef] [PubMed]

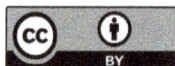

nutrients

MDPI

Article

Postprandial Glycaemic, Hormonal and Satiety Responses to Rice and Kiwifruit Preloads in Chinese Adults: A Randomised Controlled Crossover Trial

Alex Lubransky [1], John Monro [2,*], Suman Mishra [2], Hui Yu [1], Jillian J. Haszard [1] and Bernard J. Venn [1]

[1] Department of Human Nutrition, University of Otago, P.O. Box 56, Dunedin 9054, New Zealand; alex.lubransky@gmail.com (A.L.); yuev5129@student.otago.ac.nz (H.Y.); jill.haszard@otago.ac.nz (J.J.H.); bernard.venn@otago.ac.nz (B.J.V.)

[2] New Zealand Institute for Plant & Food Research Ltd., Private Bag 11600, Palmerston North 4442, New Zealand; Suman.Mishra@plantandfood.co.nz

* Correspondence: John.Monro@plantandfood.co.nz; Tel.: +64-6355-6137

Received: 26 July 2018; Accepted: 14 August 2018; Published: 17 August 2018

check for updates

Abstract: Controlling postprandial glycaemia helps to prevent and manage non-communicable diseases. One strategy in controlling glycaemia may be to consume meals in two parts; a preload, followed by the remainder of the meal. Our aim was to test preloading a rice meal given for breakfast and lunch on different days, either by splitting the meal (rice preload followed by rice meal) or by using kiwifruit as a preload compared with consuming the rice meal in one sitting. Primary outcomes were glycaemic and insulinaemic responses with secondary outcomes of other hormonal responses, subjective satiety, and subsequent energy intake. Following breakfast, postprandial glycaemic peak concentration was 0.9 (95% CI: 0.2, 1.6) mmol/L lower for the kiwifruit preload compared with the rice meal eaten in one sitting. Following lunch, glycaemic peak concentrations were 1.0 (0.7, 1.4) and 1.1 (0.5, 1.7) mmol/L lower for the rice-split and kiwifruit preload compared with the rice meal alone, respectively. Postprandial insulinaemia area-under-the-curve was 1385 (87, 2684) mU/L·min less for the kiwifruit preload compared with the rice-split. There were no differences among treatments for subsequent energy intake. Meal splitting is useful for lowering postprandial glycaemia, and replacing part of a meal with kiwifruit may help with insulin efficiency without detriment to subsequent energy intake.

Keywords: fructose; glycaemia; insulinaemia; preload; kiwifruit; fruit

1. Introduction

Given the worldwide prevalence of prediabetes and diabetes mellitus, there is interest in managing postprandial blood glucose concentration [1]. One strategy has been to advise people to eat fatty or high protein foods before eating the carbohydrate portion of a meal [2]. The rationale for this is that a fat preload delays gastric emptying and dampens glycaemia [3,4], and a protein preload reduces glycaemia by stimulating insulin [5,6]. However, the type of fatty acids ingested with carbohydrate has health implications, as diets enriched with *trans*- and saturated fatty acids increased postprandial insulinaemia relative to a baseline diet containing an equivalent amount of fat, a metabolic state indicative of post-meal insulin resistance [7]. Although co-ingestion of fat and carbohydrate may effectively reduce glycaemia, consumer knowledge about the types of fatty acids is poor, and the consumer perception of dietary fat as being unhealthy may preclude widespread uptake of this strategy [8]. While carbohydrate co-ingested with 25 g protein contained in beef, turkey, gelatin, egg white, cottage cheese, fish, or soy foods has been found to reduce postprandial glycaemia, in each case, this was accompanied by a 2- to 4-fold increase in postprandial insulin [9]. Increases in postmeal insulin may be undesirable, as postprandial hyperinsulinemia has been found to be independently associated with coronary artery disease risk among women without diabetes [10]. For people with type 2 diabetes, the use of an insulin-stimulating drug has been associated with adverse cardiovascular outcomes [11] and there is evidence to suggest that protein restriction may slow the progression of diabetic kidney disease [12]. Thus, the use of protein to increase postprandial insulin may be contraindicated in people with and without diabetes [10,12].

Other options for controlling glycaemia include manipulating the frequency of meals [13]. It has been found that compared with three larger meals, smaller meals consumed throughout the day reduced glycaemic and insulinaemic fluctuations and improved postprandial insulin sensitivity [14,15]. The inclusion of fruit (raisins) in a starchy meal (oats) had no deleterious effect on postprandial glycaemia and insulinaemia in people with type 2 diabetes [16]. The addition or introduction of fruit into diets may be useful because whole-fruit consumption has been associated with a lower risk of type 2 diabetes [17]. Fruit consumption is consistent with dietary advice, as given by health authorities across Europe and North America [18–20]. Despite these recommendations, the inclusion of sugars in the diet has attracted negative publicity, with fructose being of particular concern [21]. Thus, an apparent contradiction arises in that fruit (containing fructose) is healthy, while the metabolism of fructose is suggestive of potentially harmful effects [22]. This has led to commentary that fructose is only a problem when consumed in excess from processed foods as a component of sucrose or high fructose corn syrup, and that fruit can be tolerated by humans in large quantities [23].

These observations led us to speculate that splitting a predominantly carbohydrate-containing meal (white rice) might have glycaemic benefit over consuming the rice in one sitting; in effect, creating a carbohydrate preload of rice followed by the remainder of the rice meal. An expansion of this concept involved the replacement of the rice preload on an equi-carbohydrate basis with kiwifruit. The purpose of replacing rice starch with kiwifruit sugars derives from the fructose component of kiwifruit, as fructose is less glycaemic and less insulinaemic compared with glucose [24]. Additional benefits from substituting kiwifruit for cereal may be obtained from kiwifruit properties that retard physical processes of carbohydrate digestion in vitro [25]. In vivo, it has been found that kiwifruit co-ingested with cereal reduces postprandial glycaemic responses in comparison to the cereal ingested alone, by more than could be explained by simple fructose substitution of starch [26]. Neither the acute effects of meal-splitting nor kiwifruit-for-starch preload substitution on postprandial glycaemic, hormonal, and satiety responses have been tested. From previously published work, an appropriate time interval between the preload and the remainder of the meal is 30 min, a time lapse that has been recommended to investigate gastrointestinal and satiety effects [27]. Indeed, the compensation of energy intake compared with no preload was most precise when a 30 min interval was used, compared with longer time intervals [28]. A priori, the study was designed for Chinese participants, as postprandial glycaemia has been found to be higher in Chinese people compared with people of European descent [29].

Hence, the primary aims of this research were to establish whether meal-splitting and incorporating kiwifruit into a starchy meal by carbohydrate exchange would be beneficial in terms of postprandial glycaemic and insulinaemic responses compared to a single rice meal, with secondary aims of measuring other postprandially affected hormones and monitoring the satiety of the meals in healthy adults. In practice, people might split a meal or substitute a preload at different meals; thus, the experiment was to be carried out both at breakfast time and at lunch time on separate days, with a two-day washout.

2. Materials and Methods

2.1. Ethics and Design

The study was approved by the University of Otago Human Ethics Committee (Health), reference H16/066, dated 9th June, 2016. This study has been registered with the Australian and New Zealand Clinical Trials Registry ACTRN12616000771459.

The trial used an unblinded, randomised, repeated measures cross-over design with 30 participants (Figure 1). Participants were allocated randomly to undertake the breakfast or lunch testing first. The treatment order was then randomised separately for breakfast and lunch testing.

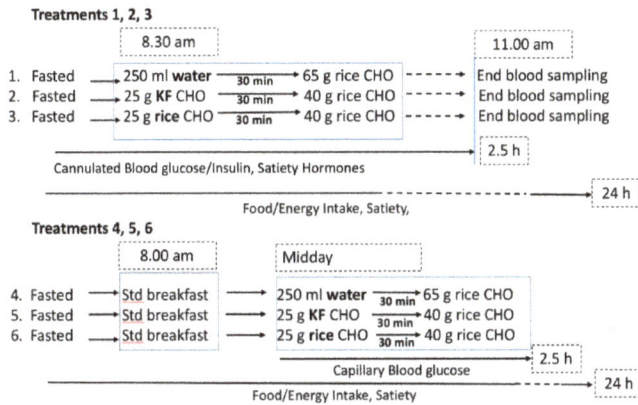

Figure 1. Summary of experimental design. KF = kiwifruit; CHO = carbohydrate, Std breakfast = standard breakfast.

2.2. Meal Components

Kiwifruit (*Actinidia chinensis* var. *chinensis* 'Zesy002', marketed as Zespri®SunGold Kiwifruit) of export quality were provided in a ready-to-eat state of ripeness by Zespri International Limited, Tauranga, New Zealand. The carbohydrate content of the kiwifruit was determined by standard colourimetric methods from the fructose and glucose content after preliminary amyloglucosidase and invertase hydrolysis. Zespri International Ltd provided the nutritional composition of kiwifruit (Table 1) except that the available carbohydrate content was measured directly on the fruit used in the trial at the Plant and Food Research Laboratories by extraction with 80% ethanol, hydrolyzing an aliquot with invertase, and measuring total reducing sugars and fructose colorimetrically (Glucose:fructose 0.94:1) Starch was not measured, as previous analyses have shown that it constitutes only about 1% of available carbohydrate in ripe SunGold kiwifruit [30].

The rice meal consisted of a rice porridge served in a chicken-flavoured broth as the traditional Asian food known as congee, for which all ingredients were obtained from a local supermarket. The congee was prepared in the metabolic kitchen of the Human Nutrition department at the University of Otago in the hour prior to participants arriving for testing (between 0700–0800 h for breakfast; between 1100–1200 h for lunch). Jasmine rice (SunRice, Sydney, Australia) was cooked in a rice cooker with water and chicken stock until the desired consistency was reached. Boiled shredded chicken breast, fresh chopped spring onion, fried shallots, and sesame oil were added to the top of the cooked rice before it was served.

On lunch testing days, a standard breakfast consisting of two steamed pork buns and a cup of Chinese green tea was provided to participants. The compositions of the congee and steamed bun were determined using standard food analytical methods by Cawthron Analytical Services, Nelson, New Zealand (Table 1).

The weight of congee provided in a complete meal was 468 g. The split congee meal was given as 180 g preload followed thirty minutes later by a 288 g serving size. The congee given as a split meal (rice preload) or as eaten in one sitting (water preload) had an energy content of 1797 kJ and a carbohydrate content of 65 g. The carbohydrate content of the preload (both rice and kiwifruit) was 25 g. The overall energy content of the kiwifruit preload and congee meal was 1583 kJ.

Table 1. Composition of foods consumed.

Component	Kiwifruit	Rice Porridge (Congee)	Steamed Bun
Energy (kJ/100 g)	238	384	911
Protein (g/100 g)	1.02	4.1	6.6
Fat (g/100 g)	0.28	2.1	3.2
Carbohydrate (g/100 g)	13.1	13.9	40
Moisture (g/100 g)	82.4	79.7	49.1
Ash (g/100 g)	0.47	0.2	1.1

2.3. Participants

The inclusion criteria were adults aged 18–75 years, self-identified as being ethnically Chinese. Recruitment was by posters and flyers placed around the campus of the University of Otago, New Zealand, and at adjacent workplaces. Respondents were assessed according to the inclusion and exclusion criteria for the study. Exclusion criteria were inability to speak English, self-reported disease of the digestive system (coeliac, Crohn's diseases), having had gastrointestinal surgical procedures, an allergy to kiwifruit, and pregnancy. Diagnosis of other chronic diseases (diabetes mellitus, cardiovascular disease) did not exclude participation. Respondents that were potentially eligible to take part were provided with an information sheet to take away and consider. People willing to participate were booked in for an initial visit, during which a screening questionnaire was filled in, eligibility criteria were rechecked, and people were given an opportunity to ask questions. When satisfied, participants signed a consent form, filled out a personal information questionnaire, and had their height and weight measured. Reimbursement of $150 in supermarket vouchers was given for a complete set of six tests (or pro rata if participants withdrew).

2.4. Blood Sampling

Participants were asked to fast overnight and to avoid any strenuous exercise before testing. Blood samples were taken at baseline and at 15, 30, 45, 60, 75, 90, 120, and 150 min thereafter.

2.4.1. Breakfast Test

For the breakfast tests, blood samples were withdrawn into K EDTA-treated blood collection tubes by a cannula inserted into a vein in the cubital fossa by a research nurse. An initial (baseline) sample was taken before ingesting any food, after which the participants consumed a pre-randomised preload within 10 min. Further blood was drawn at 15 and 30 min. At 30 min, participants were given breakfast and asked to consume this within 15 min. Blood samples were taken at 45, 60, 75, 90, 120, and 150 min following baseline, making a total of nine blood draws. At each time point, participants filled out a satiety questionnaire that involved making marks on four visual analogue scales to indicate that person's degree of satiety. The questionnaire was used on each of the six days of testing (Figure 1). The questions and the extremes (in brackets) were:

How hungry do you feel at this moment? (Not at all hungry ——— Extremely hungry)
How full does your stomach feel at this moment? (Not at all full ——— Extremely full)
How strong is your desire to eat at this moment? (Very weak ——— Very strong)

How much food do you think you could eat at this moment? (Nothing at all —— A very large amount).

All questions were combined into a total appetite scale by taking the mean of the four questions, after reverse scoring the "How full does your stomach feel at this moment?" item. The total appetite score ranged from a possible 0 to 10 cm, with 10 indicating a high level of hunger.

2.4.2. Lunch Test

On lunch test days, participants attended the clinic at 0800 h to eat a standard breakfast, which consisted of two steamed pork buns and hot green tea; participants were then free to leave the clinic but were requested to return four hours later without meanwhile consuming any other food. The steamed buns were purchased from a local Asian supermarket in frozen packs of 10. The buns were stored frozen and steamed until hot before serving to participants. For lunch, the same rice preparation and preload procedure as the breakfast test was used, but blood glucose was measured as capillary blood glucose collected via finger prick rather than by cannula. The purpose of giving a standard breakfast was to standardise the meal prior to lunch to reduce variation in a possible 'second-meal effect', a phenomenon by which the glycaemic response to a meal is influenced by the preceding meal.

2.5. Blood Analysis

Blood glucose in plasma samples from the cannula draws at breakfast were measured using a Cobas c311 analyser (Roche, Germany). At lunch, capillary blood glucose concentration was measured using a HemoCue (Ängelholm, Sweden) blood glucose analyser. The glycaemic data were compared using measures of incremental area under the blood glucose response curve (iAUC; mmol/L·min) and for glucose, peak height (BGRmax; mmol/L·min).

Blood hormones (insulin, ghrelin, glucagon, and GLP-1) were determined by Multiplex Elisa analysis (Thermo Fisher Scientific, Waltham, MA). The data are expressed as mean concentration over the 150 min period following commencement of the breakfast test.

2.6. Energy Intake

Participants were given a set of electronic kitchen scales and instructed to weigh all of their food and beverage intake consumed for the remainder of the day following the tests. Participants recorded the name, brand, and weight of the food or beverage, and the time of eating. For homemade food, participants were asked to record each raw ingredient and preparation method. The food diary entries were entered into a nutrient analysis software program (Kai-calculator version v1.15s, Department of Human Nutrition, University of Otago) that sources its nutritional information from the New Zealand food composition database [30].

2.7. Statistical Methods

Based on data derived from a pilot study, 25 participants would be sufficient to detect a clinically significant difference in blood glucose response of 25% (approximately the difference between a low and a high glycaemic index food) using a significance level (α) of 0.05 and with a power of 0.9. We over-recruited ($n = 30$) to allow for dropouts. Stata 15.1 (StataCorp, College Station, TX, USA) was used for all statistical analyses. Differences in treatments were determined using mixed effects regression models with participant id as a random effect, robust standard errors, and adjusted for randomised order. Mean differences, 95% confidence intervals, and p-values were calculated.

3. Results

Thirty healthy Chinese participants, 25 female and 5 male, aged 19–41 years with a mean (SD) body mass index of 21.8 (3.8) kg/m^2, were enrolled in the study. Twenty-eight participants completed all three treatment arms at breakfast, and 29 completed at lunch. One female completed the lunch treatments only, and another female withdrew without providing any data. Participants were randomised to the order in which they received the treatments, as shown in Figure 2.

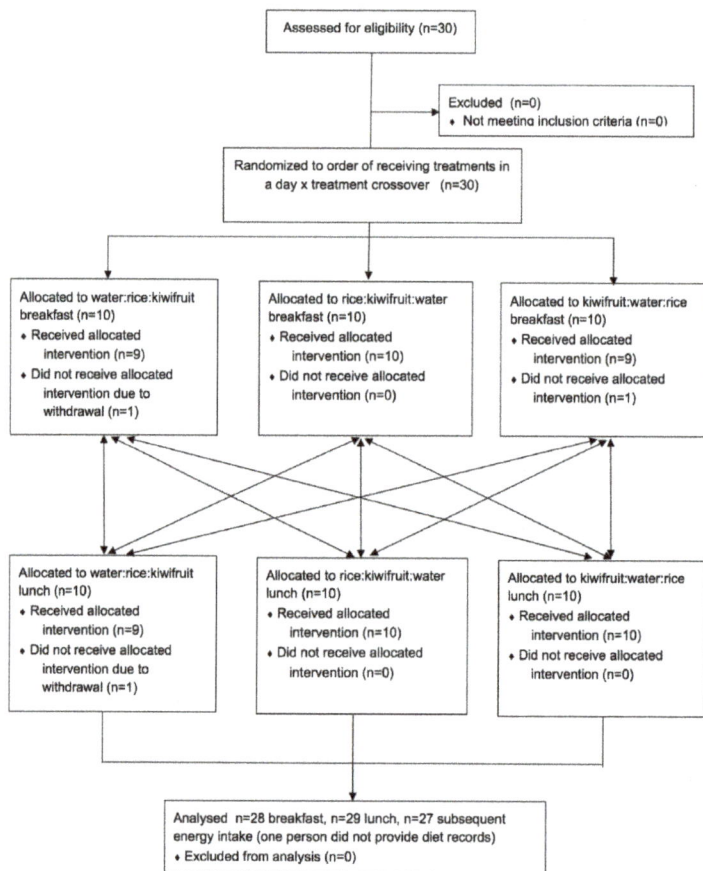

Figure 2. Participant flowchart.

3.1. Blood Glucose

The mean (SD) baseline blood glucose concentrations at breakfast were 5.2 (0.7), 5.2 (0.5), and 5.3 (0.6) mmol/L, and at lunch, 4.6 (0.5), 4.6 (0.6), and 4.4 (0.6) mmol/L for the water, rice, and kiwifruit treatments, respectively. The mean incremental rise in blood glucose concentration over time is plotted in Figure 3.

Water given as a preload half an hour before the rice meals resulted in no rise in blood glucose concentration whereas when rice and kiwifruit were given as preloads, there was a continuous rise in blood glucose throughout the first 45–60 min. Although the rice meals were identical in nutrient content, the postprandial rise in capillary blood glucose response (iAUC) was considerably larger at lunch compared with venous blood collected at breakfast ($p < 0.05$ for all treatments).

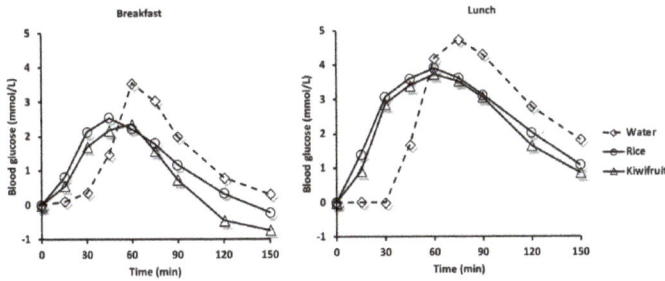

Figure 3. Mean incremental change in blood glucose concentrations at breakfast (n = 28) and at lunch (n = 29) given on different days from baseline (time 0), at which time preloads of water, rice, or kiwifruit were followed at 30 min by the remainder of the rice meal.

Incremental areas-under-the-glucose-curves (iAUC), peak glucose concentration, time to peak and comparisons of these factors among treatments are given in Table 2 for both breakfast and lunch. Peak capillary blood glucose concentration after lunch generally occurred at the 75 and 90 min timepoints and exceeded 10 mmol/L in nine, three, and three participants, following the water preload, split meal and kiwifruit preload, respectively.

Table 2. Postprandial blood glucose responses to treatments (preloads and meals combined) over 150 min.

Blood Glucose	Mean (SD)			Mean Difference (95% CI)		
	Water Preload + Rice	Rice Preload + Rice	Kiwifruit Preload + Rice	Rice vs. Water	Kiwifruit vs. Water	Kiwifruit vs. Rice
Breakfast iAUC [1] (mmol/L·min)	218 (171)	191 (125)	153 (93)	−26 (−82, 30) $p = 0.357$	−65 (−129, −1) $p = 0.047$	−39 (−80, 2) $p = 0.063$
Lunch iAUC (mmol/L·min)	365 (185)	371 (156)	336 (146)	6 (−38, 50) $p = 0.788$	−29 (−76, 19) $p = 0.237$	−35 (−82, 12) $p = 0.147$
Breakfast peak (mmol/L)	9.1 (2.0)	8.4 (1.4)	8.1 (1.1)	−0.7 (−1.4, 0.1) $p = 0.107$	−0.9 (−1.6, −0.2) $p = 0.010$	−0.3 (0.2, −0.8) $p = 0.264$
Lunch peak (mmol/L)	9.7 (1.6)	8.7 (1.1)	8.6 (1.5)	−1.0 (−1.4, −0.7) $p < 0.001$	−1.1 (−1.7, −0.5) $p < 0.001$	−0.1 (−0.5, 0.4) $p = 0.761$

[1] iAUC = incremental area-under-the-curve.

The treatments comprised a preload of water, rice or kiwifruit ingested 30 min before the same rice meal eaten for breakfast on three days and for lunch on another three days: n = 28 at breakfast; n = 29 at lunch.

At breakfast, the kiwifruit preload resulted in a smaller glucose iAUC compared with the water preload; there was no difference in glucose iAUC among treatments at lunch. Peak glucose was lower following the kiwifruit compared with the water preload at breakfast, and both the rice and the kiwifruit preloads resulted in lower peak glucose at lunch compared with water. Time to peak was shorter at breakfast and at lunch for the rice and kiwifruit preloads, compared with water. There was no difference for any of these factors between the rice and kiwifruit treatments.

3.2. Hormones

The mean (SD) baseline plasma insulin concentrations at breakfast were 7.6 (5.8), 6.8 (6.3), and 6.4 (4.5) mU/L for the water, rice, and kiwifruit treatments, respectively. The mean incremental rise in plasma insulin concentration over time is plotted in Figure 4.

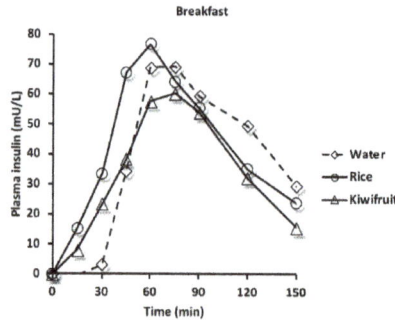

Figure 4. Mean incremental change in plasma insulin concentrations at breakfast from baseline (time 0) at which time preloads of water, rice, or kiwifruit were followed at 30 min by the remainder of the rice meal.

Water given as a preload half an hour before the rice meals resulted in a minimal rise in plasma insulin concentration, whereas when rice and kiwifruit were given as preloads, there was a continuous rise in plasma insulin throughout the first 60 min. Postprandial incremental areas-under-the-insulin-curves (iAUC) and mean concentration of plasma ghrelin, glucagon, and GLP-1 over 150 min after breakfast are given in Table 3.

Table 3. Mean postprandial hormonal responses to breakfast treatments (preloads and meals combined) over 150 min ($n = 28$).

Hormone	Mean (SD)			Mean Difference (95% CI)		
	Water Preload + Rice	Rice Preload + Rice	Kiwifruit Preload + Rice	Rice vs. Water	Kiwifruit vs. Water	Kiwifruit vs. Rice
Insulin iAUC [1] (mU/L·min)	5962 (2858)	6552 (3437)	5167 (2779)	498 (−688, 1685) $p = 0.296$	−887 (−1894, 119) $p = 0.152$	−1385 (−2684, −87) $p = 0.036$
Ghrelin (pg/mL)	32.9 (25.6)	35.1 (34.7)	32.3 (21.2)	2.2 (−2.5, 6.8) $p = 0.359$	−0.6 (−5.3, 4.0) $p = 0.787$	−2.8 (−7.4, 1.8) $p = 0.235$
Glucagon (pg/ml)	25.3 (10.8)	24.3 (10.8)	26.9 (14.9)	−1.0 (−3.0, 1.1) $p = 0.353$	1.6 (−0.5, 3.6) $p = 0.134$	2.5 (0.5, 4.6) $p = 0.015$
GLP-1 (pg/mL)	149 (44)	137 (47)	142 (41)	−12 (−18, −5) $p < 0.001$	−6 (−13, 0.3) $p = 0.063$	5 (−1, 12) $p = 0.100$

[1] iAUC = incremental area-under-the-curve.

The kiwifruit preload resulted in a smaller plasma insulin iAUC compared with the rice preload. There was no difference among treatments for mean plasma ghrelin concentration. The mean plasma glucagon concentration was higher for the kiwifruit compared with the rice preload; and for GLP-1, the concentration was lower for the rice compared with the water preload.

3.3. Satiety and Subsequent Energy Intake

Subjective appetite for a duration of 150 min after breakfast and lunch, and subsequent energy intake throughout the remainder of the days are given in Table 4. One male participant did not provide diet records following the tests.

Following breakfast, a greater appetite was reported after the kiwifruit compared with the water and the rice preloads. Following lunch, a smaller appetite was reported after the rice compared with the water preload; and a greater appetite after the kiwifruit compared with the rice preloads. There was no difference among treatments in the subsequent energy intake for the rest of the day following breakfast or lunch.

Table 4. Appetite responses via visual analogue scales, and subsequent energy intake following treatments (note: the breakfast and the lunch tests were on different days).

Satiety and Energy Intake	Mean (SD)			Mean Difference (95% CI)		
	Water Preload + Rice	Rice Preload + Rice	Kiwifruit Preload + Rice	Rice vs. Water	Kiwifruit vs. Water	Kiwifruit vs. Rice
Appetite after breakfast cm·min	593 (177)	605 (226)	687 (218)	12 (−39, 63) $p = 0.650$	94 (39, 149) $p = 0.001$	82 (26, 138) $p = 0.004$
Appetite after lunch cm·min	690 (229)	631 (242)	724 (261)	−59 (−103, −15) $p = 0.009$	34 (−19, 86) $p = 0.208$	93 (28, 157) $p = 0.005$
Energy intake after breakfast (MJ)	6.08 (2.02)	5.99 (2.44)	6.08 (2.34)	−0.09 (−0.94, 0.76) $p = 0.836$	0.00 (−0.88, 0.89) $p = 0.995$	0.09 (−0.72, 0.90) $p = 0.823$
Energy intake after lunch (MJ)	4.22 (2.20)	4.41 (1.87)	4.32 (1.54)	0.19 (−0.58, 0.96) $p = 0.629$	0.10 (−0.63, 0.83) $p = 0.788$	−0.09 (−0.74, 0.56) $p = 0.786$

Appetite scale combined all four items, with the 'how full do you feel' item reversed. A higher score indicates a greater appetite. Appetite $n = 28$ at breakfast; $n = 29$ at lunch; Energy intake $n = 27$.

4. Discussion

The main findings of the study are that a predominantly carbohydrate preload given 30 min before the remainder of the meal changes the shape of the glycaemic response curve by suppressing the peak concentration. This effect was found after breakfast and after lunch for both the rice and kiwifruit preloads, compared with the water preload treatment. Consistent with the literature, postprandially venous blood has lower glucose concentrations than capillary blood [31]. However, our main outcome was a comparison among treatments and the pattern of response was similar between breakfast and lunch, despite the different blood pools sampled (venous at breakfast and capillary at lunch).

Controlling peak glucose may be important, as postprandial glycaemic peaks have been associated with higher glycated haemoglobin concentrations and with thicker carotid intima-media thickness in people with type 2 diabetes [32]. Due to evidence of increased cardiovascular risk, maintaining a peak postprandial capillary blood glucose concentration below a threshold of 10 mmol/L is a recommendation of the American Diabetes Association [33]. Three participants exceeded 10 mmol/L following the split meal and the kiwifruit preload meal, compared with nine following the meal eaten in one sitting, a finding consistent with a glycaemic benefit of spreading the time-course of consuming a meal.

This study has shown that consuming fruit, recommended for multiple health benefits, need not cause high postprandial glycaemic responses due to fruit sugars. Reasons for this are firstly, that fructose is intrinsically less glycaemic than cooked starch in most cereal products [34]. This quality is consistent with the concept that when used in an equicarbohydrate exchange format, as in the present study, glycaemic response is likely to be reduced. Secondly, increasing meal frequency from three to six per day spreads the ingestion period, and using this approach, it has been found that fluctuations in postprandial glycaemic and insulinaemic responses are evened out [15], and that postprandial insulin sensitivity is improved [14]. Splitting the meal into a preload and a main meal without increasing carbohydrate, as in the present study, is an example of an extended ingestion period in which realistic intakes of preload and main meal were used. In the present study, 25 g of available carbohydrate in a total of 65 g carbohydrate was ingested in the preload, that is, 38% of the carbohydrate. However, as the kiwifruit sugars yield about 50% glucose and 50% fructose, the fructose alone would have substituted about 19% of the rice starch, so the contribution of substitution by fructose to any overall effects could be expected to be modest. Nevertheless, the study has shown that consuming kiwifruit as a preload did reduce glycaemic response—at breakfast, the kiwifruit preload reduced iAUC by about 30% compared with 12% for the rice preload, possibly reflecting the combined effect of fructose substitution and the gut-level action of other kiwifruit components at digestion, as found previously [26]. The results indicate the safety of consuming fruit in a carbohydrate exchange format, particularly when carbohydrate loading is attenuated by preloading.

Drugs have been developed to target postprandial glycaemia, and there are dietary strategies that have been tested, including adding protein and fat to carbohydrate, limiting carbohydrate intake, and reducing the carbohydrate load by making food choices based on the glycaemic index. Suppression of peak glucose has been reported previously with protein preloads [6,35]. The mechanism by which a protein preload has a moderating effect on glycaemia is by stimulating a greater insulin response [6]. This strategy for reducing glycaemia may not be ideal, as total and animal protein intakes have been associated with increased risk of developing type 2 diabetes [36]. Additionally, drugs designed to stimulate insulin have been associated with major adverse events in people with type 2 diabetes [11,37]. Another method used to reduce postprandial glycaemia is to limit carbohydrate intake by increasing the fat content of the diet. When applied for one or two days, this strategy has been found to be effective at reducing postprandial glycaemia but unless this dietary pattern is maintained, a return to more usual carbohydrate intakes results in exaggerated postprandial glucose excursions [38,39]. When low carbohydrate diets have been followed for up to three months, some improvement in glycaemic control in people with type 2 diabetes has been found [40,41], but it has been difficult to show maintenance of glycaemic benefit in the longer-term [42–44]. The concept of the glycaemic index has been used to reduce postprandial glycaemia. In this scenario, the macronutrient composition of the diet can be maintained whilst choosing foods on the basis of imparting low glycaemic responses [45]. Peak glucose concentration has been reduced when low, compared with high glycaemic index foods, have been chosen [46]. This strategy does rely on people being able to choose appropriate foods, and when applied over a number of weeks or months, has not always shown glycaemic benefit [47–49].

Co-ingestion of fat and carbohydrate has been found to reduce postprandial glycaemia, but this may not be a healthy strategy, as fat is calorically more dense than protein and carbohydrate; triglycerides and insulin were found to be raised by the combination of macronutrients indicative of fat intake, potentiating insulin secretion to the detriment of insulin sensitivity [50]. Similarly, the ability of ingested protein to potentiate insulin secretion under euglycaemic clamp conditions is indicative of peripheral insulin resistance [51]. The strength of a carbohydrate preload approach to lower peak glucose is that insulin concentrations were not increased compared with a single meal. Additionally, usual foods can be consumed, albeit with a 30-min time gap as in our study, between the preload and the remainder of the meal. Peak glucose was reduced when the rice meal was split and when kiwifruit was given as a preload. An advantage of using kiwifruit compared with the split rice meal was a lower insulin demand with the kiwifruit preload. Despite the lower insulin demand, the blood glucose concentration fell below baseline with the kiwifruit treatment, perhaps indicating a higher mean glucagon concentration to correct for this undershoot. An undershoot might have been expected, given that this is a characteristic of consuming foods containing fructose, including fruit [52]. However, the lower peak glucose, together with the reduced insulin demand, are potentially beneficial, as postprandial glycaemia and resultant insulin responses are positively associated with postprandial arterial stiffness [53].

The rice and kiwifruit preload meals were associated with a greater appetite score over the postprandial period compared with when the rice meal was eaten in one sitting. However, despite this subjective difference, there was no difference among treatments in subsequent energy intake throughout the test days. Our data are consistent with the use of water and fruit preloads in a weight loss setting; the preload concept being equally effective among treatments [54]. However, an advantage of using kiwifruit as a preload over the rice and water preloads was a lower energy content of the overall meal compared with using rice alone. The strategy of providing a low energy dense fruit as a preload to a starchy meal appears to be beneficial in these Chinese participants.

Although potentially beneficial effects on glycaemia and insulinaemia have been found in an acute setting, a limitation of the work described here is whether people would be willing to habitually adopt the concept of spreading a meal over a longer duration. Some people may not have the time, some may, and others might be able to reorganise their schedule to fit. It may be useful to test shorter time periods between preloading and the remainder of a meal. Other considerations would be the types of foods and mealtimes that people would be willing to apply the concept to. Splitting a rice meal, as was done here would require keeping the rice warm over an extended period, and this may be unacceptable to some people. The use of kiwifruit as a preload has the advantage over splitting a heated meal in that the fruit and the main meal are separate items. Kiwifruit has qualities that may make it particularly suitable for use in this way [25], but kiwifruit may be unobtainable throughout the year, and it would be informative in future research to compare the metabolic potential of other fruits. Our work is also limited in its demographic generalisability. Our participants were Chinese because postprandial glycaemia has been found to be higher in Chinese people compared with people of European descent [29,55]. It would be of interest to prepare meals containing other carbohydrate-rich foods to test the generalisability of findings among foods and other population groups, including by age, ethnicity and glucose tolerance.

5. Conclusions

Splitting the congee meal (rice preload) or using kiwifruit as a preload resulted in lower glycaemic responses compared with the congee eaten in one sitting, suggestive of a glycaemic advantage. Additional benefits of the kiwifruit preload were lower insulinaemia compared with the split meal and a lower energy content of the kiwifruit/congee combination compared with the congee alone, with no difference among meals in subsequent energy intake.

Author Contributions: Conceptualization, J.M.; Data curation, A.L., H.Y. and B.J.V.; Formal analysis, J.J.H.; Funding acquisition, J.M.; Investigation, A.L. and H.Y.; Methodology, A.L., S.M., J.J.H. and B.J.V.; Project administration, A.L., J.M., S.M., H.Y. and B.J.V.; Resources, A.L., J.M. and B.J.V.; Supervision, J.M.; Writing—original draft, A.L., J.M. and B.J.V.; Writing—review & editing, A.L., J.M., S.M., H.Y., J.J.H. and B.J.V.

Funding: This research was funded by The New Zealand National Science Challenge (subcontract UOAX1421), and The New Zealand Institute for Plant & Food Research Limited (Contract no. 33115).

Acknowledgments: We acknowledge our research nurse Margi Bryant for her skill in the cannulation procedure, and our laboratory technicians Ashley Duncan and Michelle Harper for their technical assistance in the analysis of blood samples.

Conflicts of Interest: The authors declare no conflict of interest.

References

1. Ceriello, A.; Colagiuri, S. International Diabetes Federation guideline for management of postmeal glucose: A review of recommendations. *Diabet. Med.* **2008**, *25*, 1151–1156. [CrossRef] [PubMed]
2. Trico, D.; Filice, E.; Trifiro, S.; Natali, A. Manipulating the sequence of food ingestion improves glycemic control in type 2 diabetic patients under free-living conditions. *Nutr. Diabetes* **2016**, *6*, e226. [CrossRef] [PubMed]
3. Stacher, G.; Bergmann, H.; Gaupmann, G.; Schneider, C.; Kugi, A.; Hobart, J.; Binder, A.; Mittelbach-Steiner, G. Fat preload delays gastric emptying: Reversal by cisapride. *Br. J. Clin. Pharmacol.* **1990**, *30*, 839–845. [CrossRef] [PubMed]
4. Gentilcore, D.; Chaikomin, R.; Jones, K.L.; Russo, A.; Feinle-Bisset, C.; Wishart, J.M.; Rayner, C.K.; Horowitz, M. Effects of fat on gastric emptying of and the glycemic, insulin, and incretin responses to a carbohydrate meal in type 2 diabetes. *J. Clin. Endocrinol. Metab.* **2006**, *91*, 2062–2067. [CrossRef] [PubMed]
5. Wu, T.; Little, T.J.; Bound, M.J.; Borg, M.; Zhang, X.; Deacon, C.F.; Horowitz, M.; Jones, K.L.; Rayner, C.K. A protein preload enhances the glucose-lowering efficacy of vildagliptin in type 2 diabetes. *Diabetes Care* **2016**, *39*, 511–517. [CrossRef] [PubMed]
6. Ma, J.; Stevens, J.E.; Cukier, K.; Maddox, A.F.; Wishart, J.M.; Jones, K.L.; Clifton, P.M.; Horowitz, M.; Rayner, C.K. Effects of a protein preload on gastric emptying, glycemia, and gut hormones after a carbohydrate meal in diet-controlled type 2 diabetes. *Diabetes Care* **2009**, *32*, 1600–1602. [CrossRef] [PubMed]
7. Christiansen, E.; Schnider, S.; Palmvig, B.; Tauber-Lassen, E.; Pedersen, O. Intake of a diet high in trans monounsaturated fatty acids or saturated fatty acids. Effects on postprandial insulinemia and glycemia in obese patients with NIDDM. *Diabetes Care* **1997**, *20*, 881–887. [CrossRef] [PubMed]
8. Diekman, C.; Malcolm, K. Consumer perception and insights on fats and fatty acids: Knowledge on the quality of diet fat. *Ann. Nutr. Metab.* **2009**, *54*, 25–32. [CrossRef] [PubMed]

9. Nuttall, F.Q.; Gannon, M.C. Metabolic response of people with type 2 diabetes to a high protein diet. *Nutr. Metab. (Lond.)* **2004**, *1*, 6. [CrossRef] [PubMed]

10. Baltali, M.; Korkmaz, M.E.; Kiziltan, H.T.; Muderris, I.H.; Ozin, B.; Anarat, R. Association between postprandial hyperinsulinemia and coronary artery disease among non-diabetic women: A case control study. *Int. J. Cardiol.* **2003**, *88*, 215–221. [CrossRef]

11. Douros, A.; Dell'Aniello, S.; Yu, O.H.Y.; Filion, K.B.; Laurent, A.; Suissa, S. Sulfonylureas as second line drugs in type 2 diabetes and the risk of cardiovascular and hypoglycaemic events: Population based cohort study. *Br. Med. J.* **2018**, *362*. [CrossRef] [PubMed]

12. Robertson, L.; Waugh, N.; Robertson, A. Protein restriction for diabetic renal disease. *Cochrane Database Syst. Rev.* **2007**, *4*. [CrossRef] [PubMed]

13. Holmstrup, M.E.; Owens, C.M.; Fairchild, T.J.; Kanaley, J.A. Effect of meal frequency on glucose and insulin excursions over the course of a day. *e-SPEN Eur. e-J. Clin. Nutr. Metab.* **2010**, *5*, e277–e280. [CrossRef]

14. Papakonstantinou, E.; Kechribari, I.; Mitrou, P.; Trakakis, E.; Vassiliadi, D.; Georgousopoulou, E.; Zampelas, A.; Kontogianni, M.D.; Dimitriadis, G. Effect of meal frequency on glucose and insulin levels in women with polycystic ovary syndrome: A randomised trial. *Eur. J. Clin. Nutr.* **2016**, *70*, 646. [CrossRef] [PubMed]

15. Munsters, M.J.; Saris, W.H. Effects of meal frequency on metabolic profiles and substrate partitioning in lean healthy males. *PLoS ONE* **2012**, *7*, e38632. [CrossRef] [PubMed]

16. Rasmussen, O.; Winther, E.; Hermansen, K. Postprandial glucose and insulin responses to rolled oats ingested raw, cooked or as a mixture with raisins in normal subjects and type 2 diabetic patients. *Diabet. Med.* **1989**, *6*, 337–341. [CrossRef] [PubMed]

17. Muraki, I.; Imamura, F.; Manson, J.E.; Hu, F.B.; Willett, W.C.; van Dam, R.M.; Sun, Q. Fruit consumption and risk of type 2 diabetes: Results from three prospective longitudinal cohort studies. *BMJ* **2013**, *347*, f5001. [CrossRef] [PubMed]

18. Montagnese, C.; Santarpia, L.; Buonifacio, M.; Nardelli, A.; Caldara, A.R.; Silvestri, E.; Contaldo, F.; Pasanisi, F. European food-based dietary guidelines: A comparison and update. *Nutrition* **2015**, *31*, 908–915. [CrossRef] [PubMed]

19. Government of Canada. Canada's Food Guides. Available online: https://www.canada.ca/en/health-canada/services/canada-food-guides.html (accessed on 18 July 2018).

20. U.S. Department of Health and Human Services; U.S. Department of Agriculture. *2015–2020 Dietary Guidelines for Americans*, 8th ed.; U.S. Department of Health and Human Services: Washington, DC, USA, December 2015. Available online: http://health.gov/dietaryguidelines/2015/guidelines/ (accessed on 18 July 2018).

21. Lustig, R.H.; Schmidt, L.A.; Brindis, C.D. Public health: The toxic truth about sugar. *Nature* **2012**, *482*, 27–29. [CrossRef] [PubMed]

22. Tappy, L.; Le, K.A. Metabolic effects of fructose and the worldwide increase in obesity. *Physiol. Rev.* **2010**, *90*, 23–46. [CrossRef] [PubMed]

23. Ludwig, D.S. Examining the health effects of fructose. *JAMA* **2013**, *310*, 33–34. [CrossRef] [PubMed]

24. Teff, K.L.; Grudziak, J.; Townsend, R.R.; Dunn, T.N.; Grant, R.W.; Adams, S.H.; Keim, N.L.; Cummings, B.P.; Stanhope, K.L.; Havel, P.J. Endocrine and metabolic effects of consuming fructose- and glucose-sweetened beverages with meals in obese men and women: Influence of insulin resistance on plasma triglyceride responses. *J. Clin. Endocrinol. Metab.* **2009**, *94*, 1562–1569. [CrossRef] [PubMed]

25. Mishra, S.; Monro, J. Kiwifruit remnants from digestion in vitro have functional attributes of potential importance to health. *Food Chem.* **2012**, *135*, 2188–2194. [CrossRef] [PubMed]

26. Mishra, S.; Edwards, H.; Hedderley, D.; Podd, J.; Monro, J. Kiwifruit non-sugar components reduce glycaemic response to co-ingested cereal in humans. *Nutrients* **2017**, *9*. [CrossRef] [PubMed]

27. Livingstone, M.B.E.; Robson, P.J.; Welch, R.W.; Burns, A.A.; Burrows, M.S.; McCormack, C. Methodological issues in the assessment of satiety. *Scand. J. Nutr.* **2000**, *44*, 98–103. [CrossRef]

28. Rolls, B.J.; Kim, S.; McNelis, A.L.; Fischman, M.W.; Foltin, R.W.; Moran, T.H. Time course of effects of preloads high in fat or carbohydrate on food intake and hunger ratings in humans. *Am. J. Physiol.* **1991**, *260*, R756–R763. [CrossRef] [PubMed]

29. Kataoka, M.; Venn, B.J.; Williams, S.M.; Te Morenga, L.A.; Heemels, I.M.; Mann, J.I. Glycaemic responses to glucose and rice in people of Chinese and European ethnicity. *Diabet. Med.* **2013**, *30*, e101–e107. [CrossRef] [PubMed]

30. The New Zealand Institute of Plant and Food Research; The New Zealand Ministry of Health. New Zealand food composition database: New Zealand Food Files 2012 Version 01. Available online: http://www.foodcomposition.co.nz (accessed on 30 April 2013).

31. Yang, C.; Chang, C.; Lin, J. A comparison between venous and finger-prick blood sampling on values of blood glucose. *Int. Conf. Nutr. Food Sci.* **2012**, *39*, 206–210.

32. Esposito, K.; Ciotola, M.; Carleo, D.; Schisano, B.; Sardelli, L.; Di Tommaso, D.; Misso, L.; Saccomanno, F.; Ceriello, A.; Giugliano, D. Post-meal glucose peaks at home associate with carotid intima-media thickness in type 2 diabetes. *J. Clin. Endocrinol. Metab.* **2008**, *93*, 1345–1350. [CrossRef] [PubMed]

33. American Diabetes Association. Standards of medical care in diabetes-2018 abridged for primary care providers. *Clin. Diabetes* **2018**, *36*, 14–37.

34. Atkinson, F.S.; Foster-Powell, K.; Brand-Miller, J.C. International tables of glycemic index and glycemic load values: 2008. *Diabetes Care* **2008**, *31*, 2281–2283. [CrossRef] [PubMed]

35. Clifton, P.M.; Galbraith, C.; Coles, L. Effect of a low dose whey/guar preload on glycemic control in people with type 2 diabetes—A randomised controlled trial. *Nutr. J.* **2014**, *13*, 103. [CrossRef] [PubMed]

36. Tian, S.; Xu, Q.; Jiang, R.; Han, T.; Sun, C.; Na, L. Dietary protein consumption and the risk of type 2 diabetes: A systematic review and meta-analysis of cohort studies. *Nutrients* **2017**, *9*. [CrossRef] [PubMed]

37. Holman, R.R.; Haffner, S.M.; McMurray, J.J.; Bethel, M.A.; Holzhauer, B.; Hua, T.A.; Belenkov, Y.; Boolell, M.; Buse, J.B.; Buckley, B.M.; et al. Effect of nateglinide on the incidence of diabetes and cardiovascular events. *N. Engl. J. Med.* **2010**, *362*, 1463–1476. [PubMed]

38. Numao, S.; Kawano, H.; Endo, N.; Yamada, Y.; Konishi, M.; Takahashi, M.; Sakamoto, S. Short-term low carbohydrate/high-fat diet intake increases postprandial plasma glucose and glucagon-like peptide-1 levels during an oral glucose tolerance test in healthy men. *Eur. J. Clin. Nutr.* **2012**, *66*, 926–931. [CrossRef] [PubMed]

39. Kanamori, K.; Ihana-Sugiyama, N.; Yamamoto-Honda, R.; Nakamura, T.; Sobe, C.; Kamiya, S.; Kishimoto, M.; Kajio, H.; Kawano, K.; Noda, M. Postprandial glucose surges after extremely low carbohydrate diet in healthy adults. *Tohoku J. Exp. Med.* **2017**, *243*, 35–39. [CrossRef] [PubMed]

40. Tay, J.; Luscombe-Marsh, N.D.; Thompson, C.H.; Noakes, M.; Buckley, J.D.; Wittert, G.A.; Yancy, W.S., Jr.; Brinkworth, G.D. Comparison of low- and high-carbohydrate diets for type 2 diabetes management: A randomized trial. *Am. J. Clin. Nutr.* **2015**, *102*, 780–790. [CrossRef] [PubMed]

41. Saslow, L.R.; Kim, S.; Daubenmier, J.J.; Moskowitz, J.T.; Phinney, S.D.; Goldman, V.; Murphy, E.J.; Cox, R.M.; Moran, P.; Hecht, F.M. A randomized pilot trial of a moderate carbohydrate diet compared to a very low carbohydrate diet in overweight or obese individuals with type 2 diabetes mellitus or prediabetes. *PLoS ONE* **2014**, *9*. [CrossRef] [PubMed]

42. Guldbrand, H.; Dizdar, B.; Bunjaku, B.; Lindstrom, T.; Bachrach-Lindstrom, M.; Fredrikson, M.; Ostgren, C.J.; Nystrom, F.H. In type 2 diabetes, randomisation to advice to follow a low-carbohydrate diet transiently improves glycaemic control compared with advice to follow a low-fat diet producing a similar weight loss. *Diabetologia* **2012**, *55*, 2118–2127. [CrossRef] [PubMed]

43. Iqbal, N.; Vetter, M.L.; Moore, R.H.; Chittams, J.L.; Dalton-Bakes, C.V.; Dowd, M.; Williams-Smith, C.; Cardillo, S.; Wadden, T.A. Effects of a low-intensity intervention that prescribed a low-carbohydrate vs. a low-fat diet in obese, diabetic participants. *Obesity (Silver Spring)* **2010**, *18*, 1733–1738. [CrossRef] [PubMed]

44. Davis, N.J.; Tomuta, N.; Schechter, C.; Isasi, C.R.; Segal-Isaacson, C.J.; Stein, D.; Zonszein, J.; Wylie-Rosett, J. Comparative study of the effects of a 1-year dietary intervention of a low-carbohydrate diet versus a low-fat diet on weight and glycemic control in type 2 diabetes. *Diabetes Care* **2009**, *32*, 1147–1152. [CrossRef] [PubMed]

45. Jenkins, D.J.; Wolever, T.M.; Taylor, R.H.; Barker, H.; Fielden, H.; Baldwin, J.M.; Bowling, A.C.; Newman, H.C.; Jenkins, A.L.; Goff, D.V. Glycemic index of foods: A physiological basis for carbohydrate exchange. *Am. J. Clin. Nutr.* **1981**, *34*, 362–366. [CrossRef] [PubMed]

46. Kaur, B.; Quek Yu Chin, R.; Camps, S.; Henry, C.J. The impact of a low glycaemic index (GI) diet on simultaneous measurements of blood glucose and fat oxidation: A whole body calorimetric study. *J. Clin. Transl. Endocrinol.* **2016**, *4*, 45–52. [CrossRef] [PubMed]

47. Shikany, J.M.; Phadke, R.P.; Redden, D.T.; Gower, B.A. Effects of low- and high-glycemic index/glycemic load diets on coronary heart disease risk factors in overweight/obese men. *Metabolism* **2009**, *58*, 1793–1801. [CrossRef] [PubMed]

48. Das, S.K.; Gilhooly, C.H.; Golden, J.K.; Pittas, A.G.; Fuss, P.J.; Cheatham, R.A.; Tyler, S.; Tsay, M.; McCrory, M.A.; Lichtenstein, A.H.; et al. Long-term effects of 2 energy-restricted diets differing in glycemic load on dietary adherence, body composition, and metabolism in CALERIE: A 1-y randomized controlled trial. *Am. J. Clin. Nutr.* **2007**, *85*, 1023–1030. [CrossRef] [PubMed]

49. Wolever, T.M.; Gibbs, A.L.; Mehling, C.; Chiasson, J.L.; Connelly, P.W.; Josse, R.G.; Leiter, L.A.; Maheux, P.; Rabasa-Lhoret, R.; Rodger, N.W.; et al. The Canadian Trial of Carbohydrates in Diabetes (CCD), a 1-y controlled trial of low-glycemic-index dietary carbohydrate in type 2 diabetes: No effect on glycated hemoglobin but reduction in C-reactive protein. *Am. J. Clin. Nutr.* **2008**, *87*, 114–125. [CrossRef] [PubMed]

50. Collier, G.; O'Dea, K. The effect of coingestion of fat on the glucose, insulin, and gastric inhibitory polypeptide responses to carbohydrate and protein. *Am. J. Clin. Nutr.* **1983**, *37*, 941–944. [CrossRef] [PubMed]

51. Smith, G.I.; Yoshino, J.; Stromsdorfer, K.L.; Klein, S.J.; Magkos, F.; Reeds, D.N.; Klein, S.; Mittendorfer, B. Protein ingestion induces muscle insulin resistance independent of leucine-mediated mTOR activation. *Diabetes Care* **2015**, *64*, 1555–1563. [CrossRef] [PubMed]

52. Brand-Miller, J.C.; Stockmann, K.; Atkinson, F.; Petocz, P.; Denyer, G. Glycemic index, postprandial glycemia, and the shape of the curve in healthy subjects: Analysis of a database of more than 1000 foods. *Am. J. Clin. Nutr.* **2009**, *89*, 97–105. [CrossRef] [PubMed]

53. Greenfield, J.R.; Samaras, K.; Chisholm, D.J.; Campbell, L.V. Effect of postprandial insulinemia and insulin resistance on measurement of arterial stiffness (augmentation index). *Int. J. Cardiol.* **2007**, *114*, 50–56. [CrossRef] [PubMed]

54. Silver, H.J.; Dietrich, M.S.; Niswender, K.D. Effects of grapefruit, grapefruit juice and water preloads on energy balance, weight loss, body composition, and cardiometabolic risk in free-living obese adults. *Nutr. Metab. (Lond.)* **2011**, *8*. [CrossRef] [PubMed]

55. Dickinson, S.; Colagiuri, S.; Faramus, E.; Petocz, P.; Brand-Miller, J.C. Postprandial hyperglycemia and insulin sensitivity differ among lean young adults of different ethnicities. *J. Nutr.* **2002**, *132*, 2574–2579. [CrossRef] [PubMed]

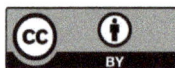

nutrients

MDPI

Article

Carbohydrate Knowledge and Expectations of Nutritional Support among Five Ethnic Groups Living in New Zealand with Pre- and Type 2 Diabetes: A Qualitative Study

Zhuoshi Zhang [1], John Monro [2] and Bernard J. Venn [1,*]

[1] Department of Human Nutrition, University of Otago, PO Box 56, Dunedin 9054, New Zealand; zhuoshi.zhang@gmail.com
[2] New Zealand Institute for Plant & Food Research Ltd., Private Bag 11600, Palmerston North 4442, New Zealand; John.Monro@plantandfood.co.nz
* Correspondence: bernard.venn@otago.ac.nz; Tel.: +643-479-5068

check for updates

Received: 26 July 2018; Accepted: 3 September 2018; Published: 4 September 2018

Abstract: Despite availability of diabetes and nutrition information for people with pre- and type 2 diabetes, the uptake and understanding of these resources may differ among ethnic groups. Our objective was to explore dietary knowledge and diabetes experiences amongst Māori, European, Pacific Island, Indian and East Asian people living in New Zealand with a focus on carbohydrate-containing foods. A registered diabetes dietitian led ethnic-specific discussions in groups involving 29 people with pre- or type 2 diabetes. Discussions were audio-recorded, fully transcribed and coded independently by two investigators. Themes were developed using deductive and inductive techniques. Five themes emerged: knowledge, concerns, achievements, simplicity and self-determination. Nutritional knowledge was lacking and a greater awareness of trustworthy dietary resources was needed. There were concerns about diabetes complications and appropriate carbohydrate-containing foods and portions. Contrary to this, people felt proud when achieving dietary goals and grateful for support from health care providers and family. Participants were willing to engage in self-care if advice from health professionals was given in plain language, and in a culturally appropriate manner. Given the desire to take an active role in diabetes self-management and willingness to use electronic devices, an ethnic-specific nutrition education resource could be a valuable tool.

Keywords: diabetes; ethnicity; knowledge; discussion groups; qualitative

1. Introduction

Diabetes is one of the fastest growing chronic conditions in the world [1–3]. In 2014, an estimated 422 million adults were living with diabetes compared to 108 million in 1980 [4]. To provide the best diabetes care, a structured multidisciplinary team input is required [5,6]. However, the reality for many countries is a general lack of resources to cater for the growing number of people with diabetes, resulting in a knowledge gap for people both recently diagnosed and for those with a longstanding diagnosis [7,8]. To fill the knowledge gap, people with pre- and type 2 diabetes can obtain information on their condition from healthcare professionals and also from less regulated sources such as the internet or from other people [9]. However, information obtained from unregulated sources can lead to misunderstanding, frustration and anxiety [10–12], poor compliance in treatment [12–15] and unnecessary food avoidance [12,16,17]. In questioning people with diabetes, there was confusion about the effect of macronutrients on glucose metabolism with carbohydrates being particularly misunderstood to the extent that some people were avoiding fruit due to the sugar content [17].

Psychological stresses for people with diabetes including fear, worry and perceived discrimination have been found in the second Diabetes Attitudes, Wishes and Needs (DAWN2) study [10].

Negative emotions and lack of knowledge could be even more pronounced in ethnic minorities living in Caucasian counties, who tend to receive less diabetes education [18], have less diabetes and nutritional knowledge [19], are less engaged with diabetes services [20,21], and have higher emotional distress [22,23] compared with the ethnic majority. Compounding these inequalities is a tendency for ethnic minority groups to have a higher prevalence of type 2 diabetes and to have poorer health outcomes compared with the ethnic majority group [18,24,25].

Identifying barriers and expectations to diabetes care and nutrition education is important if ethnic inequalities are to be addressed. Little work has been carried out comparing differences among ethnicities regarding diabetes nutrition management [10,12,13,17]. New Zealand is a country in which ethnic experiences can be explored because it has indigenous and immigrant minority groups living in a predominantly Caucasian population, reflecting ethnic diversity in many other countries [26]. The research described herein was aimed at exploring experiences and emotions among Māori, European, Pacific Island, Indian, and East Asian people living with diabetes or pre-diabetes using ethnic-specific discussion groups. The purpose was to ascertain participants knowledge and beliefs pertaining to diabetes and nutrition management with an emphasis on carbohydrate-containing foods, and expectations of diabetes care.

2. Materials and Methods

2.1. Ethics and Recruitment

Discussion groups were recruited through verbal referral from general practitioners' practices, primary health organisations and community health support services; and via advertisements in local medical centres, libraries, community centres, sports facilities and supermarkets within Auckland city, New Zealand. A Māori group was recruited in Palmerston North, New Zealand through contacts with funders of the study. Adults with pre- and type 2 diabetes who expressed interest were asked for their consent to receive a telephone call regarding the study. Eligible participants were invited to attend one discussion group based on their ethnicity. The inclusion criteria were: A diagnosis of pre-diabetes or type 2 diabetes confirmed by medical records, New Zealand residency and the ability to communicate in English. The exclusion criteria were people with severe speech or hearing difficulties, inability to speak English or over 79 years of age. The Ngāi Tahu Research Consultation Committee was consulted and the study was approved by the University of Otago Human Ethics Committee (Reference no. 14/179).

Of the 71 referrals and respondents (19 Europeans, 10 Māori, 11 Pacific Islanders, 14 East Asian and 17 Indian), 13 people could not be contacted and 22 declined. Of the remaining 36 people confirmed, seven did not show up on the day. Thus, 29 participants (six Europeans, five Māori, four Pacific Islanders, eight East Asians and six Indians) attended separate ethnic-specific discussion groups. Prior to the discussion group meetings, an information sheet was given to each participant, queries were answered and consent was obtained.

2.2. Procedures

The discussion groups were designed and conducted in accordance with a published protocol [27]. The discussions were held onsite in Auckland and via Skype® in Palmerston North with Māori participants, a method of synchronous interviewing that is becoming more widely used [28]. The duration of each discussion group was approximately 1 h, and was conducted in a safe and comfortable environment with each session audio-recorded. An interviewer guide was used to facilitate each discussion.

Predefined questions were open-ended and designed to avoid wording suggestive of a 'correct' answer. All participants were encouraged to speak freely, whilst the facilitator (Z.Z.) ensured that the discussion moved at an appropriate pace and finished on time. Sentence completion exercises and brainstorming on a whiteboard were used during the discussion. At the end of the session, the purpose of the discussion was repeated and final questions from participants were answered. The predefined questions were as follows:

- What do you know about pre-diabetes and type 2 diabetes?
- What diabetes support have you received?
- What nutrition for diabetes advice have you been given by clinicians?
- Where do you seek for diabetes and nutrition information and how accurate is it?
- What do you want to know about nutrition for diabetes?
- Have you seen a dietitian for pre- and type 2 diabetes?
- What foods do you think affect your blood glucose?
- What foods do you think are healthy or unhealthy?
- Would an electronic diabetes nutritional education resource be useful for you?

2.3. Data Analysis

A published thematic approach involving deductive and inductive techniques was used [29]. A priori, the broad code categories of knowledge, experience and desire were selected. All audio recordings were transcribed verbatim by the facilitator (Z.Z.) and checked by a second investigator (B.J.V.). Photographs were taken to record notes written on a whiteboard during discussions. Two researchers (Z.Z. and B.J.V.) independently coded the transcript. Potentially important words and phrases were identified through both inductive and deductive analysis. These two sets of coding phrases were compared. Any discrepancies were discussed through reviewing of the transcript and the meaning of a code until consensus was reached. Coding phrases were further developed into themes through creating a coding manual.

3. Results

Participant characteristics are given in Table 1. The average time since diagnosis for the nine people with pre-diabetes was 2.6 years and for those with type 2 diabetes, 13.7 years. Of the 29 participants, six participants were not on any diabetes medication. Of those on medication; 19 were prescribed metformin; eight sulfonylureas; one dipeptidyl peptidase-4 inhibitor and four used insulin with or without oral medications.

Table 1. Characteristics of the study participants.

	Total	European	Māori	PI	East Asian	Indian
	(*n* = 29)	(*n* = 6)	(*n* = 5)	(*n* = 4)	(*n* = 8)	(*n* = 6)
N, pre-diabetes	9	3	1		4	1
N, type 2 diabetes	20	3	4	4	4	5
Mean years of pre-diabetes	2.6	4.3	2.0		2.0	0.5
Mean years of type 2 diabetes	13.7	3.3	27.3	10.8	14.0	11.2
Sex, *n* (Male, Female)	11M, 18F	1M, 5F	3M, 2F	1M, 3F	2M, 6F	4M, 2F
Age, n						
45–54 year	3		1		2	
55–64 year	10	2	1	2	3	2
65–74 year	15	4	3	2	3	3
74–79 year	1					1
Diabetes medication, n						
None	6	3	1		2	
Metformin	19	3	3	3	5	5
Sulfonylureas	8		2	1	2	3
Insulin	4	1	2		1	
Other	1	1				
Education, n						
University	10	1			6	3
Polytechnic	7	2	2		1	2
Secondary	1	1				
Did not answer	11	2	3	4	1	1

PI, Pacific Islander.

3.1. Knowledge

General practitioners (GPs) and registered nurses (RNs) were identified as the two main sources providing diabetes dietary advice across all discussion groups. Half of the participants felt that they had not received adequate nutrition advice. Being unaware of, and having limited access to a diabetes service was emphasised within the Māori, Pacific Island and Indian discussions. All groups voiced a strong need for adequate consultation time with health professionals to discuss their queries and concerns regarding nutrition and diabetes control.

"You don't really have a lot time, you go in there, and you just don't have time to ask some questions."—European group

"So far the lecture from diabetes centre was the only one come and discuss something (sic). We have not heard from anybody else. It will help a long way if there are more dietitian lectures."—Indian group

Apart from three people who had recently attended diabetes education classes, participants struggled when asked to describe pre- and type 2 diabetes, what the risk factors were of developing type 2 diabetes, and the reasons for pharmaceutical and lifestyle intervention. European, Māori and East Asian groups commented on the inconsistency of medical and nutritional information obtained from the Internet, and of more concern, among health professionals. Confusion due to lack of diabetes knowledge or being exposed to conflicting information was apparent within all ethnic groups. Animated discussions on suitable food and beverage options, and how to interpret laboratory test results, occurred in all discussions.

"You go on to the Internet and you can find that this is good. Do this and do that, and you can also go to another parts and it says this is all wrong."—European group

Identifying "good" and "bad" dietary choices was another key discussion point in all discussions. Most participants were restricting foods and beverages that were perceived by them to be bad for diabetes whilst increasing the intake of so-called good foods. Although all participants understood foods and drinks with added sugar increased blood glucose concentrations, the majority failed to recognise or understand that other carbohydrate in food has blood glucose raising potential.

"Eat less potatoes, we are not allowed to eat potatoes, only once a week."—Indian group
"These three fruits are deadly for diabetes. They are very high in sugar."—Māori group

The foods in Table 2 were identified within the groups as raising blood glucose concentration. Foods identified as raising blood sugar among all groups were sugar and rice. Bread was not specifically referred to by any group and only the Indian group mentioned potato. Some ethnic-specific starchy foods were identified; taro by the Pacific Island group and noodles by the East Asian group. Three out of four Pacific Island and half of the European and East Asian participants believed that fatty foods raised blood glucose. In conclusion, half of the participants across all ethnic groups considered that they had received inadequate nutrition information from the health system. Conflicting messages from various official, online and lay sources led to misunderstanding, confusion and unnecessary dietary restriction. Māori, Pacific Island and Indian participants were less likely to have accessed specialist diabetes and dietetic services in both primary and secondary care.

3.2. Concerns

All participants were fearful and worried about diabetes complications, medication side effects, eating unhealthy foods and having inappropriate portion sizes. Suspicion regarding the credibility of information obtained from health professionals and other sources was expressed by all except the Indian group who relied heavily upon the information provided by general practitioners and practice nurses. The Indian participants were less aware of specific diabetes education services compared with the other groups. A lack of involvement in diabetes management decision making left the majority of Māori and Pacific Island participants feeling powerless over their own health destiny. One Māori and one East Asian participant also described feelings of embarrassment in discussing their diabetes with friends and family.

Table 2. Foods thought by participants to affect blood glucose.

	Europeans	Māori	PI [1]	East Asian	Indian
Carbohydrate foods or foods containing a substantial proportion of carbohydrate	Bakery food	Banana	Chocolate	Muffins	Beetroot
	Biscuits	Corn	Lollies	Fruit	Cola
	Cakes	Fruit	Rice	Instant noodles	Rice
	Chocolate	Refined sugar	Sugar	Rice	Soft drinks
	Pasta	Rice	Takeaways (e.g., sweet and sour)	Rice cakes	Potato
	Rice	Sprite	Taro	Sugar	
	Processed foods [2]				
Foods containing little carbohydrate	Bacon		Fatty foods	Alcohol	Alcohol
	Butter			Cheese	
	Nuts				
	Sausages				

[1] PI, Pacific Islander; [2] Processed foods may or may not contain substantial amounts of carbohydrate.

"How do you know that we got diabetes? Because I don't know I have diabetes, until I had a stroke."—Pacific Island group

"It says it affect the heart, kidneys, eyes and foot. We've told it starts with eyes, heart, kidney and sensation of the foot. Sensation of the foot starts lose, any disease on the foot is difficult to get cured."—Indian group

Participants of all ethnicities, except Indian, expressed aversion to a top-down nutrition consultation style in which health providers were viewed as judgemental. With regard to food, there was some confusion and resentment expressed in all groups with health care providers making incorrect assumptions, giving mixed messages, and imposing unexplained dietary restrictions.

"The practice nurse assumed that I drank a lot of juice and coke. And I said, No! I don't!"—Māori group

"My GP tells me the same thing, keep doing some exercise, eat these and don't eat that. But I said, the food is just food. What you just told me not to eat is not fair."—Pacific Island group

"What about apple? Red apple or granny smith? Just one apple? What about rock melon? Yoghurt?"—Indian group

"My GP asked me to go back to Korean diet like rice and soup. I am kind of confused, cause I eat so much rice."—East Asian group

"You tend to not like suddenly a whole lot of restrictions coming from middle of nowhere, telling you that you can't eat this bread roll, you can't drink this, you can't do this, you can't do that. And you rebel."—European group

Frustration was expressed that some of the nutrition advice was conflicting both among health care providers and between the advice received and what they had read or believed. One Pacific Island and one Indian participant were angry with themselves for relapsing into unhealthy eating habits and not paying enough attention to their own health.

Concern was expressed in the Māori, Pacific Island and Indian groups regarding self-adjustment of medication and treatment. The main drivers were doubt about their understanding of best practice and fear of diabetes complications.

"I started to feel shaking of my hands. Then I take some sugar or any foods. Once I okay with it, I stop. If I am outside, the best thing I do is buy bananas, two or three bananas, and one or two lollies."—Indian group

"Knowing that the insulin should have not been starting at two units. I raised it up myself to straight up to 20, 30 units. My sugar level was too high and I can sense things going wrong in the eyes. I've just started to deal with it myself."—Māori group

In summary, participants were fearful about diabetes complications. Doubt, confusion, embarrassment, powerlessness, frustration and anger were all negative emotions expressed by different ethnic groups.

3.3. Achievements

All ethnic groups stated an interest in understanding diabetes, diabetes medications, diet, lifestyle, and how to make changes. Several participants in the European, Māori and Pacific Island groups expressed strong desires to halt the progression of diabetes and to stay healthy. Several participants from each ethnic group described feeling satisfied and even delighted when achieving goals such as achieving recommended blood glucose and maintaining dietary change. Some participants described their sense of gratitude towards families, friends, healthcare professionals, and other people with diabetes for psychosocial and medical support. Although this was mentioned in all group discussions, appreciation of family involvement was specifically highlighted by the majority of the Māori and Pacific Island participants.

"Sometimes, I get frustrated. I didn't want to take any more medicine, but my wife talk me out of it. That's why I need my family, because they are the part taking care of you when you are at home."—Pacific Island group

Recognising the need for good diabetes control and the setting of life goals, such as preventing diabetes complications and spending quality time with families, served as inspiration. Many participants expressed satisfaction from having discovered ways to change diet and lifestyle, being able to sustain these changes, avoiding temptation, and ultimately improving blood glucose control. Although the Indian group expressed determination to make change, the sense of achievement conveyed by the other groups was absent from the Indian group discussion.

"I felt really good now. I said I feel I have to do something for myself, and I will see a real change, even up until now, I am a really changed person."—Pacific Island group

"You need to have a reason to want to live in a long healthy life. For me, I want to see my grandchildren."—East Asian group

"I realise in the end it is the weight. I just concentrated on the quantity that I eat, and when I eat. I stopped the night snacking. I love chocolate, but I can now go to the fridge and look at the chocolate and then just walk away."—European group

Overall, all ethnic groups showed positive attitudes such as feeling motivated and satisfied when good diabetes control was attained. Family support was a highlight for Māori and Pacific Island groups.

3.4. Simplicity

All groups wanted simple explanations regarding appropriate food choices. A pictorial or video format illustrated with 'hands' and 'plate' models were favoured over text-based advice, particularly if text incorporated scientific jargon. Some European, East Asian and Indian participants were also receptive to advice in numerical form for ease of compliance, for example, 30 min of exercise.

"Dietitian said I could have enough potatoes like 3 small eggs, so that's how I used to measure my carbohydrate portions. It's like 3 small egg size."—East Asian Group

"Plate is plate. Half, quarter, quarter simple (for vegetables, protein and carbohydrate)."—Māori Group

Participants wanted advice to be practical, especially around home cooking methods and dietary patterns. Participants discussed how simple, practical advice that they had received had increased their confidence in trying and maintaining dietary and lifestyle changes. Being culturally appropriate was also highlighted by East Asian and Pacific Island groups. Although European, Māori and Indian groups felt comfortable with English-language-based education, being able to receive information in their own language was preferred by some participants in East Asian and Pacific Island groups.

"With diabetes, I want to know how to cook from what you have in your cupboards rather than buy all these lovely things, which is not realistic for your diabetes."—Māori group

"Beans, corn, and nuts . . . See we've never eaten these good foods. We weren't brought up with it."
—Pacific Island group

"It will be nice if you can speak Samoan."—Pacific Island group

All ethnic groups expressed a desire for simple, visual and practical dietary advice. Some participants wanted dietary advice to include cultural foods and to be presented in their familiar language.

3.5. Self-Determination

Māori, Pacific Island and Indian participants expressed a willingness to make lifestyle changes but felt overly dependent on treatment plans assigned by health professionals. Several participants described frustration at the lack of involvement in decision-making around their own diabetes care, citing poor communication with their healthcare provider. All groups indicated reluctance in making dietary and lifestyle changes because they felt inadequately informed as to the need for change as well as perceived difficulties in avoiding temptation and fitting additional self-monitoring tasks into their life.

"It's more peace of mind, actually explaining what the medication is, instead of, go it's one of these."—Māori group

"The chemist said, Oh! You don't need this medication anymore. It is not on the prescription. You are on this. I turned around and said, what do you mean? It isn't inside of what I have been taking? They've changed that, and I never knew."—Pacific Island group

Most participants supplemented the advice of their health professionals by taking initiatives to improve their diabetes knowledge by reading books, searching online, attending diabetes classes, making dietary changes and self-monitoring blood glucose.

"You would look it on the computer, because the information is there."—Māori group

"I read all about the diabetes myself from library books."—East Asian group

All ethnic groups wanted to have ongoing support and reminders to achieve and maintain a healthy diet and to increase compliance with medication. Peer support was valued by several Māori, Pacific Island and European participants who found sharing their experiences with other people with diabetes helpful and reassuring.

"Diabetes, diet is the main issue. Required to be reminded it again and again."—Indian group

"Being around with people got the same illness as myself, it's like a support group (sic). What they said was exactly what I am going through. And I think, none of us has been perfect. We all did the same thing."—Pacific Island group

The use of new technology to search for health-related information and recipes, and to create meal plans was clearly shown in all discussions. Convenience and immediate information feedback were highly regarded attributes, although reliability of this information was a major concern. Only five out of 29 participants said they would probably not use online learning resources, with cost and age identified as barriers.

"When we went on the Internet, we have to depend on it. Sometimes there is different information on one topic."—Indian group

"You cut back on the portions of your meal and then finish with a piece of fruit. You don't really know if it is the right thing or not. If you have a website that you could look at would be quite good."—European group

4. Discussion

The main findings of the discussion groups were a recognised lack of knowledge and confusion regarding diet and medication, fear of diabetes complications, a willingness to participate in the management of their condition, the need to keep advice practical, the use of simple language, avoidance of medical jargon, and engagement with self-directed searching for information despite some level of mistrust and confusion with Internet sites. All ethnic groups expressed willingness to modify diet and carbohydrate sources given reliable and culturally appropriate guidance. Ethnic-specific issues included Māori, Pacific Island and Indian participants discussing lack of group education and access to specialist diabetes services. Explanation as to why dietary modification and medication treatment was needed would provide motivation for change in the Māori and Pacific Island groups. Some Māori, Pacific Island and East Asian participants thought it desirable that information be made available in their own language. Some participants were self-checking blood glucose and body weight but there was a general feeling among the Indian participants that this should be monitored by clinicians rather than by themselves. The Māori and Pacific Island groups discussed family support more prominently than other ethnic groups.

One theme common to all groups was dietary restriction, a topic that was discussed with some resentment. In the United States, dietary restriction has been associated with diabetes distress, in part because it affected other members of the family [30]. To what extent carbohydrate foods should be restricted by people with type 2 diabetes is questionable, as carbohydrate intake has not been associated with long-term glycaemic control [31]. Food avoidance can be restrictive, but a positive idea that emerged from our Māori group was the desire to learn about food and nutrition in order to pass that knowledge onto the next generation. However, sourcing reliable dietary information was problematic for all groups. The European group cited 'on-going referrals' from health care providers to diabetes educational classes, whilst the other ethnic groups mentioned engagements in formal education sessions only sporadically. Our data are consistent with those obtained in Australia in which non-European ethnicity was associated with a lessened likelihood of having received formal diabetes education [18], highlighting the need to promote diabetes support services to non-European ethnic communities.

Participants regarded the quality of diabetes information to be variable. The Internet was challenging as it provided instantly accessible information but conflicting messages. In other work it has been found that the quality of information is dependent on various factors including whether people are seeking factual information and advice on a course of action or subjective opinion [32]. The 'hit' rates for correct, complete or appropriate responses were low, typically around 50%, with lower scores for the advice type questions [32]. Hence, the frustration and confusion expressed by our participants is entirely consistent with other people's experiences with the Internet [33]. The quality and safety of online diabetes information has been queried, with misinformation, promotional material, poor readability, lack of evidence-based recommendations and lack of medical disclaimers of concern [34–36]. Despite drawbacks, use of the Internet as a source of information will continue for all ethnicities as it is a resource that has broad reach and ease of access [37].

In contrast, there were differences among the ethnic groups for engagement and experience with health professionals. The European group discussed on-going interactions with healthcare services whereas Pacific Island participants seemed unaware of such services. The Indian group respected and trusted clinicians' knowledge and judgment similar to British Indian patients [38,39] favouring clinicians' guidance over self-care [40]. However, diabetes management requires a considerable component of self-care and advising Indian patients of the importance of this is essential [40]. The East Asian group reported positive experiences of healthcare providers despite lack of consultation time, reflecting experiences of Vietnamese women with gestational diabetes [41]. Our Māori participants were less trusting of the advice that they had received from health professionals. It has been documented that Māori and Pacific Island people are more likely to miss hospital appointments compared with Europeans [42]. Perhaps these sentiments and behaviours partly explain the reliance that Māori and Pacific Island participants placed on family for emotional and practical support, consistent with being more likely to live in multi-generational households and taking care of family members [43]. In South Africa, black African patients were found to be frequently receiving incorrect and inappropriate dietary advice from health educators [44]. In our participants, lack of dietary knowledge, confusion and mistrust in sources of dietary information identifies a clear need for reliable dietary education and advice.

Cumulatively, the views expressed by our participants encompassed those found in Canada where limited consulting time, excessive workload and insufficient trust in physicians advice led to patients' poor motivation and compliance [45]. It has been suggested that health systems set up to deal with acute care are poorly configured to cater to the needs of people with chronic conditions and that strategies are needed within those systems to foster self-management in people with diabetes [46]. A move away from an authoritarian approach to one of an equal partnership between health professionals and those with chronic conditions has been advocated [46]. Aspirational goals of partnership in disease management are in agreement with the views expressed by our participants who objected to a 'top-down' approach. To encourage partnership, communication with patients should be designed to answer their queries and to fit in with individuals' goals and culture [46,47]. A patient-centred partnership program has facilitated patient participation and shared decision-making with health care providers [48]. Although trials designed to enhance patient-practitioner partnership may have positive outcomes in terms of patient engagement, more studies are needed to assess clinical outcomes following such intervention trials [49].

The present article describes novel research in which the experiences and expectations of diabetes management has been explored by a diabetes dietitian in participants representing five ethnic groups living in New Zealand. Sample numbers for each ethnic group were small and this poses a problem for generalisability within ethnicities as factors such as urban/rural; country of origin; cultural background; socioeconomic status; and education are underlying variables to the experiences and expectations of the individuals that participated. Nevertheless, the themes described herein were expressed in all discussion groups, suggestive that at least these themes may have commonality. In that context, the findings may have generalisability to other predominantly Caucasian countries whose population includes ethnic minority groups. In Australia, language, level of education and indigenous ethnicity were associated with lower diabetes knowledge and reduced likelihood of having received diabetes education and dietetic advice [18]. In the United States, immigrant and indigenous people experience diet-related disparities in which poorer diets are consumed by minority groups compared with the white populous [50]. Limitations to the generalizability of our study are that only participants who spoke English and who had an interest in diabetes management were involved. Potentially, our information is optimistic as people with a lesser command of the English language may struggle even more with accessing reliable information. Lack of knowledge of a country's main language has been identified as disadvantaging access to health care [51]. Another limitation may be a small sample with participant numbers ranging from four to eight, although five has been suggested as an appropriate number for conducting group discussions [52]. Nevertheless, there are still limits on the generalisability of the discussions both within New Zealand, a geographically diverse country, and among other countries. Some issues though are likely to be common around the world, particularly with regard to ethnic minority groups living in Westernised countries. In summary, for people of various ethnicities with pre-diabetes and type 2 diabetes living in New Zealand, we have found heterogeneity in dietary knowledge and experience of the health care system. An overarching sentiment expressed by all ethnic groups was a desire for reliable dietary information to assist with self-management of the disease.

Our participants expressed a need to access trustworthy sources of dietary information, a view consistent with previous work in which participants with pre- or type 2 diabetes were wary of some of the dietary information that they had accessed [53]. A general feeling was expressed that the nutrition advice of primary care providers was reliable although some reservations were expressed regarding inconsistency of messages and many participants supplemented the advice of their health professionals from other sources. Confusion around food and general dietary advice expressed by our participants is perhaps not surprising given that there is still uncertainty and controversy in the best dietary approaches for the prevention and management of type 2 diabetes [54].

It has been recommended that nutritional advice be given by a registered dietitian or by referral to a diabetes self-management education (DSME) program [55]. However, success in weight loss and diabetes remission over 1 year has been reported when participants were guided by general practitioners [56]. Nevertheless, it is unclear how well long-term nutrition goals and sustained weight loss can be maintained outside of the study setting, or whether it is feasible or necessary for continuing general practitioner involvement in dietary management. In a focus group survey of general practitioners practicing in Belgium, a sentiment expressed was that dieticians could give more adequate and more varied food advice than the general practitioners themselves [57]. Indeed, dietitian advice has been found to improve clinical outcomes in people with type 2 diabetes [58,59]. However, dietary advice is time-consuming and for many countries there are too few dietitians to adequately cater to the service demand [5].

5. Conclusions

It is telling that despite a plethora of electronic devices, websites and software applications, our participants struggled to find reliable information given in a practical and culturally appropriate manner. From the participants' perspective, dietary advice needed to be consistent and to have been derived from a solid evidence base. With the challenge of an increasing prevalence of diabetes and limited health care resources, development of a professional organisation-endorsed, evidence-based, electronic resource using lay language, in video or pictorial format and available in different languages could be a highly sought after instructional tool. Consumer acceptance and performance of such a multi-ethnic resource would need to be monitored for efficacy.

Author Contributions: Conceptualization, Z.Z., B.J.V.; Methodology, Z.Z., J.M., B.J.V.; Transcription and analysis, Z.Z., B.J.V.; Draft manuscript, Z.Z., B.J.V.; Funding acquisition, J.M.; Final draft, Z.Z., B.J.V., J.M.

Funding: This research was funded by a New Zealand Ministry of Business Innovation and Employment grant to the New Zealand Institute of Plant & Food Research Ltd under the 'Foods for Health' research programme.

Conflicts of Interest: The authors declare no conflicts of interest.

References

1. Whiting, D.R.; Guariguata, L.; Weil, C.; Shaw, J. IDF diabetes atlas: Global estimates of the prevalence of diabetes for 2011 and 2030. *Diabetes Res. Clin. Pract.* **2011**, *94*, 311–321. [CrossRef] [PubMed]
2. Wild, S.; Roglic, G.; Green, A.; Sicree, R.; King, H. Global prevalence of diabetes: Estimates for the year 2000 and projections for 2030. *Diabetes Care* **2004**, *27*, 1047–1053. [CrossRef] [PubMed]
3. International Diabetes Federation. IDF Diabetes Atlas, 8th edition. Available online: http://www.diabetesatlas.org/ (accessed on 26 July 2018).
4. World Health Organization. *Global Report on Diabetes*; WHO Press: Geneva, Switzerland, 2016.
5. Segal, L.; Leach, M.J.; May, E.; Turnbull, C. Regional primary care team to deliver best-practice diabetes care: A needs-driven health workforce model reflecting a biopsychosocial construct of health. *Diabetes Care* **2013**, *36*, 1898–1907. [CrossRef] [PubMed]
6. Goenka, N.; Turner, B.; Vora, J. Commissioning specialist diabetes services for adults with diabetes: Summary of a Diabetes UK Task and Finish group report. *Diabet. Med.* **2011**, *28*, 1494–1500. [CrossRef] [PubMed]
7. Nobel, J. Bridging the knowledge-action gap in diabetes: Information technologies, physician incentives and consumer incentives converge. *Chronic Illn.* **2006**, *2*, 59–69. [PubMed]
8. Saleh, F.; Ara, F.; Afnan, F. Assessment of Gap between Knowledge and Practices among Type 2 Diabetes Mellitus Patients at a Tertiary-Care Hospital in Bangladesh. Available online: http://dx.doi.org/10.1155/2016/4928981 (accessed on 16 July 2018).
9. Cantaro, K.; Jara, J.A.; Taboada, M.; Mayta-Tristan, P. Association between information sources and level of knowledge about diabetes in patients with type 2 diabetes. *Endocrinol. Nutr.* **2016**, *63*, 202–211. [CrossRef] [PubMed]
10. Stuckey, H.L.; Mullan-Jensen, C.B.; Reach, G.; Kovacs Burns, K.; Piana, N.; Vallis, M.; Wens, J.; Willaing, I.; Skovlund, S.E.; Peyrot, M. Personal accounts of the negative and adaptive psychosocial experiences of people with diabetes in the second diabetes attitudes, wishes and needs (DAWN2) study. *Diabetes Care* **2014**, *37*, 2466–2474. [CrossRef] [PubMed]
11. Benroubi, M. Fear, guilt feelings and misconceptions: Barriers to effective insulin treatment in type 2 diabetes. *Diabetes Res. Clin. Pract.* **2011**, *93* (Suppl. 1), S97–S99. [CrossRef]
12. Badruddin, N.; Basit, A.; Hydrie, M.Z.I.; Hakeem, R. Knowledge, attitude and practices of patients visiting a diabetes care unit. *Pak. J. Nutr.* **2002**, *1*, 99–102.
13. Al-Qazaz, H.; Sulaiman, S.A.; Hassali, M.A.; Shafie, A.A.; Sundram, S.; Al-Nuri, R.; Saleem, F. Diabetes knowledge, medication adherence and glycemic control among patients with type 2 diabetes. *Int. J. Clin. Pharm.* **2011**, *33*, 1028–1035. [CrossRef] [PubMed]
14. Al-Qazaz, H.K.; Hassali, M.A.; Shafie, A.A.; Syed Sulaiman, S.A.; Sundram, S. Perception and knowledge of patients with type 2 diabetes in Malaysia about their disease and medication: A qualitative study. *Res. Soc. Adm. Pharm.* **2011**, *7*, 180–191. [CrossRef] [PubMed]
15. Puder, J.J.; Keller, U. Quality of diabetes care: Problem of patient or doctor adherence? *Swiss Med. Wkly.* **2003**, *133*, 530–534. [PubMed]
16. Spronk, I.; Kullen, C.; Burdon, C.; O'Connor, H. Relationship between nutrition knowledge and dietary intake. *Br. J. Nutr.* **2014**, *111*, 1713–1726. [CrossRef] [PubMed]
17. Breen, C.; Ryan, M.; Gibney, M.J.; O'Shea, D. Diabetes-related nutrition knowledge and dietary intake among adults with type 2 diabetes. *Br. J. Nutr.* **2015**, *114*, 439–447. [CrossRef] [PubMed]
18. Bruce, D.G.; Davis, W.A.; Cull, C.A.; Davis, T.M. Diabetes education and knowledge in patients with type 2 diabetes from the community: The fremantle diabetes study. *J. Diabetes Complicat.* **2003**, *17*, 82–89. [CrossRef]
19. Hawthorne, K.; Robles, Y.; Cannings-John, R.; Edwards, A.G. Culturally appropriate health education for type 2 diabetes mellitus in ethnic minority groups. *Cochrane Database Syst. Rev.* **2008**. [CrossRef]
20. Kristensen, J.K.; Bak, J.F.; Wittrup, I.; Lauritzen, T. Diabetes prevalence and quality of diabetes care among Lebanese or Turkish immigrants compared to a native Danish population. *Prim. Care Diabetes* **2007**, *1*, 159–165. [CrossRef] [PubMed]
21. Ferguson, W.J.; Candib, L.M. Culture, language, and the doctor-patient relationship. *Fam. Med.* **2002**, *34*, 353–361. [PubMed]

22. Delahanty, L.; Grant, R.W.; Wittenberg, E.; Bosch, J.; Wexler, D.; Cagliero, E.; Meigs, J. Association of diabetes-related emotional distress with diabetes treatment in primary care patients with Type 2 diabetes. *Diabet. Med.* **2007**, *24*, 48–54. [CrossRef] [PubMed]

23. Spencer, M.S.; Kieffer, E.C.; Sinco, B.R.; Palmisano, G.; Guzman, J.R.; James, S.A.; Graddy-Dansby, G.; Two Feathers, J.; Heisler, M. Diabetes-specific emotional distress among African Americans and Hispanics with type 2 diabetes. *J. Health Care Poor Underserved* **2006**, *17*, 88–105. [CrossRef] [PubMed]

24. Lanting, L.C.; Joung, I.M.A.; Mackenbach, J.P.; Lamberts, S.W.J.; Bootsma, A.H. Ethnic differences in mortality, end-stage complications, and quality of care among diabetic patients: A review. *Diabetes Care* **2005**, *28*, 2280–2288. [CrossRef] [PubMed]

25. Mukhopadhyay, B.; Forouhi, N.G.; Fisher, B.M.; Kesson, C.M.; Sattar, N. A comparison of glycaemic and metabolic control over time among South Asian and European patients with type 2 diabetes: Results from follow-up in a routine diabetes clinic. *Diabet. Med.* **2006**, *23*, 94–98. [CrossRef] [PubMed]

26. Fearon, J.D. Ethnic and cultural diversity by country. *J. Econ. Growth* **2003**, *8*, 195–222. [CrossRef]

27. Stewart, D.W.; Shamdasani, P.N. *Focus Groups: Theory and Practice*, 3rd ed.; SAGE Publications Inc.: Thousand Oaks, CA, USA, 2015.

28. Janghorban, R.; Latifnejad Roudsari, R.; Taghipour, A. Skype interviewing: The new generation of online synchronous interview in qualitative research. *Int. J. Qual. Stud. Health Well-Being* **2014**, *9*. [CrossRef] [PubMed]

29. Fereday, J.; Muir-Cochrane, E. Demonstrating rigor using thematic analysis: A hybrid approach of inductive and deductive coding and theme development. *Int. J. Qual. Methods* **2006**, *5*, 1–11. [CrossRef]

30. Egede, L.E.; Funnell, M.M.; Hsu, W.C.; Ruggiero, L.; Siminerio, L.M.; Stuckey, H.L. Ethnic differences in family member diabetes involvement and psychological outcomes: Results from the second Diabetes Attitudes, Wishes and Needs (DAWN2) study in the USA. *Curr. Med. Res. Opin.* **2015**, *31*, 1297–1307.

31. Snorgaard, O.; Poulsen, G.M.; Andersen, H.K.; Astrup, A. Systematic review and meta-analysis of dietary carbohydrate restriction in patients with type 2 diabetes. *BMJ Open Diabetes Res. Care* **2017**, *5*. [CrossRef] [PubMed]

32. Kanthawala, S.; Vermeesch, A.; Given, B.; Huh, J. Answers to health questions: Internet search results versus online health community responses. *J. Med. Internet Res.* **2016**, *18*. [CrossRef] [PubMed]

33. Arora, N.K.; Hesse, B.W.; Rimer, B.K.; Viswanath, K.; Clayman, M.L.; Croyle, R.T. Frustrated and confused: The American public rates its cancer-related information-seeking experiences. *J. Gen. Intern. Med.* **2008**, *23*, 223–228. [CrossRef] [PubMed]

34. Greene, J.; Choudhry, N.; Kilabuk, E.; Shrank, W. Online social networking by patients with diabetes: A qualitative evaluation of communication with facebook. *J. Gen. Intern. Med.* **2011**, *26*, 287–292. [CrossRef] [PubMed]

35. Weitzman, E.R.; Cole, E.; Kaci, L.; Mandl, K.D. Social but safe? Quality and safety of diabetes-related online social networks. *J. Am. Med. Inform. Assoc.* **2011**, *18*, 292–297. [CrossRef] [PubMed]

36. Chomutare, T.; Fernandez-Luque, L.; Årsand, E.; Hartvigsen, G. Features of mobile diabetes applications: Review of the literature and analysis of current applications compared against evidence-based guidelines. *J. Med. Internet Res.* **2011**, *13*. [CrossRef] [PubMed]

37. Fox, S.; Duggan, M. PewInternet: Health online 2013. Available online: http://www.pewinternet.org/2013/01/15/health-online-2013/ (accessed on 4 September 2018).

38. Lawton, J.; Ahmad, N.; Hanna, L.; Douglas, M.; Hallowell, N. Diabetes service provision: A qualitative study of the experiences and views of Pakistani and Indian patients with type 2 diabetes. *Diabet. Med.* **2006**, *23*, 1003–1007. [CrossRef] [PubMed]

39. Lawton, J.; Ahmad, N.; Hallowell, N.; Hanna, L.; Douglas, M. Perceptions and experiences of taking oral hypoglycaemic agents among people of Pakistani and Indian origin: Qualitative study. *BMJ* **2005**, *330*. [CrossRef] [PubMed]

40. Sohal, T.; Sohal, P.; King-Shier, K.M.; Khan, N.A. Barriers and facilitators for type-2 diabetes management in South Asians: A systematic review. *PLoS ONE* **2015**, *10*. [CrossRef] [PubMed]

41. Hirst, J.E.; Tran, T.S.; Do, M.A.; Rowena, F.; Morris, J.M.; Jeffery, H.E. Women with gestational diabetes in Vietnam: A qualitative study to determine attitudes and health behaviours. *BMC Pregnancy Childbirth* **2012**, *12*. [CrossRef] [PubMed]

42. Milne, V.; Kearns, R.; Harrison, A. Patient age, ethnicity and waiting times determine the likelihood of non-attendance at a first specialist rheumatology assessment. *Int. J. Rheum. Dis.* **2014**, *17*, 19–25. [CrossRef] [PubMed]

43. Ministry of Social Development. In *New Zealand Families Today: A Briefing for the Families Commision*; Ministry of Social Development: Wellington, New Zealand, 2004.

44. Nthangeni, G.; Steyn, N.P.; Alberts, M.; Steyn, K.; Levitt, N.S.; Laubscher, R.; Bourne, L.; Dick, J.; Temple, N. Dietary intake and barriers to dietary compliance in black type 2 diabetic patients attending primary health-care services. *Public Health Nutr.* **2002**, *5*, 329–338. [CrossRef] [PubMed]

45. Brez, S.; Rowan, M.; Malcolm, J.; Izzi, S.; Maranger, J.; Liddy, C.; Keely, E.; Ooi, T.C. Transition from specialist to primary diabetes care: A qualitative study of perspectives of primary care physicians. *BMC Fam. Pract.* **2009**, *10*. [CrossRef] [PubMed]

46. Funnell, M.M.; Anderson, R.M. Empowerment and Self-Management of Diabetes. *Clin. Diabetes* **2004**, *22*, 123–127. [CrossRef]

47. Bains, S.S.; Egede, L.E. Associations between health literacy, diabetes knowledge, self-care behaviors, and glycemic control in a low income population with type 2 diabetes. *Diabetes Technol. Ther.* **2011**, *13*, 335–341. [CrossRef] [PubMed]

48. Varming, A.R.; Hansen, U.M.; Andresdottir, G.; Husted, G.R.; Willaing, I. Empowerment, motivation, and medical adherence (EMMA): The feasibility of a program for patient-centered consultations to support medication adherence and blood glucose control in adults with type 2 diabetes. *Patient Prefer. Adherence* **2015**, *9*, 1243–1253. [PubMed]

49. Griffin, S.J.; Kinmonth, A.L.; Veltman, M.W.; Gillard, S.; Grant, J.; Stewart, M. Effect on health-related outcomes of interventions to alter the interaction between patients and practitioners: A systematic review of trials. *Ann. Fam. Med.* **2004**, *2*, 595–608. [CrossRef] [PubMed]

50. Satia, J.A. Diet-related disparities: Understanding the problem and accelerating solutions. *J. Am. Diet. Assoc.* **2009**, *109*, 610–615. [CrossRef] [PubMed]

51. Attridge, M.; Creamer, J.; Ramsden, M.; Cannings-John, R.; Hawthorne, K. Culturally appropriate health education for people in ethnic minority groups with type 2 diabetes mellitus. *Cochrane Database Syst. Rev.* **2014**, *9*. [CrossRef] [PubMed]

52. Krueger, R.A.; Casey, M.A. *Focus Groups: A Practical Guide for Applied Research*, 4th ed.; SAGE Publications Inc.: Thousand Oaks, CA, USA, 2009.

53. Lawrence, H.; Nathan Reynolds, A.; Joseph Venn, B. Perceptions of the healthfulness of foods of New Zealand adults living with prediabetes and type 2 diabetes: A pilot study. *J. Nutr. Educ. Behav.* **2017**, *49*, 339–345.e1. [CrossRef] [PubMed]

54. Forouhi, N.G.; Misra, A.; Mohan, V.; Taylor, R.; Yancy, W. Dietary and nutritional approaches for prevention and management of type 2 diabetes. *BMJ* **2018**, *361*. [CrossRef] [PubMed]

55. Gray, A. Nutritional Recommendations for Individuals with Diabetes. Available online: https://www.ncbi.nlm.nih.gov/pubmed/25905243 (accessed on 23 August 2018).

56. Unwin, D.; Unwin, J. Low carbohydrate diet to achieve weight loss and improve HbA1c in type 2 diabetes and pre-diabetes: Experience from one general practice. *Pract. Diabetes* **2014**, *31*, 76–79. [CrossRef]

57. Wens, J.; Vermeire, E.; Royen, P.V.; Sabbe, B.; Denekens, J. GPs' perspectives of type 2 diabetes patients' adherence to treatment: A qualitative analysis of barriers and solutions. *BMC Fam. Pract.* **2005**, *6*. [CrossRef] [PubMed]

58. Franz, M.J.; Monk, A.; Barry, B.; McClain, K.; Weaver, T.; Cooper, N.; Upham, P.; Bergenstal, R.; Mazze, R.S. Effectiveness of medical nutrition therapy provided by dietitians in the management of non-insulin-dependent diabetes mellitus: A randomized, controlled clinical trial. *J. Am. Diet. Assoc.* **1995**, *95*, 1009–1017. [CrossRef]

59. Coppell, K.J.; Kataoka, M.; Williams, S.M.; Chisholm, A.W.; Vorgers, S.M.; Mann, J.I. Nutritional intervention in patients with type 2 diabetes who are hyperglycaemic despite optimised drug treatment—Lifestyle Over and Above Drugs in Diabetes (LOADD) study: Randomised controlled trial. *BMJ* **2010**, *341*. [CrossRef] [PubMed]

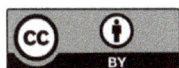

nutrients

MDPI

Article

The Effect of White Rice and White Bread as Staple Foods on Gut Microbiota and Host Metabolism

Fumika Mano, Kaori Ikeda, Erina Joo, Yoshihito Fujita, Shunsuke Yamane, Norio Harada and Nobuya Inagaki *

Department of Diabetes, Endocrinology and Nutrition, Graduate School of Medicine, Kyoto University, Kyoto 606-8507, Japan; fumanou@kuhp.kyoto-u.ac.jp (F.M.); krikeda@kuhp.kyoto-u.ac.jp (K.I.); erinajoo@kuhp.kyoto-u.ac.jp (E.J.); yfujita9@kuhp.kyoto-u.ac.jp (Y.F.); shyamane@kuhp.kyoto-u.ac.jp (S.Y.); nharada@kuhp.kyoto-u.ac.jp (N.H.)
* Correspondence: inagaki@kuhp.kyoto-u.ac.jp; Tel.: +81-757-513-562

Received: 10 August 2018; Accepted: 17 September 2018; Published: 18 September 2018

check for updates

Abstract: The purpose of this study was to examine the influence of two kinds of major Japanese staple foods, white rice and white bread, on gut microbiota against the background in which participants eat common side dishes. Seven healthy subjects completed the dietary intervention with two 1-week test periods with a 1-week wash-out period in cross-over design (UMIN registration UMIN000023142). White bread or white rice and 21 frozen prepared side dishes were consumed during the test periods. At baseline and at the end of each period, fasting blood samples, breath samples, and fecal samples were collected. For fecal samples, 16S rRNA gene sequencing was used to analyze the gut microbiota. After the bread period, the abundance of fecal *Bifidobacterium* genus (19.2 ± 14.5 vs. 6.2 ± 6.6 (%), $p = 0.03$), fasting glucagon-like peptide 1 (GLP-1) (13.6 ± 2.0 vs. 10.5 ± 2.9 (pg/mL), $p = 0.03$), and breath hydrogen (23.4 ± 9.9 vs. 8.2 ± 5.5 (ppm), $p = 0.02$) were significantly higher than those of after the rice period. Plasma SCFAs also tended to be higher after the bread period. White bread contains more dietary fiber than refined short grain rice. These findings suggest that indigestible carbohydrate intake from short grain rice as a staple food may be smaller than that of white bread.

Keywords: Japanese diet; dietary pattern; intestinal biota; prebiotics; rice consumption

1. Introduction

Rice is a traditional staple food of the Japanese diet, but per capita rice consumption in Japan has decreased during the past 50 years [1,2]. Meanwhile, bread consumption in Japan has increased, and rice and bread are now the two major staple foods that supply the main proportion of Japanese energy intake [3].

The dietary pattern of eating rice as a staple food includes lower intake of fat and saturated fat and higher intake of dietary fiber compared with eating wheat flour products as staple foods [4]. A previous cross-sectional study indicates that higher intake of rice and the lower intake of bread are associated with lower prevalence of functional constipation [5]. However, it remains unclear whether this effect is mainly due to the difference of staple foods or dietary constituents including side dishes.

Approximately 10% of the carbohydrates ingested resist pancreatic amylase and escape digestion in the small intestine and remain a main substrate for fermentation in the colon [6]. During the fermentation of these indigestible carbohydrates, the gut microbiota produces short-chain fatty acids (SCFAs) [7,8]. According to some previous studies, SCFAs produced by gut microbiota are associated with lipid metabolism [9] and glucose metabolism in humans [10–12].

In our everyday meals, side dishes are different from meal to meal, but staple foods are consumed repeatedly. We hypothesized that dietary intake of indigestible carbohydrates derived from staple foods would have effects on host metabolism via the composition of the gut microbiota. In the current pilot study, we focus on the difference of staple foods and their influence on gut microbiota composition and glucose and lipid metabolism in a two-period crossover design using a commercially available package of side dishes.

2. Method

2.1. Subjects

Healthy volunteers from our research department (students, technical and research staff) were recruited for this study. Inclusion criteria were the following: (1) those who were not currently taking any medication; (2) those who had no abnormality in physical checkup in the past year. Subjects who had a fever, diarrhea or upper respiratory inflammation during the research period were excluded from analysis. The protocol (UMIN registration UMIN000023142) was approved by Kyoto University Graduate School and Faculty of Medicine, Ethics Committee. The study was conducted at Kyoto University Hospital according to the principles of the Declaration of Helsinki. All subjects gave written informed consent.

2.2. Study Design

The study was a randomized, crossover trial. Following a 1-week run-in period, the subjects were randomized in a 1:1 fashion to one of two intervention sequences: A bread period with supplied side dishes for 1 week followed by a rice period with supplied side dishes for 1 week or a rice period with supplied side dishes for 1 week followed by a bread period with supplied side dishes for 1 week (Figure 1). A 1-week washout period was incorporated between the two test periods. At the baseline and the end of each test period, the blood, breath and fecal samples were collected (Figure 1).

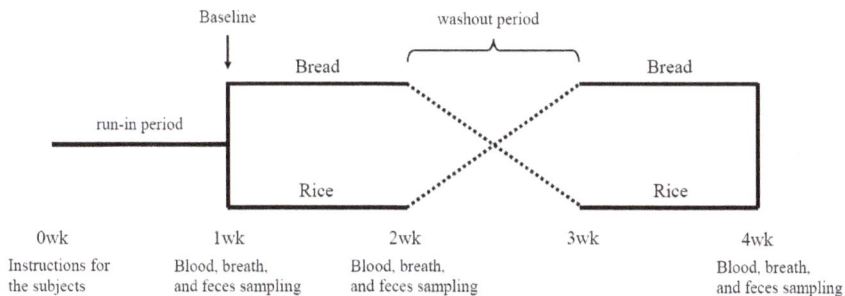

Figure 1. Study design.

In the run-in and washout periods, the subjects were instructed to avoid eating probiotics, yogurt, oligosaccharides and cultured milk drink. During the test periods, the subjects consumed nothing other than staple food (white bread or white rice) and the supplied side dishes. White bread and white rice on the market were prepared by each subject. The supplied side dishes were a package of the frozen prepared 21 sets of side dishes (TOKATSU FOODS Corporation, Yokohama, Japan). The subjects chose one set of side dishes for each meal in the order they liked during the first 6 days, but on the last day, three sets of side dishes were fixed in both periods. The subjects recorded the amount of bread or rice they ate in the first test period, and they ate the equivalent energy of rice or bread in the second test period. Nutritional content of bread and rice was calculated based on the Food Composition Database published by the Ministry of Education, Culture, Sports, Science and Technology, Japan [13], and nutritional content of side dishes were provided by the manufacturer.

2.3. Assessment of Fecal Samples

The fecal samples were collected by subjects at home. The subjects were instructed to put fecal samples in the tubes and put them into boxes with dry ice (−78 °C) immediately after collection, and to bring the boxes to the laboratory. The collected fecal samples were stored at −80 °C until analysis.

16S rRNA gene sequencing analyses of microbial community structure in fecal samples was conducted using a MiSeq (Illumina, San Diego, CA, USA) at TechnoSuruga Laboratory Co., Ltd. (Shizuoka, Japan) according to the method previously described [14]. In brief, PCR amplification was performed by using 341F (5′-CCTACGGGAGGCAGCAG-3′) [15] and 806R (5′-GGACTACH VGGGTWTCTAAT-3′) [16], which were primers for amplifying the V3–V4 region in bacterial 16S rDNA. In addition to the V3–V4 specific priming regions, these primers were complementary to standard Illumina forward and reverse primers. The reverse primer also contained a 6-bp indexing sequence (CAGATC, ACTTGA, GATCAG, TAGCTT, GGCTAC, CTTGTA, ATCACG, CGATGT, TTAGGC and TGACCA) to allow for multiplexing. The touchdown PCR method for thermal cycling was used with a GeneAmp PCR system 9700 (ABI, Foster City, CA, USA). Each PCR reaction mixture (25 μL) contained 20 ng genomic DNA, 2× MightyAmp Buffer Ver.2 (Takara, Otsu, Japan), 0.25 μM of each primer, and 1.25 units of MightyAmp DNA Polymerase (Takara, Otsu, Japan). Each PCR reaction and preparation of amplicon pool were performed as previously described [14].

Each multiplexed library pool was spiked with 12.5% phiX control to improve base calling during sequencing, as recommended by Illumina for the pooling of two libraries [14]. Sequencing was conducted using a paired-end, 2 × 281-bp cycle run on an Illumina MiSeq sequencing system and MiSeq Reagent Kit version 2 (500 Cycle) chemistry. Paired-end sequencing with read lengths of 281 bp was performed. After demultiplexing, a clear overlap in the paired-end reads was observed. This overlap allowed paired reads to be joined together with the fastq-join program (http://code. google.com/p/ea-utils/). The method of quality filtering of sequences was as follows: Only reads that had quality value (QV) scores of ≥20 for more than 99% of the sequence were extracted for further analyses.

Metagenome@KIN software (World Fusion Co., Ltd., Tokyo, Japan) was used to perform homology searching with the determined 16S rDNA sequences, against the TechnoSuruga Lab Microbial Identification Databese DB-BA10.0 (TechnoSuruga Laboratory, Co., Ltd., Tokyo, Japan) which contains only bacteria with standing in the taxonomic nomenclature [17,18]. Bacterial species were identified based on data from 97% similarity cut-off with DB-BA 10.0 [17,18].

2.4. Measurement of Blood Samples

The blood samples were drawn after an overnight fast (12 h). At all points, blood samples for measurement of plasma glucose were collected into tubes containing sodium fluoride (NaF) and Ethylenediamine tetraacetic acid (EDTA); blood samples for serum insulin, serum-free fatty acids (FFA) and serum triglyceride (TG) were collected into tubes containing blood coagulation accelerant; and blood samples for incretin were collected into tubes containing dipeptidyl peptidase-4 (DPP-4) inhibitor (BD P800; Becton Dickinson, San Jose, CA, USA). These blood samples were centrifuged (3000 rpm, 20 min, 4 °C), and the collected plasma and serum samples were stored at −80 °C until analysis. Blood samples for short-chain fatty acids (SCFA) were collected into ice-cooled tubes containing EDTA, and were immediately centrifuged (3000 rpm, 10 min, 4 °C). The collected plasma samples were frozen instantly in liquid nitrogen and were stored at −80 °C until analysis.

Plasma glucose was measured by ultraviolet absorption spectrophotometry at SRL, Inc., Tokyo, Japan. Serum insulin was determined using chemiluminescent enzyme immune assay at SRL, Japan. Serum FFA and serum triglyceride were determined using enzymatic colorimetric kits and glycerol-3-phosphate oxidase method, respectively, at SRL, Japan. Total glucagon-like peptide 1 (GLP-1) was measured by human total GLP-1 (ver. 2) assay kit (K150JVC-1; Mesoscale Discovery, Gaithersburg, MD, USA); total glucose-dependent insulinotropic polypeptide (GIP) was measured by human GIP (total) ELISA (EZHGIP-54K; Merck Millipore, Darmstadt, Germany). Plasma SCFA was measured by liquid chromatography coupled with tandem mass spectrometry (LC-MS/MS) at LSI Medience Corporation, Tokyo, Japan.

2.5. Analyses of Breath Hydrogen

Endtidal breath samples were collected into aluminum bags at the same occasion as blood sampling in order to measure breath hydrogen, which is an indicator of colonic fermentation [10,11,19–21]. Breath hydrogen was measured by simple gas chromatograph (Breath Gas Analyzer BGA1000D) at Laboratory for Expiration Bio-chemistry Nourishment Metabolism Co., Ltd., Nara, Japan [22,23].

2.6. Statistical Analysis

The sample size calculation was based on a standardized effect size of 2.5 (breath hydrogen) estimated from a previous study [10]. A sample size of five was needed to provide 80% power to detect this difference at a two-tailed significance level of 0.05.

All data are expressed as mean with standard deviation. Comparisons between samples at the end of bread periods and those at the end of rice periods were performed using paired *t* test. Two-tailed $p < 0.05$ was considered statistically significant. Statistical analyses were performed with JMP version 13 (SAS Institute, Cary, NC, USA).

3. Results

3.1. Characteristic of Subjects

Ten healthy volunteers participated in this study. Three subjects had a fever or diarrhea in the test period and were excluded from the analysis. Seven healthy subjects (two males and five females; mean (±standard deviation (SD)) age 36.7 ± 4.0 years (range 31–42) and body mass index (BMI) (kg/m^2) 21.0 ± 1.5 (range 18.6–23.1)) were analyzed. Plasma glucose and serum insulin of all subjects were within normal limits (91.2 ± 2.9 mg/dL, 5.2 ± 1.6 µIU/mL, respectively) (Table 1). Five of the seven subjects (two males and three females; mean (±SD) age 36.2 ± 3.9 years and BMI (kg/m^2) 20.4 ± 1.3) were analyzed for plasma SCFA, breath hydrogen and intestinal microbiota.

Table 1. Characteristics of the subjects at baseline.

Subjects (*n*)	7
Glucose (mg/dL)	91.2 ± 2.9
Insulin (µIU/mL)	5.2 ± 1.6
GIP (pg/mL)	56.6 ± 31.6
GLP-1 (pg/mL)	15.7 ± 7.5
TG (mg/dL)	64.4 ± 22.3
FFA (µEq/L)	646.3 ± 250.0
Short-chain fatty acids	
Acetate (µg/mL)	6.64 ± 6.14
Propionate (µg/mL)	0.07 ± 0.02
Butyrate (µg/mL)	0.04 ± 0.02
Breath H$_2$ (ppm)	15.8 ± 12.0

All values are means ± SD.

3.2. Energy Intake and Dietary Composition

The provided sets of frozen side dishes were composed of three side dishes (one main dish and two small side dishes). Main dishes were made with meat, fish or egg, and two small side dishes were mainly made with vegetables. Further information on the typical Japanese side dishes used in this study can be seen in Supplemental Table S1. The mean energy content of 21 sets of side dishes was 294.7 ± 66.8 (kcal/meal), and the mean energy intake from white bread and white rice were 270.6 ± 43.5 (kcal/meal) and 272.7 ± 32.9 (kcal/meal), respectively (Table 2). In both periods, all subjects consumed the staple foods and supplied side dishes completely. White bread, however, has more protein, fat and fiber, and less carbohydrate compared with the equivalent energy of white rice. The calculated energy composition of protein, carbohydrate and fat were 16.4%, 54.1% and 29.5% in the bread period and 12.8%, 63.8% and 23.5% in the rice period, respectively.

Table 2. Nutritional composition of bread, rice and side dish per one meal.

	Energy (kcal)	Protein (g)	Carbohydrate (g)	Fat (g)	Fiber (g)
Bread (*n* = 7)	270.6 ± 43.5	9.5 ± 1.5	47.9 ± 7.7	4.5 ± 0.7	2.4 ± 0.4
Rice (*n* = 7)	272.7 ± 32.9	4.1 ± 0.5	60.2 ± 7.3	0.5 ± 0.1	0.5 ± 0.1
Side dish (*n* = 7)	294.7 ± 66.8	13.7 ± 3.2	28.5 ± 7.4	14.0 ± 5.0	4.3 ± 1.0

All values are Means ± SD.

3.3. Intestinal Microbiota Composition

An average of 40,754 reads were obtained for each sequencing reaction. The minimum and maximum number of sequencing reads were 35,791 and 46,687, respectively. The abundance was a percentage of each number of read in all sequencing reads.

Bacteroidetes, Firmicutes and *Actinobacteria* were the major three *phyla*, and dietary interventions did not make any significant difference in the abundance of *Bacteroidetes* and *Firmicutes*. (Figure 2). However, the abundance of *Actinobacteria* was significantly higher after the bread period compared with that after the rice period (18.0 ± 9.8 vs. 7.9 ± 5.1 (%), $p = 0.02$). Class-level analyses revealed that the abundance of *Actinobacteria* was significantly higher after the bread period compared with that after the rice period (18.0 ± 9.8 vs. 7.9 ± 2.3 (%), $p = 0.02$). No significant difference was observed in other classes. The abundance of *Bifidobacteriales* at order-level (14.7 ± 9.9 vs. 5.4 ± 5.5 (%), $p = 0.02$), and the abundance of *Bifidobacteriaceae* at family-level (14.7 ± 9.9 vs. 5.4 ± 5.5 (%), $p = 0.02$) were significantly higher after the bread period than those after the rice period. No significant difference was observed in other orders and families. Genus-level analyses determined that the abundance of *Bifidobacterium* was significantly higher after the bread period than after the rice period (19.2 ± 14.5 vs. 6.2 ± 6.6 (%), $p = 0.03$) (Table 3). Although there was individual difference in the abundance of *Biffidobacterium* at the baseline, four of the five subjects showed higher abundance of *Bifidobacterium* after the bread period compared with those after the rice period (Figure 3). No significant difference was observed in other genera. At species level, the abundance of *Bifidobacterium longum* was significantly higher after the bread period compared with that after the rice period (3.3 ± 3.1 vs. 2.3 ± 3.3 (%), $p < 0.01$). The abundance of *Blautia faecis* was significantly higher after the rice period compared with that after the bread period (0.6 ± 0.4 vs. 1.0 ± 0.7 (%), $p = 0.046$; the abundance at the baseline = 0.8 ± 0.4 (%)). No significant difference was observed in other species.

Table 3. Mean value of genera of the *Actinobacteria phylum* identified in fecal samples at baseline, and after bread and rice periods.

	Baseline (*n* = 7)	Bread (*n* = 7)	Rice (*n* = 7)
Bifidobacterium (%)	15.3 ± 13.2	19.2 ± 14.5 *	6.2 ± 6.6
Collinsella (%)	3.2 ± 3.9	3.5 ± 4.5	2.3 ± 2.8
Eggerthella (%)	0.3 ± 0.3	0.1 ± 0.1	0.3 ± 0.3
Actinomyces (%)	0.1 ± 0.05	0.1 ± 0.1	0.1 ± 0.05

All values are Means ± SD. After bread period: Bread; After rice period: Rice. *p* values are derived by two-tailed paired *t* test. *p* * < 0.05 for Bread versus Rice.

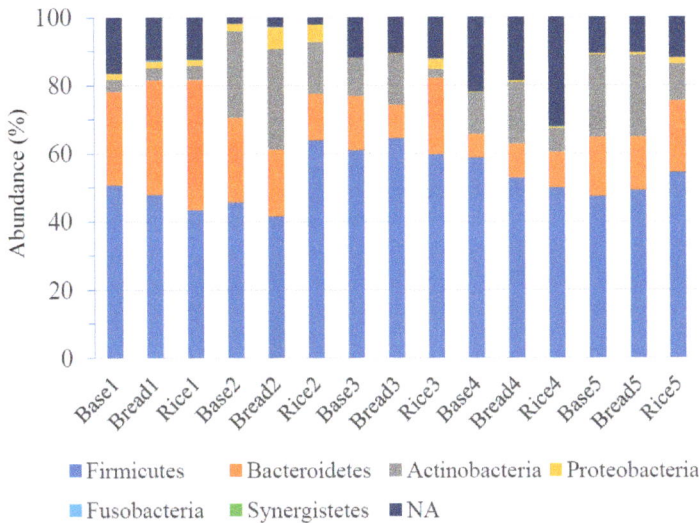

Figure 2. *Phylum*-level classification of bacteria identified in fecal samples of five subjects. The *phyla* represented by the different colors are shown below the figure. Baseline: Base; After bread period: Bread; After rice period: Rice.

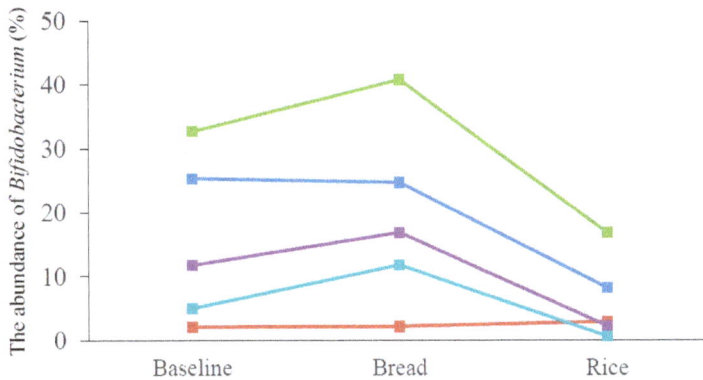

Figure 3. The abundance of *Bifidobacterium* of five subjects at baseline, after bread period and after rice period. After bread period: Bread; After rice period: Rice. Each color indicates each subject.

3.4. Hormonal and Metabolic Changes in Blood and Breath

The plasma GLP-1 level after the bread period was significantly higher than that after the rice period (13.6 ± 2.0 vs. 10.5 ± 2.9 (pg/mL), $p = 0.03$) (Table 4). Glucose, insulin, GIP, triglyceride and free fatty acids showed no significant differences. Plasma propionate and butyrate levels tended to be higher after the bread period compared with those after the rice period (0.11 ± 0.09 vs. 0.06 ± 0.03 (µg/mL), $p = 0.16$, 0.06 ± 0.04 vs. 0.02 ± 0.01 (µg/mL), $p = 0.12$, respectively). Breath hydrogen was significantly higher after the bread period than after the rice period (23.4 ± 9.9 vs. 8.2 ± 5.5 (ppm), $p = 0.02$).

Table 4. Plasma or serum concentration of metabolites, and breath hydrogen after bread and rice periods.

	Bread (*n* = 7)	Rice (*n* = 7)	*p* Value
Glucose (mg/dL)	86.2 ± 5.0	87.4 ± 6.9	0.52
Insulin (μIU/mL)	4.0 ± 0.9	3.5 ± 1.1	0.34
GIP (pg/mL)	55.2 ± 18.9	43.8 ± 21.1	0.11
GLP-1 (pg/mL)	13.6 ± 2.0	10.5 ± 2.9	0.03 *
TG (mg/dL)	58.4 ± 16.4	73.9 ± 29.4	0.20
FFA (μEq/L)	619.6 ± 149.1	561.6 ± 281.6	0.63
Short-chain fatty acids			
Acetate (μg/mL)	5.34 ± 4.08	4.12 ± 3.06	0.70
Propionate (μg/mL)	0.11 ± 0.09	0.06 ± 0.03	0.16
Butyrate (μg/mL)	0.06 ± 0.04	0.02 ± 0.01	0.12
Breath H_2 (ppm)	23.4 ± 9.9	8.2 ± 5.2	0.02 *

All values are means ± SD. After bread period: Bread; After rice period: Rice; *p* values are derived by two-tailed paired *t* test. * *p* < 0.05 for Bread versus Rice.

4. Discussion

In the current study, we examined the influence of staple foods on gut microbiota against the background in which subjects consumed fixed sets of side dishes. Many previous studies on the effect of dietary intervention on gut microbiota were conducted by using foods with a large difference in dietary fiber content [8,10–12,20,21] or by adding specific non-digestible carbohydrates to daily meals [24–27]. The strength of the current study is that the test meals used were very similar to everyday meals of Japanese people; we used two major staple foods, white rice and white bread together with ordinary kinds of side dishes. After the bread period, abundance of fecal *Bifidobacterium*, fasting plasma GLP-1 level, and breath hydrogen were significantly higher than those of after the rice period. Dietary fiber and resistant starch are prebiotics, which act as a fermentation substrate within the colon and stimulate preferential growth and activity of specific microbial species (e.g., *Bifidobacterium*) and confer health benefits on the host [27,28]. The major products of fermentable carbohydrate in gut microbiota are SCFAs (e.g., acetate, propionate, butyrate) and gases (e.g., hydrogen and carbon dioxide) [29]. In this study, 7-days intake of bread containing a higher amount of dietary fiber than rice induced higher abundance of *Bifidobacterium* and higher excretion of hydrogen. At species level, the abundance of *Blautia faecis* which belongs to the genus *Blautia* was significantly higher after the rice period compared with that after the bread period. A previous study reported that the composition of the Japanese gut microbiome showed more abundance in the genus *Bifidobacterium* and *Blautia* compared with those of Western and other Asian people [30]. However, to our knowledge, there is no report that dietary intervention affects the abundance of *Blautia faecis*.

GLP-1 is an incretin secreted by intestinal endocrine L cells located mainly in the ileum and colon [31]. SCFAs produced by fermentation in gut microbiota can directly enhance L cells' release of GLP-1 through the SCFA receptors, GPR41 and GPR43 [29,32,33]. GPR41 are activated by propionate and butyrate and GPR43 are activated by acetate and propionate [32,34,35]. In our study, plasma propionate and butyrate levels after the bread period tended to be higher than those after the rice period. These facts support the higher fasting GLP-1 observed after the bread period.

One limitation of this study is that resistant starch content of bread and rice was not measured. Murphy et al. reported in her review article that the mean value of resistant starch content of white bread and white rice was almost the same [36], but in that review, rice included long grain rice cultivars. In Japan, the *japonica* rice cultivars (short grain rice), which contain lesser resistant starch than long grain rice cultivars, are popular [37,38]. In the current study, one possibility is that the resistant starch content of bread was higher than that of rice.

Another limitation of this study is that food records of the subjects' usual diet before the test periods were not obtained. The baseline values of fecal *Bifidobacterium*, plasma GLP-1, and breath hydrogen were generally higher than those after the rice period. It is possible that the intake of indigestible carbohydrate during the washout period was larger than that during the rice period. The mean amount of dietary fiber consumed in the rice period was calculated to be about 14.4 (g/day), which was comparable to the average amount of the dietary fiber intake of Japanese people, 14.2 (g/day) [3].

Given that the Japanese diet is almost always composed of one staple food and side dishes [2], the choice of staple foods has considerable influence on the intake volume of indigestible carbohydrate. This study suggests that people who consume rice as a staple food (especially short grain rice) may need to consume more dietary fiber from side dishes.

5. Conclusions

Against the background of people eating common side dishes, 7 days intake of white bread induced significantly higher abundance of fecal *Bifidobacterium*, fasting GLP-1, and breath hydrogen compared with 7 days intake of white rice.

Supplementary Materials: The following are available online at http://www.mdpi.com/2072-6643/10/9/1323/s1, Table S1: Menu and food ingredients of the side dish sets on the 7th day of both test periods (bread and rice).

Author Contributions: The authors' contributions were as follows: F.M., K.I. and E.J. designed the research; F.M., K.I. and E.J. conducted research; F.M., K.I., E.J., Y.F., S.Y., N.H. and N.I. analyzed data; and F.M. and K.I. wrote the paper. N.I. had primary responsibility for final content. None of the authors had any conflicts of interest related to this study. All authors read and approved the final manuscript.

Funding: This research was supported by Integration research for agriculture and interdisciplinary fields, Ministry of Agriculture, Fisheries and Forests, Japan, and Japan Agency for Medical Research and Development (AMED) under Grant Number JP17ek0210079. They had no role in the design, analysis or writing of this article.

Conflicts of Interest: The authors declare no conflict of interest.

References

1. Maff~close to your daily life. Available online: http://www.maff.go.jp/e/data/publish/maff_2016.html (accessed on 4 April 2018).
2. Suzuki, N.; Goto, Y.; Ota, H.; Kito, K.; Mano, F.; Joo, E.; Ikeda, K.; Inagaki, N.; Nakayama, T. Characteristics of the Japanese diet described in epidemiologic publications: A qualitative systematic review. *J. Nutr. Sci. Vitaminol.* **2018**, *64*, 129–137. [CrossRef] [PubMed]
3. Ministry of Health, Labor and Welfare. The national health nutrition survey in japan, 2016. Available online: http://www.nibiohn.go.jp/eiken/kenkounippon21/en/eiyouchousa/koumoku_eiyou_chousa.html (accessed on 6 April 2018).
4. Batres-Marquez, S.P.; Jensen, H.H.; Upton, J. Rice consumption in the United States: Recent evidence from food consumption surveys. *J. Am. Diet. Assoc.* **2009**, *109*, 1719–1727. [CrossRef] [PubMed]
5. Okubo, H.; Sasaki, S.; Murakami, K.; Kim, M.K.; Takahashi, Y.; Hosoi, Y.; Itabashi, M. Dietary patterns associated with functional constipation among Japanese women aged 18 to 20 years: A cross-sectional study. *J. Nutr. Sci. Vitaminol.* **2007**, *53*, 232–238. [CrossRef] [PubMed]
6. Cummings, J.H.; Englyst, H.N. Measurement of starch fermentation in the human large intestine. *Can. J. Physiol. Pharmacol.* **1991**, *69*, 121–129. [CrossRef] [PubMed]
7. Tan, J.; McKenzie, C.; Potamitis, M.; Thorburn, A.N.; Mackay, C.R.; Macia, L. The role of short-chain fatty acids in health and disease. *Adv. Immunol.* **2014**, *121*, 91–119. [PubMed]
8. Nilsson, A.C.; Ostman, E.M.; Knudsen, K.E.; Holst, J.J.; Bjorck, I.M. A cereal-based evening meal rich in indigestible carbohydrates increases plasma butyrate the next morning. *J. Nutr.* **2010**, *140*, 1932–1936. [CrossRef] [PubMed]
9. Teixeira, T.F.; Grzeskowiak, L.; Franceschini, S.C.; Bressan, J.; Ferreira, C.L.; Peluzio, M.C. Higher level of faecal SCFA in women correlates with metabolic syndrome risk factors. *Br. J. Nutr.* **2013**, *109*, 914–919. [CrossRef] [PubMed]

10. Johansson, E.V.; Nilsson, A.C.; Ostman, E.M.; Bjorck, I.M. Effects of indigestible carbohydrates in barley on glucose metabolism, appetite and voluntary food intake over 16 h in healthy adults. *Nutr. J.* **2013**, *12*, 46. [CrossRef] [PubMed]

11. Nilsson, A.C.; Ostman, E.M.; Holst, J.J.; Bjorck, I.M. Including indigestible carbohydrates in the evening meal of healthy subjects improves glucose tolerance, lowers inflammatory markers, and increases satiety after a subsequent standardized breakfast. *J. Nutr.* **2008**, *138*, 732–739. [CrossRef] [PubMed]

12. Kovatcheva-Datchary, P.; Nilsson, A.; Akrami, R.; Lee, Y.S.; De Vadder, F.; Arora, T.; Hallen, A.; Martens, E.; Bjorck, I.; Backhed, F. Dietary fiber-induced improvement in glucose metabolism is associated with increased abundance of *prevotella*. *Cell MeTab.* **2015**, *22*, 971–982. [CrossRef] [PubMed]

13. Standard tables of food composition in Japan-2015-(seventh revised version). Available online: http://www. mext.go.jp/en/policy/science_technology/policy/title01/detail01/1374030.htm (accessed on 4 April 2018).

14. Takahashi, S.; Tomita, J.; Nishioka, K.; Hisada, T.; Nishijima, M. Development of a prokaryotic universal primer for simultaneous analysis of bacteria and archaea using next-generation sequencing. *PLoS ONE* **2014**, *9*, e105592. [CrossRef] [PubMed]

15. Muyzer, G.; de Waal, E.C.; Uitterlinden, A.G. Profiling of complex microbial populations by denaturing gradient gel electrophoresis analysis of polymerase chain reaction-amplified genes coding for 16s rRNA. *Appl. Environ. Microbiol.* **1993**, *59*, 695–700. [PubMed]

16. Caporaso, J.G.; Lauber, C.L.; Walters, W.A.; Berg-Lyons, D.; Lozupone, C.A.; Turnbaugh, P.J.; Fierer, N.; Knight, R. Global patterns of 16s rRNA diversity at a depth of millions of sequences per sample. *Proc. Natl. Acad. Sci. USA* **2011**, *108*, 4516–4522. [CrossRef] [PubMed]

17. Hisada, T.; Endoh, K.; Kuriki, K. Inter- and intra-individual variations in seasonal and daily stabilities of the human gut microbiota in Japanese. *Arch. Microbiol.* **2015**, *197*, 919–934. [CrossRef] [PubMed]

18. Kasai, C.; Sugimoto, K.; Moritani, I.; Tanaka, J.; Oya, Y.; Inoue, H.; Tameda, M.; Shiraki, K.; Ito, M.; Takei, Y.; et al. Comparison of the gut microbiota composition between obese and non-obese individuals in a Japanese population, as analyzed by terminal restriction fragment length polymorphism and next-generation sequencing. *BMC Gastroenterol.* **2015**, *15*, 100. [CrossRef] [PubMed]

19. Ibrugger, S.; Vigsnaes, L.K.; Blennow, A.; Skuflic, D.; Raben, A.; Lauritzen, L.; Kristensen, M. Second meal effect on appetite and fermentation of wholegrain rye foods. *Appetite* **2014**, *80*, 248–256. [CrossRef] [PubMed]

20. Nilsson, A.C.; Ostman, E.M.; Granfeldt, Y.; Bjorck, I.M. Effect of cereal test breakfasts differing in glycemic index and content of indigestible carbohydrates on daylong glucose tolerance in healthy subjects. *Am. J. Clin. Nutr.* **2008**, *87*, 645–654. [CrossRef] [PubMed]

21. Nilsson, A.C.; Johansson-Boll, E.V.; Bjorck, I.M. Increased gut hormones and insulin sensitivity index following a 3-d intervention with a barley kernel-based product: A randomised cross-over study in healthy middle-aged subjects. *Br. J. Nutr.* **2015**, *114*, 899–907. [CrossRef] [PubMed]

22. Oku, T.; Nakamura, S. Evaluation of the relative available energy of several dietary fiber preparations using breath hydrogen evolution in healthy humans. *J. Nutr. Sci. Vitaminol.* **2014**, *60*, 246–254. [CrossRef] [PubMed]

23. Nakamura, S.; Tanabe, K.; Morita, S.; Hamaguchi, N.; Shimura, F.; Oku, T. Metabolism and bioavailability of newly developed dietary fiber materials, resistant glucan and hydrogenated resistant glucan, in rats and humans. *Nutr. MeTab.* **2016**, *13*, 13. [CrossRef] [PubMed]

24. Mudgil, D.; Barak, S. Composition, properties and health benefits of indigestible carbohydrate polymers as dietary fiber: A review. *Int. J. Biol. Macromol.* **2013**, *61*, 1–6. [CrossRef] [PubMed]

25. Gibson, G.R.; Roberfroid, M.B. Dietary modulation of the human colonic microbiota: Introducing the concept of prebiotics. *J. Nutr.* **1995**, *125*, 1401–1412. [PubMed]

26. Ramirez-Farias, C.; Slezak, K.; Fuller, Z.; Duncan, A.; Holtrop, G.; Louis, P. Effect of inulin on the human gut microbiota: Stimulation of *bifidobacterium adolescentis* and *faecalibacterium prausnitzii*. *Br. J. Nutr.* **2009**, *101*, 541–550. [CrossRef] [PubMed]

27. Slavin, J. Fiber and prebiotics: Mechanisms and health benefits. *Nutrients* **2013**, *5*, 1417–1435. [CrossRef] [PubMed]

28. Gibson, G.R.; Probert, H.M.; Loo, J.V.; Rastall, R.A.; Roberfroid, M.B. Dietary modulation of the human colonic microbiota: Updating the concept of prebiotics. *Nutr. Res. Rev.* **2004**, *17*, 259–275. [CrossRef] [PubMed]

29. Everard, A.; Cani, P.D. Gut microbiota and GLP-1. *Rev. Endocr. Metab. Disord.* **2014**, *15*, 189–196. [CrossRef] [PubMed]

30. Nishijima, S.; Suda, W.; Oshima, K.; Kim, S.; Hirose, Y.; Morita, H.; Hattori, M. The gut microbiome of healthy Japanese and its microbial and functional uniqueness. *DNA Res.* **2016**, *23*, 125–133. [CrossRef] [PubMed]

31. Seino, Y.; Fukushima, M.; Yabe, D. GIP and GLP-1, the two incretin hormones: Similarities and differences. *J. Diabetes Investig.* **2010**, *1*, 8–23. [CrossRef] [PubMed]

32. Tolhurst, G.; Heffron, H.; Lam, Y.S.; Parker, H.E.; Habib, A.M.; Diakogiannaki, E.; Cameron, J.; Grosse, J.; Reimann, F.; Gribble, F.M. Short-chain fatty acids stimulate glucagon-like peptide-1 secretion via the G-protein-coupled receptor FFAR2. *Diabetes* **2012**, *61*, 364–371. [CrossRef] [PubMed]

33. Psichas, A.; Sleeth, M.L.; Murphy, K.G.; Brooks, L.; Bewick, G.A.; Hanyaloglu, A.C.; Ghatei, M.A.; Bloom, S.R.; Frost, G. The short chain fatty acid propionate stimulates GLP-1 and PYY secretion via free fatty acid receptor 2 in rodents. *Int. J. Obes.* **2015**, *39*, 424–429. [CrossRef] [PubMed]

34. Brown, A.J.; Goldsworthy, S.M.; Barnes, A.A.; Eilert, M.M.; Tcheang, L.; Daniels, D.; Muir, A.I.; Wigglesworth, M.J.; Kinghorn, I.; Fraser, N.J.; et al. The orphan g protein-coupled receptors GPR41 and GPR43 are activated by propionate and other short chain carboxylic acids. *J. Biol. Chem.* **2003**, *278*, 11312–11319. [CrossRef] [PubMed]

35. Le Poul, E.; Loison, C.; Struyf, S.; Springael, J.Y.; Lannoy, V.; Decobecq, M.E.; Brezillon, S.; Dupriez, V.; Vassart, G.; Van Damme, J.; et al. Functional characterization of human receptors for short chain fatty acids and their role in polymorphonuclear cell activation. *J. Biol. Chem.* **2003**, *278*, 25481–25489. [CrossRef] [PubMed]

36. Murphy, M.M.; Douglass, J.S.; Birkett, A. Resistant starch intakes in the United States. *J. Am. Diet. Assoc.* **2008**, *108*, 67–78. [CrossRef] [PubMed]

37. Hu, P.; Zhao, H.; Duan, Z.; Linlin, Z.; Wu, D. Starch digestibility and the estimated glycemic score of different types of rice differing in amylose contents. *J. Cereal Sci.* **2004**, *40*, 231–237. [CrossRef]

38. Nakamura, S.; Satoh, H.; Ohtsubo, K. Development of formulae for estimating amylose content, amylopectin chain length distribution, and resistant starch content based on the iodine absorption curve of rice starch. *Biosci. Biotechnol. Biochem.* **2015**, *79*, 443–455. [CrossRef] [PubMed]

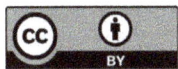

nutrients

MDPI

Review

Relevance of the Glycemic Index and Glycemic Load for Body Weight, Diabetes, and Cardiovascular Disease

Sonia Vega-López [1,*], Bernard J. Venn [2] and Joanne L. Slavin [3]

[1] College of Health Solutions and Southwest Interdisciplinary Research Center, Arizona State University, Phoenix, AZ 85004, USA

[2] Department of Human Nutrition, University of Otago, Dunedin 9054, New Zealand; Bernard.Venn@otago.ac.nz

[3] Department of Food Science and Nutrition, University of Minnesota, St. Paul, MN 55108, USA; jslavin@umn.edu

* Correspondence: Sonia.Vega.Lopez@asu.edu; Tel.: +1-602-827-2268

check for updates

Received: 16 August 2018; Accepted: 20 September 2018; Published: 22 September 2018

Abstract: Despite initial enthusiasm, the relationship between glycemic index (GI) and glycemic response (GR) and disease prevention remains unclear. This review examines evidence from randomized, controlled trials and observational studies in humans for short-term (e.g., satiety) and long-term (e.g., weight, cardiovascular disease, and type 2 diabetes) health effects associated with different types of GI diets. A systematic PubMed search was conducted of studies published between 2006 and 2018 with key words glycemic index, glycemic load, diabetes, cardiovascular disease, body weight, satiety, and obesity. Criteria for inclusion for observational studies and randomized intervention studies were set. The search yielded 445 articles, of which 73 met inclusion criteria. Results suggest an equivocal relationship between GI/GR and disease outcome. The strongest intervention studies typically find little relationship among GI/GR and physiological measures of disease risk. Even for observational studies, the relationship between GI/GR and disease outcomes is limited. Thus, it is unlikely that the GI of a food or diet is linked to disease risk or health outcomes. Other measures of dietary quality, such as fiber or whole grains may be more likely to predict health outcomes. Interest in food patterns as predictors of health benefits may be more fruitful for research to inform dietary guidance.

Keywords: body weight; carbohydrates; glycemic index; glycemic load; glycemic response; satiety; type 2 diabetes; chronic disease risk

1. Introduction

The appearance of glucose in the bloodstream following eating—the glycemic response (GR)—is a normal physiological occurrence that depends on the rate of glucose entry into the circulation, the amount of glucose absorbed, the rate of disappearance from the circulation due to tissue uptake, and hepatic regulation of glucose release [1]. Foods containing carbohydrates have a wide range of effects on the GR, with some resulting in a rapid rise followed by rapid fall in blood glucose concentrations, while others show an extended rise and slow extended fall in blood glucose. The Glycemic Index (GI) was created in 1981 as a tool for people with diabetes to select foods [2]. GI provides information on the GR that might be expected when a person consumes the quantity of a food containing a fixed amount of carbohydrate (usually 50 g). In this system, GR is defined as the increase in the blood glucose concentration following eating, expressed as the incremental area-under-the-blood-glucose-curve (iAUC) over a period of two hours. The GI value is actually given as a relative GR; the GR of the food is expressed as a percentage of the GR of a reference food (usually a glucose solution or white bread):

$$GI = (iAUC_{test\ food} / iAUC_{reference\ food}) \times 100 \qquad (1)$$

To a large extent, control of the GR is governed by the amount of food eaten; that is, if a large amount of a low or a high GI food is consumed, the GR will be large and vice versa, a small amount of either a low or a high GI food will limit the GR. The concept of the glycemic load (GL) was introduced as a means of predicting the GR; it takes into account the GI and the amount of available carbohydrate in a portion of the food eaten (GL = GI × available carbohydrate in a given amount of food) [3].

Much work has been undertaken since the introduction of the concepts of GI and GL to ascertain how they relate to health and disease. In applying the concepts, foods have been classified by GI into low (GI ≤ 55), medium (GI 56–69), and high (GI ≥ 70) categories, and classified by GL as being low (GL ≤ 10), medium (GL 11–19), and high (GL ≥ 20). The GI and GL classification systems were developed arbitrarily in the sense that they did not relate to nutrient density of the food or to any risk factor for chronic disease as a consequence of consuming the food. The observational epidemiological work relating GI and GL to overweight and obesity, and to chronic disease risk has been controversial, as has been whether consuming diets with low GI translates into better health outcomes and more effective weight management for the general population. Therefore, the purpose of this review is to summarize the most recent evidence for short-term (e.g., satiety) and long-term (e.g., weight, cardiovascular disease, and type 2 diabetes) health effects associated with different types of GI diets.

2. Methods

Articles were initially selected by conducting a PubMed online search using the following keywords and combinations: glycemic index, glycemic load, diabetes, cardiovascular disease, body weight, satiety, and obesity. For purposes of this review, studies included were limited to those published in English between 2006 and 2018 conducted in adults and in which the study design allowed for a clear comparison between foods, meals, or diets with distinct GI (i.e., frank comparison of low GI foods, meals, or diets with their high GI counterparts). PubMed was last searched on 20 July 2018; data were extracted and summarized into tables for content review.

Cross-sectional studies were included if they had body weight or BMI, type-2 diabetes diagnosis, or a cardiovascular event as an endpoint. For intervention studies, only those with a randomized design were included in an attempt to assess evidence only from studies with greater internal validity than those using a quasi-experimental design. Studies aimed at assessing the effects of specific foods as part of a low GI diet (e.g., legumes or low GI fruits), those in which additional dietary components were part of one of the diet treatments (e.g., vinegar or olive oil), and those in which physical activity was part of the intervention were excluded because those additional components could have confounded the effects from the GI itself on study outcomes. Studies with a quasi-experimental design were not included. Animal studies were also excluded.

Additional considerations of inclusion criteria for studies incorporated in this review will be described within each section. Among the studies included herein, a majority focused on GI rather than GL because there has been no consensus of whether GI or GL is used in research settings. Descriptions of the studies were kept consistent with the parameter assessed (GI or GL).

Of the 445 articles retrieved from the keyword search, 278 were not relevant for this review. After reviewing the remaining 167 articles, 73 met the selection criteria and were included (Figure 1).

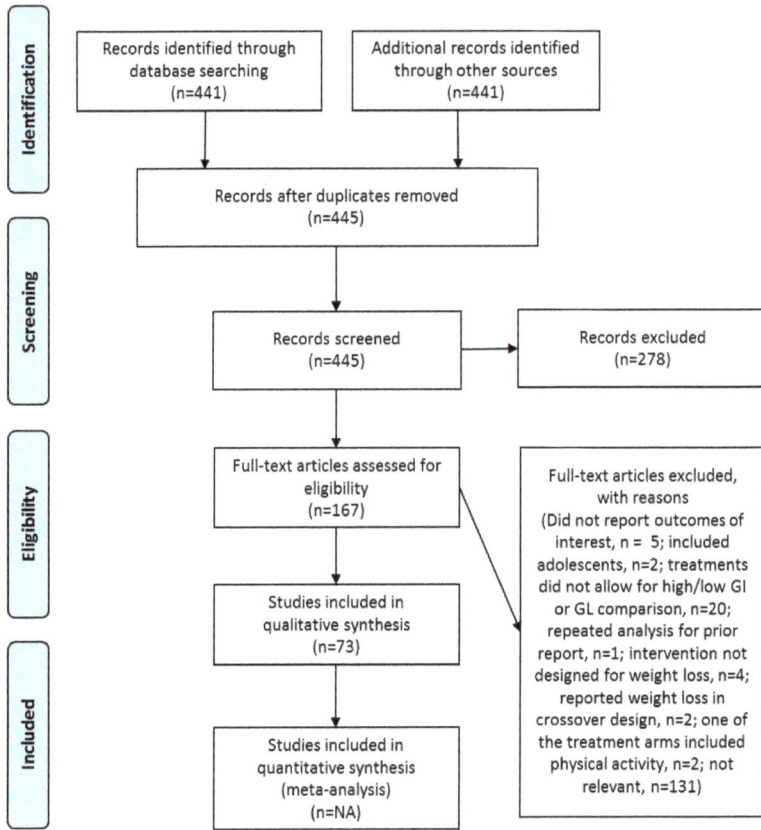

Figure 1. PRISMA Flow Diagram illustrating study selection.

3. Glycemic Index/Glycemic Load and Satiety

Classification of foods based on their GI stems from the premise that the presence of different carbohydrates within foods elicits different GRs and potential downstream metabolic responses [2,4]. Regulation of satiety is a complex mechanism dependent on multiple factors, among them satiety-related hormones such as insulin, leptin, ghrelin, cholecystokinin (CCK), glucagon-like peptide 1 (GLP-1), peptide tyrosine-tyrosine (PYY), enterostatin, amylin, and oxyntomodulin [5,6]. Thus, there is no biomarker that could serve as a single measure of satiety. Although there is increasing interest in how different dietary components affect appetite or satiety, the specific effects of GI have not been thoroughly studied, and with a few exceptions, have been assessed using subjective self-reported measures. The most commonly used instruments for subjectively assessing satiety consist of visual analog scales that prompt a responder to rate their degree of satiety on a numerical scale graph (similar to a ruler) [7].

3.1. Acute Effects of Meals with Different GI

Studies that included an assessment of the effects of different GI meals on satiety have been designed to evaluate postprandial biomarker responses after acute ingestion of meals with different composite GI values. Although the standard methodology for assessing GI of a food involves measuring the GR over a 2-h period [8], there are no standard protocols for assessing the postprandial effects of different GI foods on other outcomes. Several studies have consisted of randomized crossover assessments of responses to breakfast meals after a standardized overnight fast, followed by a postprandial observation period of 2 to 4 h in length (Table 1) [9–16]. These interventions were conducted in healthy adults [10,13,15,16], adults with type 2 diabetes [11,12], pregnant women with gestational diabetes [9], and men with type 1 diabetes [14].

Table 1. Intervention studies assessing the acute effect of low GI foods or meals on appetite/satiety [1].

Study	Sample	Design	Duration	Intervention	Treatment Effects (Low vs. High GI)	Greater Fiber (Low GI)
Louie et al. [9]	10 women w/GDM 30–32 weeks gestation 18–45 years	R; X	2 h PP responses to breakfast meal	LGI HGI	↓ PP Glucose ↔ Satiety (subj)	No
Makris et al. [10]	16 sedentary adults 38 ± 11 years 30.9 ± 3.7 kg/m²	R; X	4 h PP responses to breakfast	HGI-Hprot HGI-Lprot LGI-Hprot LGI-Lprot	↓ Glucose, insulin No protein effects No GI × protein effects ↔ Ad libitum energy intake ↔ Hunger (subj) ↔ Satiety (subj)	No
Silva et al. [11]	14 adults w/T2D 66 ± 5 years 27.2 ± 3.1 kg/m² HbA1c: 6.6 ± 0.9%	R; X	3 h PP responses to breakfast meal	HGI-HF HGI-LF LGI-HF LGI-LF	↓ Glucose LGIHF vs. HGILF ↓ Ins HGIHF vs. HGILF ↓ Ghrelin LGIHF @ 180 min ↔ Appetite (subj)	NA
Lobos et al. [12]	10 obese adults w/T2D and intensive insulin therapy 55 ± 6 years 34.7 ± 2.4 kg/m²	R; X	2 h PP responses to breakfast meal	LGI breakfast HGI breakfast	↔ Satiety (subj) ↓ Glucose	Yes
Png et al. [13]	12 Muslim adult men 28 ± 7 years 51 ± 9 kg	R; X	12 h PP after ingestion of the last meal before fast during Ramadan	LGI (37) Control (GI ~57)	↔ Satiety, appetite, fullness (all subj)	NR
Campbell et al. [14]	10 men with T1D 27 ± 1 years 25.5 ± 0.03 kg/m²	R; X	Postprandial responses to postexercise meal	LGI meal HGI meal	↓ Glucose AUC ↔ Glucose, insulin, glucagon, GLP-1 ↔ Appetite (subj)	No
Reynolds et al. [15]	12 adults 23 ± 3 years 23.1 ± 1.9 kg/m²	R; X	10 h PP responses to 4 consecutive meals	Low-GI diet High-GI diet	↓ Glucose, insulin ↔ CCK, ghrelin	No
Liu et al. [16]	26 overweight/obese adults 44 ± 15 years 29.1 ± 2.8 kg/m²	R; X	PP responses over 12 h including std breakfast/lunch/dinner	HGI-HCHO HGI-LCHO LGI-HCHO LGI-LCHO	↓ Glucose all vs. HGI-HCHO ↓ Insulin all vs. HGI-HCHO ↔ Hunger (subj)	No

[1] Abbreviations: GDM: gestational diabetes mellitus; GI: glycemic index; HCHO: high carbohydrate; HF: high fiber; HGI: high GI; Hprot: high protein; LCHO: low carbohydrate; LF: low fiber; LGI: low GI; Lprot: low protein; NA: not applicable; NR: not reported; PP: postprandial; R: randomized; subj: subjective measure; T1D: type 1 diabetes; T2D: type 2 diabetes; X: crossover design; ↓ lower; ↔ no difference.

Although, as expected, low GI meals resulted in lower glycemic [9–12] and insulinemic [10] responses, subjective assessments of appetite, satiety, hunger, fullness, or desire to eat did not differ based on the GI of the test meal. Moreover, the lower glycemic and/or insulinemic responses observed in two of the studies were observed in the context of higher dietary fiber content of the meals [11,12]. One of those studies compared low and high GI meals with low and high fiber content and documented lower postprandial ghrelin responses only under the low GI/low fiber combination [11]. Similar to what was documented in the previously described studies, subjectively-measured satiety, appetite, or fullness were not different 12 h after consumption of macronutrient (protein, carbohydrates, and fat)—matched meals with low or intermediate GI in 12 adult Muslim men who were fasting during Ramadan [13]. Moreover, in a crossover study comparing responses to postexercise meals with low or high GI in individuals with type 1 diabetes, despite the greater postprandial glucose area under the curve with the high GI meal, there were no differences in glucose, insulin, glucagon, and glucagon-like peptide-1 (GLP-1) concentrations or subjective appetite ratings between meals [14].

Another approach to evaluating the short-term effects of the GI consists of monitoring responses to consecutive standardized meals with low or high GI over 10 to 12 h during different test days (Table 1).

Two studies [15,16] that followed this approach included adult participants free of chronic conditions and reported responses as mean area under the curve for the entire follow-up period. In both studies, the amount of fiber consumed throughout the testing period was comparable. In a crossover study, 12 adult participants (23 ± 3 years old; 23.1 ± 1.9 kg/m^2) were randomized to receiving meals with low or high GI and were monitored over 10 h, during which participants consumed four consecutive meals [15]. Insulin, cholecystokinin, and ghrelin responses were monitored over time. Although consuming the low GI meals induced lower glucose and insulin areas under the curve, there were no differences in cholecystokinin and ghrelin responses relative to consuming the higher glycemic index meals. In a separate study with 26 overweight or obese adults (44 ± 15 years old; 29.1 ± 1.8 kg/m^2) participants were monitored over 12 h after consuming three consecutive low or high GI meals with low or high carbohydrate content [16]. The postprandial glucose and insulin areas under the curve were significantly greater only for the high GI/high carbohydrate combination, with no difference in subjectively assessed hunger among diets.

A study was undertaken to assess the satiety of 38 foods using the GI principle of expressing the satiating properties of a test food relative to a reference food of white bread [17]. In this scenario, a Satiety Index was created by providing servings of food containing a standardized energy intake of 1000 kJ (as opposed to a standardized amount of available carbohydrate for GI). The food with the highest SI was potato, a low energy dense food with a satiety rating of over three times that of white bread (SI 323%). Foods with lower SI tended to be high energy dense, low volume foods such as croissant (SI 47%) and cake (SI 65%). There was a positive relationship between serving weight and SI ($p < 0.001$). In effect, the food with the highest GI (potato) was the most satiating, and foods of smaller volume with lower GI (e.g., croissant and cake) were poorly satiating.

In summary, evidence regarding the short-term effect of the GI of foods or meals on satiety is drawn from randomized crossover studies that either assessed postprandial responses to a breakfast meal or monitored responses to consecutive meals over a 10 to 12 h period. Although the approach from these two types of studies is different, results have been consistent and do not support a short-term effect of the GI of foods or meals on satiety.

3.2. Effects of Chronic Intake of Diets with Different Glycemic Index

In order to assess the longer-term effects of GI on satiety, the approach has been to provide study participants with meals or diets differing in GI for an extended period of time varying from 4.5 days to 12 months, followed by an assessment of fasting biomarkers [18,19], postprandial responses to standardized meals [20,21], or physiological responses, including body weight [22–24] (Table 2).

In a crossover study, 40 adult women (20 White and 20 Black; ≥18 years old; 20 normal weight and 20 obese) consumed low or high GL diets for four days prior to a test day in which the 3-h postprandial responses to corresponding low or high GL meals were monitored [20]. The low GL diet resulted in lower glucose and insulin and higher ghrelin responses only among White participants, and no differences in self-reported desire to eat among all participants were documented. Fiber content of the diets was not reported. In contrast, a parallel study comparing the effects of consuming low or high GI diets for 10 weeks in 29 overweight women (31 ± 7 years old; 27.6 ± 1.5 kg/m^2) documented an increase in self-reported fullness and a reduction in the desire to eat "fatty foods" among women allocated to the low GI diet group [21]. Biomarker responses were assessed after consumption of test breakfast meals with comparable fiber. Despite lower 4-h postprandial glucose and insulin responses among the low relative to the high GI group, there were no differences between groups in glucagon, leptin, ghrelin, or ad libitum energy intake after the test period.

Because altering the GI of all meals may be unattainable for some individuals, some have considered only modifying select components of the diet. A crossover intervention designed to assess the effects of consuming breakfast meals with different GI for 21 days included 21 overweight and obese adults (25–65 years old) [18]. Although the prescribed breakfast meals with low GI had greater fiber content, there were no differences in self-reported energy, macronutrient, or fiber intake between groups. Relative to the high GI breakfast period, participants had lower fasting glucose and reported greater satiety after consuming the low GI breakfast. No other differences in fasting biomarkers (insulin and lipids) were reported. In a separate randomized crossover intervention, 19 obese women (34–65 years old; 25–47 kg/m²) were assigned to ad libitum diets in which the GI was manipulated by prescribing use of the lower or higher GI versions of select carbohydrate-containing foods for 12 weeks [22]. Although with this approach all participants gained weight over time, there were no differences in changes in body weight, body composition, energy intake, or subjectively-assessed hunger or fullness based on the GI of the staples.

Table 2. Intervention studies assessing the effects of chronic intake of diets with different GI on appetite/satiety [1].

Study	Sample	Design	Duration	Intervention	Treatment Effects (Low vs. High GI)	Greater Fiber (Low GI)
Pal et al. [18]	21 overweight/obese adults Age: 25–65 years	R; X	21 days	LGI breakfast replacement HGI breakfast replacement	↓ Glucose ↔ TG, insulin, LDL-C, HDL-C ↑ Satiety (subj)	Yes for breakfast replacement No for overall diet (self-reported)
Chang et al. [19]	80 overweight/obese adults 18–45 years 27.5 ± 5.9 kg/m²	R; X	4 weeks	LGL diet HGL diet	↑ Satiety (subj) ↓ Food cravings ↔ Leptin	Yes
Brownley et al. [20]	40 women 20 normal weight, 20 obese ≥18 years	R; X	4.5 days 3h PP Responses to last std meal assessed	LGL diet HGL diet	↓ Glucose, insulin ↑ Ghrelin ↔ Desire to eat (subj) Significant results only in White women	NR
Krog-Mikkelsen et al. [21]	29 overweight women 31 ± 7 years 27.6 ± 1.5 kg/m²	R; =	10 weeks 4 h PP Responses to last high or low GI breakfast assessed	LGI diet HGI diet	↓ Glucose, insulin, GLP-1 ↑ Fullness (subj) ↓ Desire to eat fatty food(sub) ↔ GLP-2, glucagon, leptin, ghrelin ↔ Ad libitum energy intake ↔ Substrate oxidation rates	No
Aston et al. [22]	19 women 34–65 years 25–47 kg/m²	R; X	12-week/phase No washout	LGI staples HGI staples Ad libitum	↔ Body wt, body composition, waist circumference ↔ Hunger, fullness (both subj) ↔ Energy intake	Yes
Das et al. [23]	34 overweight adults 24–42 years 25–30 kg/m²	R; =	12 months	LGL diet HGL diet 30% energy restriction	↔ Body wt, % Body fat ↔ Hunger, satiety (both subj)	No
Juanola-Falgarona et al. [24]	122 overweight or obese adults 30–60 years 27–35 kg/m²	R; =	6 months	LGI HGI HGI-LFat 500 kcal energy restriction	↔ BMI ↔ Hunger, satiety (both subj)	No

[1] Abbreviations: GI: glycemic index; GLP: glucagon-like peptide; HDL-C: high density lipoprotein cholesterol; HFat: high fat; HGI: high GI; LDL-C: low density lipoprotein cholesterol; LGI: low GI; NR: not reported; PP: postprandial; R: randomized; subj: subjective measure; TG: triglycerides; X: crossover design; =: parallel design; ↓: lower; ↑: higher; ↔: no difference.

The long-term effects of consuming diets with low or high GI on satiety have been reported in three studies [19,23,24]. In a randomized parallel weight-loss feeding intervention (30% energy restriction), in which 34 overweight adults were given controlled diets with low or high GL, although participants significantly reduced body weight over time, there were no differences between groups in body weight or composition and self-reported hunger or satiety [23]. Similarly, in a 6-month weight-loss intervention in which 122 overweight or obese adults were randomized to two moderate carbohydrate diets with high- or low-GI or a low-fat/high GI diet, there were no differences in reported hunger or satiety among groups [24]. In a weight maintenance randomized crossover study with 40 normal weight and 40 overweight/obese men and women, there was no difference in hunger over the 4-week study period between diets but women (not men) reported feeling more full when consuming the low- compared with the high-GL diet [19]. Leptin concentrations were not significantly different after both diet periods.

In summary, studies reporting the effects of long-term consumption of diets with low or high GI have had inconsistent findings regarding the role of the GI on satiety. With a few exceptions, data were limited to subjective assessments of satiety, appetite, hunger, or fullness using visual analog scales. Among studies that reported ghrelin concentrations, results were generally null. Over the longer term, an association between GI or GL and satiety could manifest as having an effect on daily energy intake, and one might expect to observe a relationship between dietary GI or GL and energy intake in large-population-based observational work. However, energy intake was not different across categories of dietary GI or GL among a sample of 15,258 people across Europe [25], among 59,000 black women in the USA [26], among 74,248 US women, 90,411 US women, and 40,498 US men [27], or among 64,227 Chinese women [28].

4. Glycemic Index/Glycemic Load and Body Weight

4.1. Cross-Sectional Evidence Regarding the GI/GL and Body Weight

Evidence regarding an association between dietary GI or GL with body weight stems from several cross-sectional observations in diverse populations, including adults [29–31], young Japanese women (18–20 years old) [32], adults with type 2 diabetes [33–35], and older adults [36,37] (Table 3). Among different studies, the body-weight related outcomes most frequently reported were body mass index (BMI) and waist circumference.

Table 3. Cross-sectional studies assessing the effects glycemic index or glycemic load on body weight [1].

Study	Sample	Association Trends			
		GI	GL	Fiber	CHO
Mendez et al. [29]	8195 Spanish adults 35–74 years 18.5–60 kg/m^2	↔ BMI (men) - BMI (women)	(-) BMI	(-) GI (+) GL	(+) GL (men) ↔ GI (women) (+) GL
Hosseinpour-Niazi et al. [30]	2457 adults 19–84 years	(+) BMI ↔ WC, Glucose, total-C, LDL-C, BP (-) HDL-C (among obese) (+) TG (among obese)	↔ BMI, WC, Total-C, LDL-C, HDL-C, TG, BP (-) Glucose, 2-h glucose (among non-obese)	NR	NR
McKeown et al. [31]	2941 adults 27.2 kg/m^2	+ Insulin ↔ Glucose	NR	NR	+ Fiber ↔ Glucose, insulin
Murakami et al. [32]	3931 Japanese women 18–20 years	+ Glucose, HbA1c, BMI	+ Glucose ↔ BMI	- BMI, GI, GL	NR
Wang et al. [33]	238 low income Latino adults w/T2D 45–67 years 33–36 kg/m^2	↔ WC (+) HbA1c ↔ Glucose	(+) WC ↔ Glucose, HbA1c	- GI	NR
Silva et al. [34]	175 adults w/T2D 52–71 years	(+) MetS (+) WC	NR	(+) MetS (+) WC	NR
Farvid et al. [35]	640 adults w/T2D 28–75 years	↔ Glucose ↔ HbA1c	(+) Glucose (+) HbA1c ↔ BMI	(-) Glucose ↔ HbA1c ↔ BMI	(+) Glucose (+) HbA1c (when substitutes CHO for prot or fat)
Milton et al. [36]	1152 older adults (>65 years)	↔ BMI, W/H ↔ TC, LDL-C, HDL-C, TG, BP	NR	NR	NR
Castro-Quezada et al. [37]	343 rural Spanish older adults Age: 60–74 years	↔ BMI, WC	↔ BMI, WC	NR	NR

[1] Abbreviations: BMI: body mass index; BP: blood pressure; CHO: carbohydrates; GI: glycemic index; GL: glycemic load; HbA1c: glycosylated hemoglobin; HDL-C: high density lipoprotein cholesterol; LDL-C: low density lipoprotein cholesterol; MetS: metabolic syndrome; NR: not reported; T2D: type 2 diabetes; TG: triglycerides; Total-C: total cholesterol; WC: waist circumference; W/H: waist to hip ratio; (+): positive association; (-): negative association; ↔: no association.

Findings regarding an association between GI or GL and body weight are equivocal. A cross-sectional analysis of 3931 Japanese young women (18–20 years old) reported positive associations between BMI and GI but not GL, suggesting that the type of carbohydrate-containing foods in the diet played a role in determining body weight [32]. Nevertheless, it is important to note that the difference in BMI between the highest and lowest quintile of BMI was relatively small (0.7 kg/m^2). Among older adults, a study with 1152 participants ($\geq$65 years old) reported no association between dietary GI and body weight or body mass index [36]. Similarly, a study with 343 participants from rural Spain (60–74 years old) reported no associations between dietary GI or GL and BMI or waist circumference, especially once diabetes status or hypoglycemic medications were included in the statistical model [37]. Further, a study 640 adults with type 2 diabetes reported no association between GL and body mass index [35]. In contrast, among 8,195 adults (35–74 years old) with a wide body mass index range (18.5–60 kg/m^2), there was no association between GI and BMI and a negative association between GL and BMI [29]. Differences between the lowest and highest tertiles of GI or GL ranged between 0.7 and 1.0 kg/m^2. For GI the negative association with body mass index was only statistically significant for women, not for men [29]. Whereas in larger-scale studies with healthy adults, there were no associations between GI/GL and waist circumference [30,31], the two smaller studies with type 2 diabetes patients (n = 175 and 238) reported a positive association between waist circumference and dietary GI [34] or GL [33].

Several studies also reported associations of body weight indicators with dietary fiber [29,32,34]. Among those, some reported a negative association between dietary fiber and BMI [32] or waist circumference [34].

In summary, cross-sectional data are inconsistent both in the direction and strength of association between GI or GL and body weight, and this being the case, do not support a strong role of dietary GI or GL on body weight. Among studies that reported an association between GI and body weight, the differences between extreme percentiles of BMI were small. Given that diets with lower GI often have greater fiber content, it is possible that any associations of GI with body weight are influenced by dietary fiber. These studies were not designed to assess whether specific sources of fiber (e.g., whole grains and fruits/vegetables) may impact body weight. An important limitation of cross-sectional studies is that GI or GL is calculated from self-reported diet data (often food frequency questionnaires).

4.2. Intervention Studies Assessing the Effects of GI/GL on Body Weight

For purposes of reviewing the effects of manipulating GI or GL on body weight, only studies designed as weight loss interventions were included (Table 4). These comprised eight studies ranging from 8 weeks to 18 months in duration that included overweight and obese adults [23,24,38–43]. Intervention studies with a crossover design were excluded from this review because fluctuations in body weight during an experimental period can confound results observed in a subsequent experimental phase. Studies focusing on weight maintenance after initial weight loss were also excluded.

Two studies reported significant differences in weight loss with low GI diets relative to the high GI diets [40,44]. In an 8-week intervention, 32 obese adults (36 $\pm$ 7 years old; 32.5 $\pm$ 4.3 kg/m^2) were randomly assigned to follow one of two energy-restricted diets ($-$30% of energy expenditure) for 8 weeks with low GI (40–45) or high GI (60–65) [40]. Both groups lost a significant amount of weight relative to baseline (p < 0.001). However, participants in the low GI group lost significantly more weight than those in the high GI group ($-$7.5 vs. $-$5.3 kg, respectively; p = 0.032) and had significantly greater reductions in BMI ($-$7.6 vs. $-$5.4 kg/m^2; p = 0.03). The lower GI diet was higher in fiber than the higher GI diet and the mean energy of the diets were 1495 $\pm$ 245 kcal/day and 1568 $\pm$ 225 kcal/day for the lower and higher GI diets, respectively.

In a separate study, 122 overweight and obese adults (30–60 years old; 27–35 kg/m^2) were randomized to one of three energy-restricted diets ($-$500 kcal/day) for 6 months with moderate carbohydrate (~42% of total energy intake vs. the standard 55–60% of energy) and high GI, moderate carbohydrate and low GI, or low fat and high GI [24]. Although participants in the three groups experienced weight loss throughout the intervention, changes in BMI were greater after 12 weeks for the low GI than for the low fat group. There were no differences in changes in waist circumference of body composition among groups. Among participants who completed the 6-month study (*n* = 104), participants in the low GI diet had greater reductions in body mass index than those in the other two groups.

Table 4. Intervention studies with parallel design assessing the effects of chronic intake of diets with different GI on body weight [1].

Study	Sample	Duration	Intervention	Treatment Effects (Low vs. High GI)	Greater Fiber (Low GI)
Buscemi et al. [38]	40 obese adults 20–60 years 25–49.9 kg/m^2	3 months	LGI diet, hypocaloric HGI diet, hypocaloric	↔ Weight loss ↔ WC ↔ BMI	No
Philippou et al. [39]	18 adults at risk for heart disease 35–65 years 27–35 kg/m^2	12 weeks	LGI diet HGI diet Deficit 500 kcal/day	↔ Weight loss ↔ BMI	No
Abete et al. [40]	32 obese Spanish adults 36 ± 7 years 32.5 ± 4.3 kg/m^2	8 weeks	LGI diet HGI diet 30% energy restriction	↓ Body weight	Yes
Das et al. [23]	34 overweight adults 24–42 years 25–30 kg/m^2	12 months	LGL diet HGL diet 30% energy restriction	↔ Weight loss, % Body fat ↔ Hunger, satiety (both subj)	No
Sichieri et al. [41]	203 women 25–45 years 23–30 kg/m^2	18 months	LGI diet HGI diet Deficit 100–300 kcal/day	↔ Weight loss	No
Juanola-Falgarona et al. [24]	122 overweight or obese adults 30–60 years 27–35 kg/m^2	6 months	LGI HGI HGI-LFat 500 kcal energy restriction	↔ Weight loss, WC ↔ BMI ↔ Hunger, satiety (both subj)	No
Karl et al. [42]	46 overweight adults 20–42 years 25–29.9 kg/m^2	12 months	LGL-10% energy restriction HGL-10% energy restriction LGL-30% energy restriction HGL-30% energy restriction	↔ Weight loss	No
Karl et al. [43]	91 obese adults	17 weeks	LGI-55% CHO HGI-55% CHO LGI-70% CHO HGI-70% CHO	↔ Weight loss, body composition	No

[1] Abbreviations: BMI: body mass index; CHO: carbohydrate; GI: glycemic index; HGI: high GI; HGL: high glycemic load; LFat: low fat; LGI: low GI; LGL: low glycemic load; WC: waist circumference; ↓ lower; ↑: higher; ↔: no difference.

Four interventions compared energy restricted diets with low or high GI in adults at risk for heart disease (12-week intervention; *n* = 18; 35–65 years old; 27–35 kg/m^2) [39], overweight adults (12-month intervention; *n* = 34; age 24–42 years old; 25–30 kg/m^2) [23], adult women (18-month intervention; *n* = 203; 25–45 years old; 23–30 kg/m^2) [41], and obese adults (3-month intervention; *n* = 40; 20–60 years old; 25–50 kg/m^2) [38]. Two of these interventions were controlled-feeding studies in which all meals were provided to study participants [23,38]. Consistently, these studies reported weight reductions over time for all study participants, with no differences in body weight, BMI, or waist circumference changes between low or high GI groups.

Two additional controlled feeding weight loss studies compared diets differing in GI under either different degree of caloric restriction [42] or different carbohydrate content [43]. A 12-month intervention with 46 overweight adults (20–42 years old; 25–30 kg/m^2) compared low and high GL diets with 10% or 30% energy restriction and reported no differences in body weight changes among groups [42]. Similarly, a 12-week weight loss intervention with 79 obese adults (45–65 years old; 28–38 kg/m^2) compared low and high GI diets with moderate or high carbohydrate content and reported no differences in weight loss by GI or carbohydrate content of the diets [43]. This study further assessed metabolic adaptation 12 months after the weight loss period, and suggested no differences in weight regain based on GI during the weight loss phase.

From intervention studies, there is insufficient data to support a benefit from incorporating low GI alternatives to energy restriction for weight loss. Although some shorter-term studies suggested a benefit from lowering the GI of the diet for greater weight loss [40,44], highly-controlled feeding interventions suggested that manipulating the GI does not make a difference in weight-related outcomes [23,38,42,43].

5. Glycemic Index/Glycemic Load and Cardiometabolic Disease Risk

Evidence regarding associations between GI or GL and cardiometabolic disease risk will be separately described first for type 2 diabetes, followed by cardiovascular disease risk, and then risk factors. Cardiovascular disease is a complex condition with diverse contributing factors including those associated with inflammation and oxidative stress. For purposes of this review, only studies that reported traditional cardiovascular disease risk factors (lipids, blood pressure, or C-reactive protein) were included. Reports with more specific inflammatory and oxidative stress markers are scarce thus limiting the ability to draw conclusions regarding existing evidence of the effect of the GI on those outcomes.

5.1. Epidemiological Evidence Regarding GI/GL and Markers of Glucose Homeostasis

5.1.1. Cross-Sectional Studies

The cross-sectional analyses that contribute to the evidence regarding an association between GI or GL and markers of glucose homeostasis (fasting plasma glucose, 2-h blood glucose, glycosylated hemoglobin (HbA1c), or calculated indices of insulin sensitivity such as the homeostatic model assessment of insulin resistance (HOMA-IR)), included adults with [33,35] or without [30,31,45–48] known type 2 diabetes. Notably, only one report included individuals with a range of glycemic control status (healthy, insulin resistance, and type 2 diabetes) [49] (Table 5).

In studies that included individuals with insulin resistance and diabetes, results were inconsistent. Using baseline data from an intervention among 238 obese low-income Latino adults with type 2 diabetes, GI, but not GL, was positively associated with HbA1c [33]. In an analysis of data from 640 adults with type 2 diabetes, fasting glucose and HbA1c were positively associated with GL, but not GI after adjusting for multiple potential dietary confounders [35]. In this study, HbA1c was also positively associated with total carbohydrate intake. In contrast, an analysis from the Insulin Resistance Atherosclerosis Study with 1255 adults with or without insulin resistance or diabetes reported no associations between GI or GL with fasting glucose, 2-h glucose, or HbA1c [49].

Although several studies among individuals without type 2 diabetes pointed to an association between GI or GL with markers of glucose homeostasis, some findings were still inconsistent. Among 2078 Inuit adults, logistic regression analyses suggested positive associations between GI and fasting glucose and between GL and insulin resistance (HOMA-IR) after adjustment for confounders [45]. No associations were documented for GI with 2-h glucose, HbA1c. or HOMA-IR, or for GL with fasting glucose, 2-h glucose, or HbA1c. In a study with 668 adults from the Canary Islands, insulin resistance (HOMA-IR) was positively associated with GL, but this association lost its statistical significance when fructose intake was added to the model [47]. This suggests that fructose intake plays a role in insulin resistance that is not captured by measuring the GI or GL of the diet.

Results from a study with 2457 adults indicated positive associations of GL with fasting glucose and 2-h glucose but only among non-obese individuals (BMI < 30 kg/m^2) [30]. In this study no associations between GI and fasting glucose or 2-h glucose were documented. In the Framingham

Offspring Study, dietary GI was positively associated with fasting insulin after, but not with fasting glucose [31]. A study with 878 postmenopausal women reported no associations between GL and fasting glucose, insulin, or HOMA-IR [48]. Finally, a cross-sectional analysis with 3931 Japanese young women (18–20 years old) indicated positive associations of dietary GI with fasting glucose and HbA1c and of GL with fasting glucose [46].

Table 5. Cross-sectional studies assessing the effects glycemic index or glycemic load on markers of glucose homeostasis [1].

Study	Sample	Association Trends			
		GI	GL	Fiber	CHO
Farvid et al. [35]	640 adults w/T2D 28–75 years	↔ Glucose ↔ HbA1c	(+) Glucose (+) HbA1c ↔ BMI	(-) Glucose ↔ HbA1c ↔ BMI	(+) Glucose (+) HbA1c (when substitutes CHO for prot or fat)
Wang et al. [33]	238 low income Latino adults w/T2D 45–67 years 33–36 kg/m^2	↔ WC (+) HbA1c ↔ Glucose	(+) WC ↔ Glucose, HbA1c	- GI	NR
van Aerde et al. [45]	2078 Inuit adults 28–62 years 21–33 kg/m^2	(+) Glucose ↔ 2 h-Glucose, HbA1c, HOMA	↔ Glucose, 2 h-Glucose, IGT, HbA1c (+) HOMA	NR	NR
Hosseinpour-Niazi et al. [30]	2457 adults 19–84 years	(+) BMI ↔ WC, Glucose, Total-C, LDL-C, BP (-) HDL-C (among obese) (+) TG (among obese)	↔ BMI, WC, Total-C, LDL-C, HDL-C, TG, BP (-) Glucose, 2-h glucose (among non-obese)	NR	NR
McKeown et al. [31]	2941 adults 27.2 kg/m^2	(+) Insulin, TG (-) HDL-C ↔ Glucose, Total-C, LDL-C ↔ WC	NR	NR	(+) Fiber ↔ Glucose, insulin
Murakami et al. [46]	3931 Japanese women 18–20 years	(+) Glucose, HbA1c, BMI	(+) Glucose ↔ BMI	(-) BMI, GI, GL	NR
Dominguez Coello et al. [47]	668 adults 18–75 years	↔ HOMA	(+) HOMA; null when adjusted for fructose	(+) HOMA for fruit fiber (-) HOMA for cereal and vegetable fiber	(+) HOMA for fructose
Shikany et al. [48]	878 postmenopausal women 63.8 ± 7.3 years 26.9 ± 5.2 kg/m^2	NR	(-) HDL-C (+) TG ↔ TC, LDL-C, glucose, insulin, HOMA	NR	NR
Mayer-Davis et al. [49]	1255 adults with/without IR or T2D 55.3±8.5 years 29.1±5.9 kg/m^2	↔ Glucose	↔ Glucose, 2 h-Glucose	NR	NR

[1] Abbreviations: BMI: body mass index; BP: blood pressure; CHO: carbohydrates; GI: glycemic index; GL: glycemic load; HbA1c: glycosylated hemoglobin; HDL-C: high density lipoprotein cholesterol; HOMA: homeostasis assessment model for insulin resistance; IGT: impaired glucose tolerance; IR: insulin resistance; LDL-C: low density lipoprotein cholesterol; NR: not reported; prot: protein; T2D: type 2 diabetes; TG: triglycerides; Total-C: total cholesterol; WC: waist circumference; (+): positive association; (-): negative association; ↔: no association.

In summary, results from cross-sectional studies relating GI or GL with markers of glucose homeostasis or insulin resistance are inconsistent. Studies are variable in design, data used to calculate the exposure of interest (GI/GL), and adjustments used for the statistical analysis of the data. The loss of statistical significance when models were adjusted for potential dietary confounders, such as fiber or fructose, suggests that carbohydrate-related factors other than GI and GL may play a role in glycemic control. Furthermore, diet data from which GI or GL were calculated in cross-sectional studies is based on self-report, mostly from food frequency questionnaires, limiting the validity of the data. At present, data do not support a reliably robust association between dietary GI or GL and markers of glucose homeostasis or insulin resistance.

5.1.2. Prospective Studies

Evidence published prior to 2006 regarding the association between dietary GI or GL with type 2 diabetes risk from large prospective studies provided inconclusive findings. Dietary GI was positively associated with type 2 diabetes risk in the Nurses' Health Study, the Health Professionals Follow-Up Study, and the Melbourne Collaborative Study [3,50–52]. GL was also positively associated with type 2 diabetes risk in the Nurses' Health Study [3]. However, no associations between GI or GL were documented from the Atherosclerosis Risk in Communities Study [53]. More recent publications of prospective studies assessing type 2 diabetes risk based on dietary GI or GL included studies with adult women [28,54], adult men [55,56], women and men combined [25,57–60], and older adults [61] (Table 6).

Table 6. Prospective studies assessing the effects glycemic index or glycemic load on type 2 diabetes risk [1].

Study	Sample	F/U, y	Type 2 Diabetes Risk			
			GI	GL	Fiber	CHO
Halton et al. [54]	85,059 women	20	NR	↑	NR	↑
Villegas et al. [28]	64,227 middle-aged Chinese women	4.6	↑	↑	NR	↑
Sakurai et al. [55]	1995 adult Japanese male	6	↑	↔	↔ (total fiber)	NR
Simila et al. [56]	25,943 male smokers 50–69 years	12	↔	↔	↔	↓ (total CHO)
Barclay et al. [57]	2123 Australian adults	10	↔	NR	↔ (total fiber)	↔ (total CHO, sugar, or starch)
Mosdol et al. [58]	7321 Caucasian adults	13	↔	↑	NR	NR
Sluijs et al. [59]	37,843 Netherlands adults 21–70 years	10	↑	↑	↓	↑ (starch)
Van Woudenbergh et al. [60]	4366 Netherlands adults ≥55 years	12	↔	↔	NR	NR
Sluijs et al. [25]	16,835 adults	12	↔	↔	NR	↔
Sahyoun et al. [61]	1898 older adults 70–79 years	4	↔	↔	NR	NR

[1] Abbreviations: CHO: carbohydrates; F/U: follow-up; GI: glycemic index; GL: glycemic load; NR: not reported; y: years ↑: increased risk; ↓: decreased risk; ↔: no difference in risk.

Several studies reported increased risk of type 2 diabetes diagnosis with higher dietary GI or GL. In a 20-year follow-up of the Nurses' Health Study including 85,059 women, the relative risk (RR) of type 2 diabetes diagnosis was greater with increased dietary GL (RR = 2.47; 95% CI 1.75–3.47) after adjusting for potential confounders including dietary fiber [54]. Low carbohydrate intake was associated with increased risk of type 2 diabetes (RR = 1.26; 95% CI 1.07–1.49). Type 2 diabetes risk by dietary GI was not reported. In a 4.6-year follow-up of 64,227 middle-aged Chinese women in the Shanghai Women's Health Study, type 2 diabetes risk was significantly higher among participants in the highest quintile of carbohydrate intake (RR = 1.28; 95% CI 1.09–1.50), GI (RR = 1.21; 95% CI 1.03–1.43), GL (RR = 1.34; 95% CI 1.13–1.58), and common staple consumption (mainly rice, noodles, steamed bread, and other bread; RR = 1.37; 95% CI 1.11–1.69) [28]. When participants were stratified by waist-to-hip ratio or BMI, GI was associated with higher diabetes risk only among overweight or obese participants. In this study, dietary fiber or its potential sources (e.g., whole grains and fruit/vegetables) were not considered in the analysis. In a 6-year follow-up of 1995 middle-aged Japanese men, type 2 diabetes risk was greater with increased GI (Hazard Ratio (HR) = 1.96; 95% CI 1.04–3.67), but not with increased GL, energy intake, or fiber intake [55]. Type 2 diabetes risk was also greater with increased GL (HR = 1.27; 95% CI 1.11–1.44) among 37,843 adults participating in the European Prospective Investigation into Cancer and Nutrition (EPIC) Study in the Netherlands [59]. In this study the association for GI and diabetes risk was only borderline significant (HR = 1.08; 95% CI

1.00–1.17). Moreover, the risk of diabetes was significantly greater with increased carbohydrate intake (HR = 1.20; 95% CI 1.01–1.42) and lower with increased fiber intake (HR = 0.89; 95% CI 0.82–0.98).

In contrast to the previous reports, six studies did not find an association between GI or GL and type 2 diabetes risk. These included a 4-year follow-up of 1898 older adults participating in the Health ABC study [61], a 10-year follow-up with 2123 Australian adults [57], a 13-year follow-up of 7321 Caucasian adults from the Whitehall II study [58], a 12-year follow-up of 4093 Dutch adults [60], a 12-year follow-up of 25,943 male smokers [56], and a 12-year follow-up in a random subcohort of the European Prospective Investigation into Cancer and Nutrition Study [25].

In summary, results from prospective studies continue to suggest an equivocal association between type 2 diabetes risk and GI or GL. Type 2 diabetes risk appears to have a stronger association with GL than with GI, but dietary fiber or its sources (e.g., whole grains and fruits/vegetables), and total carbohydrate intake could contribute to the array of results reported. Although these observations are generally derived from large-scale prospective studies, a limitation is that dietary GI and GL often derived from self-reported data generally obtained using food frequency questionnaires.

5.2. Intervention Studies Assessing the Effects of GI/GL on Markers of Glucose Homeostasis

Several dietary interventions were designed to compare low GI or GL diets with their high GI or GL counterparts using crossover [18,62–65] or parallel [24,38,66–70] randomized designs (Table 7). Among these studies, those with a crossover design were shorter in duration (10 days to 5 weeks per intervention phase), whereas parallel design interventions ranged from 45 days to 12 months in duration. Studies included adults with type 2 diabetes [66–68,70], healthy adults with diverse weight status [65], or overweight and/or obese but otherwise healthy adults [18,24,38,62–64,69]. Reports from interventions involving nutrition education in which the use of GI was compared to current dietary recommendations for patients with type 2 diabetes (e.g., American Diabetic Association guidelines [71]) were excluded from this review because participants in different treatment arms were given different diet recommendations, which resulted in diets with multiple incomparable factors aside from the GI or GL of the diet.

Four of the studies with a crossover design were well-controlled feeding interventions in which overweight or obese participants received all meals during the test periods in adequate amounts for weight maintenance [62–65]. In the shortest of these controlled studies, 12 overweight or obese young adults (18–35 years old) received low- or high-GI diets for 10 days each in random order [62]. Although insulin sensitivity, assessed using a frequently sampled intravenous glucose tolerance test at the end of each phase, was greater at the end of the low GI diet, there were no differences in response between interventions. In a longer intervention, 24 overweight or obese men (34.5 ± 8.1 years old; 27.8 ± 3.5 kg/m^2) were provided with low or high GI diets for four weeks in random order [64]. Although participants experienced reductions in both fasting glucose and insulin with both diets relative to baseline, changes were not significantly different between diets. In contrast, an intervention with 80 healthy adults (29.6 ± 8.2 years old; 27.4 ± 5.9 kg/m^2) resulted in lower fasting glucose and insulin-like growth factor 1 (IGF-1) concentrations after consuming a low GL diet for four weeks, relative to a high GL diet [65]. When analyzing separately based on participant body fat, the effect of the low GL diet on fasting glucose concentrations were only significant among individuals with high body fat (≥25% for males or ≥32% for females). Fasting insulin concentrations and HOMA-IR index were not different between diet phases. In a multisite study 163 overweight adults (53 ± 11 years old; 32 ± 6 kg/m^2) were provided with four different controlled diets for five weeks in random order: high carbohydrate/high GI, high carbohydrate low GI, low carbohydrate high GI, and low carbohydrate low GI [63]. Consumption of a low GI diet resulted in a lower insulin sensitivity index than the high GI diet only in the context of high carbohydrate intake (~58% of energy), with no differences observed when the diets had a low carbohydrate content (~40% of energy). In the only crossover study in which participants were not provided with all meals, 21 overweight or obese adults (25–65 years old) were given breakfast replacements with different GI for 21 days [18]. Participants had lower fasting glucose after the low GI breakfast replacement phase (88 ± 2 mg/dL) than after the high GI breakfast replacement phase (92 ± 3 mg/dL; $p < 0.05$). However, there were no differences in fasting insulin concentrations or HOMA index.

Table 7. Intervention studies with assessing the effects of diets with different GI on markers of glucose homeostasis [1].

Study	Sample	Design	Duration	Intervention	Treatment Effects (Low vs. High GI)	Greater Fiber (Low GI)
Botero et al. [62]	12 overweight and obese males 18–35 years 27–45 kg/m²	R; X	10 days/phase	LGL HGL	↓ Glucose, insulin	No
Pal et al. [18]	21 overweight and obese adults 25–65 years	R; X	21 days/phase	LGI breakfast replacement HGI breakfast replacement	↓ Glucose ↔ Insulin, HOMA	Yes
Sacks et al. [63]	163 overweight adults 53 ± 11 years 32 ± 6 kg/m²	R; X	5 weeks/phase	HGI-HCHO HGI-LCHO LGI-HCHO LGI-LCHO	↓ Glucose, insulin sensitivity (only with HCHO)	Yes
Shikany et al. [64]	24 overweight and obese men 34.5 ± 8.1 years 27.8 ± 3.5 kg/m²	R; X	4 weeks/phase	LGI/GL HGI/GL	↔ Weight, BMI ↔ Glucose, insulin ↔ CRP, IL-6, TNF-a, TNF-RII, PAI-1, Fibrinogen ↑ Total-C, LDL-C, HDL-C	No
Runchey et al. [65]	80 adults 29.6 ± 8.2 years 27.4 ± 5.9 kg/m²	R; X	4 weeks/phase	LGL HGL	↓ Glucose, IGF-1 ↔ Insulin, HOMA	Yes
Buscemi et al. [38]	40 obese adults 20–60 years 25–49.9 kg/m²	R; =	3 months	LGI diet, hypocaloric HGI diet, hypocaloric	↔ Weight loss, WC, BMI ↔ HbA1c, Glucose, HOMA	No
Jenkins et al. [66]	210 adults w/T2D HbA1c 6.5–8.0%	R; =	6 months	LGI diet High-cereal fiber diet	↓ HbA1c ↓ Glucose	Yes
Juanola-Falgarona et al. [24]	122 overweight or obese adults 30–60 years 27–35 kg/m²	R; =	6 months	LGI HGI HGI-LFat 500 kcal energy restriction	↔ Weight loss, WC, BMI ↔ Hunger, satiety (both subj) ↔ Glucose	No
Wolever et al. [67,68]	162 adults w/T2D HbA1c ≤ 130% of ULN 20–40 kg/m²	R; =	12 months	HCHO/HGI HCHO/LGI LCHO/HMUFA	↔ HbA1c, HOMA, insulinogenic index, muscle insulin sensitivity ↔ Weight loss	Yes
Pereira et al. [69]	19 healthy adults 22–38 years 27–35 kg/m²	R; =	45 days	LGI HGI	↔ Glucose, insulin, leptin (including AUCs) ↓ HOMA vs. baseline ↓ WC, W/H, body fat %	NR
Gomes et al. [70]	20 adults w/T2D 42.4 ± 5.1 years 29.2 ± 4.8 kg/m²	R; =	30 days	LGI HGI	↔ Glucose, adiponectin, CRP, total-C, LDL-C, HDL-C, TG ↑ fructosamine ↓ body weight	

[1] Abbreviations: BMI: body mass index; CRP: C-reactive protein; GI: glycemic index; HbA1c: glycosylated hemoglobin; HCHO: high carbohydrate; HDL-C: high density lipoprotein cholesterol; HGI: high GI; HGL: high glycemic load; HMUFA: high monounsaturated fatty acids; HOMA: homeostasis assessment model for insulin resistance; IL: interleukin; IGF: insulin-like growth factor; LCHO: low carbohydrate; LDL-C: low density lipoprotein cholesterol; LFat: low fat; LGI: low GI; LGL: low glycemic load; NR: not reported; PAI: plasminogen activator inhibitor; R: randomized; subj: subjective measure; T2D: type 2 diabetes; Total-C: total cholesterol; TNF: tumor necrosis factor; ULN: upper limits for normal; WC: waist circumference; W/H: waist to hip ratio; X: crossover design; =: parallel design; ↑: higher; ↓ lower; ↔ no difference.

Two parallel controlled feeding interventions compared energy restricted diets with low or high GI in obese adults (3-month intervention; $n = 40$; 20–60 years old; 25–50 kg/m²) [38] or overweight and obese adults (6-month intervention; $n = 122$; 30–60 years old; 27–35 kg/m²) [24]. Although these studies reported significant reductions in fasting glucose [38] or HOMA index [24,38] over time, changes in these markers of glucose homeostasis were not different between diets. Moreover, HbA1c did not change with either diet. Two smaller-scale parallel studies of shorter duration involved randomizing overweight or obese adults to either a low GI diet or its high GI counterpart for 30 days ($n = 20$, all with type 2 diabetes; 18–55 years old; 29.2 ± 4.8 kg/m^2) [70] or 45 days ($n = 19$; 22–38 years old; 27–35 kg/m^2) [69]. Participants consumed two of their daily meals in the laboratory, with the rest of their food consumed under free-living conditions following recommendations for food selection based on GI lists. In the shorter of these studies, participants in the high GI diet had a significant increase in fructosamine concentrations relative to baseline, but other biomarkers assessed (glucose, lipids, adiponectin, and CRP) did not change [70]. In the longer of these two studies, although participants in the low GI diet experienced small reductions in waist circumference and body fat relative to baseline, there were no differences in glucose, insulin, or leptin responses between groups [69].

The two longer-term studies conducted in patients with type 2 diabetes had a parallel design and yielded conflicting results [66–68]. In a 6-month intervention, 210 participants (HbA1c 6.5–8.0%; using hypoglycemic medications) were randomized to follow either a low GI diet or a high-cereal fiber diet that included cereal-based sources of fiber (e.g., whole wheat foods and brown rice) [66]. As part of the intervention, participants received dietary advice to comply with the diets. At the end of the intervention period, participants in the low GI group consumed a diet with 18.7 g of fiber per 1000 kcal and a GI of 69.6, whereas those in the high fiber group consumed a diet with 15.7 g of fiber per 1000 kcal and a GI of 83.5. Relative to baseline values, all participants had lower fasting glucose and HbA1c concentrations at the end of the study, but those following the low GI diet had a greater decrease in HbA1c (-0.50% with the low-GI diet vs. -0.18% with the high-cereal fiber diet; $p < 0.001$) and fasting plasma glucose (-8% with the low-GI diet vs -3% with the high-cereal fiber diet; $p = 0.02$).

In a separate 12-month intervention, 162 participants (HbA1c $\leq 130\%$ upper normal limit; BMI 20–40 kg/m^2; without medications) were randomized to follow a high-carbohydrate/high-GI diet, a high-carbohydrate/low-GI diet, or a low-carbohydrate/high-monounsaturated fat diet [67,68]. Participants received counseling by a dietitian to follow the prescribed diets and were provided different key foods to consume with the low or high GI diets. At the end of the intervention participants in the three groups reported comparable energy intake, but dietary fiber was significantly higher among participants in the low GI diet (37 ± 1.5 g/day) than among those following the high GI diet (21 ± 0.8 g/day) or the low carbohydrate diet (23 ± 0.8 g/day), mainly because the key foods provided in the low GI diet were naturally higher in fiber than the key foods provided in the other two diets. Although HbA1c and fasting glucose improved within the first three months of the intervention with the low GI diet, there were no differences among groups in these markers of glycemic homeostasis at the end of the intervention, and in fact HbA1c significantly increased in all groups relative to baseline concentrations (~0.2% from baseline; $p < 0.0001$) [68]. Moreover, participants in the low GI or low carbohydrate diet groups had a small, but significant, increase in fasting plasma glucose over time (~5% from baseline; $p < 0.0001$) [67]. Participants in the low GI diet group had the lowest 2-h glucose and a higher disposition index, an indicator of β-cell function, relative to the low-carbohydrate diet ($p = 0.036$).

In a systematic review and meta-analysis of the effects of dietary GI on glycemic control in people with type 2 diabetes, the authors concluded that a low GI diet is effective at lowering fasting blood glucose and HbA1c relative to a comparison diet [72]. This conclusion appears to be at odds with the findings reported here, but note that the meta-analysis was restricted to five studies carried out in people with type 2 diabetes and the findings were largely influenced by two of those studies, one of which was excluded from our review [73]. In that study, the low GI diet was achieved through the use of legumes, and the comparison diet contained more fiber (presumably soluble), less carbohydrate, less saturated fat, and more plant protein—factors that could contribute to the outcome independent of differences in GI.

In summary, although some intervention studies suggested favorable effects of low GI diets on fasting glucose, findings regarding effects on insulin, insulin sensitivity, or HbA1c are equivocal. In some studies, the benefit of a low GI diet may have been associated with higher fiber or lower carbohydrate consumption. Improvements in markers of glucose homeostasis were also observed in the context of energy restriction (in weight loss studies).

5.3. Epidemiological Evidence Regarding GI/GL and Cardiovascular Disease Risk Factors

5.3.1. Cross-Sectional Studies

The cross-sectional association between GI or GL and cardiovascular disease risk factors has been assessed in several cross-sectional studies (Table 8) [30,31,36,46,48,74–76]. These studies included a combination of adult men and women [30,31,75,76], adult women [46,74], postmenopausal women [48], and older adults [36,37].

Table 8. Cross-sectional studies assessing the effects glycemic index or glycemic load on cardiovascular disease risk factors [1].

Study	Sample	Association Trends	
		GI	GL
Hosseinpour-Niazi et al. [30]	2457 adults 19–84 years	(+) BMI ↔ WC, Glucose, Total-C, LDL-C, BP (-) HDL-C (among obese) (+) TG (among obese)	↔ BMI, WC, Total-C, LDL-C, HDL-C, TG, BP (-) Glucose, 2-h glucose (among non-obese)
Levitan et al. [74]	18,137 women ≥45 years	(-) HDL-C (+) LDL-C, LDL/HDL, TG, CRP	(-) HDL-C (+) LDL/HDL, TG
Liese et al. [75]	1026 middle-aged adults	↔ Total-C, LDL-C, HDL-C, TG	(+) Total-C, LDL-C, TG (-) HDL-C
McKeown et al. [31]	2941 adults 27.2 kg/m²	(+) Insulin, TG (-) HDL-C ↔ Glucose, TC, LDL-C ↔ WC	NR
Milton et al. [36]	1152 older adults (>65 years)	↔ BMI, W/H ↔ TC, LDL-C, HDL-C, TG, BP	NR
Murakami et al. [46]	3931 Japanese women 18–20 years	(+) Glucose, HbA1c, BMI, TG ↔ TC, LDL-C, HDL-C	(+) Glucose, TG (-) HDL-C ↔ BMI ↔ TC, LDL-C
Shikany et al. [48]	878 postmenopausal women 63.8 ± 7.3 years 26.9 ± 5.2 kg/m²	NR	(-) HDL-C (+) TG ↔ TC, LDL-C, glucose, insulin, HOMA
Juanola-Falagrona et al. [76]	6606 adults Men: 55–80 years Women: 60–80 years	(+) MetS (among <75 years without T2D) (+) elevated TG (among 65–74 years without T2D) ↔ other MetS components	↔ MetS or its components
Castro-Quezada et al. [37]	343 rural Spanish older adults 60–74 years	↔ BMI, WC ↔ Glucose, TC, LDL-C, HDL-C, TG, BP	↔ BMI, WC ↔ Glu, TC, LDL-C, HDL-C, TG, BP

[1] Abbreviations: BMI: body mass index; BP: blood pressure; GI: glycemic index; GL: glycemic load; HbA1c: glycosylated hemoglobin; HDL-C: high density lipoprotein cholesterol; HOMA: homeostasis assessment model for insulin resistance; LDL-C: low density lipoprotein cholesterol; MetS: metabolic syndrome; NR: not reported; T2D: type 2 diabetes; TG: triglycerides; Total-C: total cholesterol; WC: waist circumference; W/H: waist to hip ratio; (+): positive association; (-): negative association; ↔: no association.

Results regarding the association of GI or GL and blood lipids are mixed. Regarding total- and LDL-cholesterol, most studies have failed to find an association with GI [30,31,36,37,46,75] or GL [37,48]. One of the exceptions is a study in which women in the highest quintile of dietary GI had significantly higher total- and LDL-cholesterol concentrations by approximately 2 mg/dL relative to those in the lowest quintile [74]. Moreover, positive associations with total- and LDL-cholesterol were reported when the GL was used in the analysis instead of the GI Liese, Gilliard, Schulz, D'Agostino, and Wolever [75].

Although some studies have failed to find an association between dietary GI and HDL-cholesterol [36,37,46,75], some studies have documented that individuals in the highest tertile or quintile of GI have significantly lower HDL-cholesterol concentrations relative to those in the group with the lowest GI [30,31,74]. In these studies the reported HDL-cholesterol concentration difference between individuals in the extreme quintiles of GI has been small, ranging between 2 and 4 mg/dL. Some studies have also documented associations between triglyceride concentrations and dietary GI [30,31,46,74] or GL [48], with differences between extreme percentiles ranging from 11 to 21 mg/dL.

Evidence regarding the association of dietary GI with other cardiovascular disease risk factors is limited. Among studies that included results based on blood pressure, no significant associations with GI were reported [30,36,37]. Only one study conducted in adult women reported a significant positive association between dietary GI and C-reactive protein [74]. Differences between extreme quintiles were of small magnitude (0.21 mg/L based on adjusted values). A study that included men aged 55 to 80 years and women aged 60 to 80 years, with and without type 2 diabetes, suggested that greater dietary GI, but not GL, is associated with greater prevalence of metabolic syndrome in individuals <75 years old without diabetes, and with hypertriglyceridemia among individuals 65 to 74 years without diabetes [76]. GI or GL were not associated with other components of the metabolic syndrome. No associations were found among participants with type 2 diabetes.

In summary, findings from cross-sectional studies generally do not support an association between dietary GI or GL and blood lipid concentrations. Studies that reported such associations documented differences in LDL- or HDL-cholesterol concentrations of small magnitude and questionable physiological effect when comparing extreme percentiles of GI. Nevertheless, these small differences may have important implications at the public health level. The evidence regarding the association of dietary GI with other cardiovascular disease risk factors is limited.

5.3.2. Prospective Studies

Several prospective studies assessing the relationship between dietary GI or GL and cardiovascular disease risk were identified (Table 9). Those reporting on cardiovascular disease mortality [77,78] or on incident cardiovascular diseases (all combined) [79,80], coronary heart disease [81–85], stroke [80,82,85], myocardial infarction [80,86], or heart failure [87] were included herein. Most studies provided risk estimates that were adjusted for dietary factors, age, body mass index, and other potentially confounding factors. Meta-analyses were not included because they generally combined outcomes in their analysis [88].

The majority of analyses have focused on incident coronary heart disease [81–85]. Of these studies, those that reported no significant association between GI and incident coronary heart disease included an 11.9-year follow-up of 8855 men and 10,753 women [82], a 7.9-year follow-up of 44,132 adults [84], and a 9.8-year follow-up of 117,366 Chinese adults [81]. In this last study, coronary heart disease risk was positively associated with GL (HR = 1.87; 95% CI 1.00–3.53), refined grains intake (HR = 1.80; 95% CI 1.01–3.17), and total carbohydrate intake (HR = 2.88; 95% CI 1.44–5.78). Notably, about 68% of energy was provided by dietary carbohydrate in this population. A separate 17-year follow up of 13,051 White and African American adults reported an increased risk for coronary heart disease only among African American individuals (HR = 1.16; 95% CI 1.01–1.33) [83]. However, this association was no longer significant when individuals with diabetes were excluded from the analysis. In the same study, the significant association between coronary heart disease risk and GL was only significant among Whites (HR = 1.11; 95% CI 1.01–1.21), but the association was no longer significant when individuals with diabetes were excluded. Finally, a 9-year follow-up of 15,714 Dutch women resulted in significant associations of incident coronary heart disease with GI (HR = 2.88; 95% CI 1.44–5.78), but not GL [85].

The relationship between dietary GI or GL with incident cardiovascular diseases (all combined) was assessed in a 6-year follow-up of Swedish men 45–79 years of age [80] and in a subsequent analysis of 4167 participants from the same study with established cardiovascular disease [79]. Both analyses resulted in no significant associations. Additional analyses resulted in no significant associations of GI or GL with risk of stroke [80,82,85], myocardial infarction [86], or heart failure [87].

Table 9. Prospective studies assessing the effects glycemic index or glycemic load on cardiovascular disease risk [1].

Study	Sample	F/U, y	Outcome	Type 2 Diabetes Risk			
				GI	GL	Fiber	CHO
Nagata et al. [77]	28,356 Japanese adults	16	CVD mortality	↑ (women)	↔	NR	NR
Burger et al. [78]	6192 adults with T2D	9.2	CVD mortality	↔	↔	↓	↔ CHO, sugar or starch
Levitan et al. [79]	4617 men with prior CVD 45–79 years	6	CVD mortality	↔	↔	NR	NR
Levitan et al. [80]	36,246 Swedish men 45–79 years	6	MI Stroke CVD mortality	↔ ↔ ↔	↔ ↔ ↔	NR	NR
Yu et al. [81]	117,366 Chinese adults 40–74 years	9.8 years for women 5.4 years for men	CHD	↔	↑	↑ (refined grains)	↑
Burger et al. [82]	8855 men 10,753 women 21–64 years	11.9	Stroke CHD	↑ (men) ↔	↔ ↔	NR	↔ ↑ (men; CHO, starch)
Hardy et al. [83]	13051 adults 45–64 years	17	CHD	↑ (African Americans) ↔ (when excluding participants w/T2D)	↑ (Whites) ↔ (when excluding participants w/T2D)	NR	NR
Sieri et al. [84]	44,132 adults	7.9	CHD	↔	↑ (women)	NR	↑ (women) ↔ sugar or starch
Beulens et al. [85]	15,714 Dutch women	9	CHD Stroke Combined	↑ ↔ ↑	↔ ↔ ↑	NR	NR
Levitan et al. [86]	36,234 Swedish women 48–83 years	9	MI	↔	↔	NR	NR
Levitan et al. [87]	36,019 women 48–83 years	9	HF	↔	↔	NR	NR

[1] Abbreviations: CHD: coronary heart disease; CHO: carbohydrates; CVD: cardiovascular disease; F/U: follow-up; GI: glycemic index; GL: glycemic load; HF: heart failure; MI: myocardial infarction; NR: not reported; T2D: type 2 diabetes; y: years; ↑: increased risk; ↓: decreased risk; ↔: no difference in risk.

Two studies assessed the relationship between GI or GL and cardiovascular disease mortality. In a 9.2 year follow-up among 6192 adults with type 2 diabetes, neither GI nor GL were associated with risk of cardiovascular mortality [78]. Furthermore, greater fiber intake was associated with lower risk for cardiovascular mortality (HR = 0.76; 95% CI 0.64–0.89). Similarly, a 16-year follow-up of 28,356 Japanese adults did not result in an association between GL and cardiovascular mortality [77]. The association between GI and cardiovascular mortality was only significant in women (HR = 1.56; 95% CI 1.15–2.13).

From prospective studies, the evidence regarding the association between dietary GI or GL and cardiovascular disease incidence or mortality is equivocal and may suggest that other dietary factors such as fiber and total carbohydrates may play a role. Although these observations are generally derived from large-scale studies, a limitation is that dietary GI and GL often derived from self-reported data generally obtained using food frequency questionnaires.

5.4. Intervention Studies Assessing the Effects of GI/GL on Cardiovascular Disease Risk Factors

The long-term effects of consuming diets with low or high GI have been assessed in several randomized interventions (Table 10). Most studies with a crossover design were well-controlled feeding studies in which overweight or obese participants received all meals during the test periods in adequate amounts for weight maintenance [62–64,89].

The shortest of these interventions provided the controlled meals to 12 overweight or obese young adults (18–35 years old) for 10 days and reported no differences in fasting lipids or C-reactive protein at the end of the low or high GL diet periods [62]. In contrast, consumption of a low GI/lGL diet for four weeks increased total- and LDL-cholesterol concentrations by approximately 8 and 6 mg/dL, respectively, among 24 overweight or obese adults [64]. In this study, consumption of the high GL diet reduced total-, LDL-, and HDL-cholesterol concentrations by approximately 14, 13, and 4 mg/dL, respectively. No changes in C-reactive protein and other inflammatory markers occurred with either of the diets. Similarly, in a multisite study with 163 overweight adults, consumption of low GI diets for five weeks resulted in increased LDL-cholesterol concentrations relative to the high GI diet period by approximately 6% (from 139 to 147 mg/dL), but only in the context of high carbohydrate intake (~58% of energy) [63]. No differences in lipid responses to low or high GI diets were observed when the diets had a low carbohydrate content (~40% of energy). There were no effects on other markers of cardiovascular disease risk, including HDL-cholesterol, triglycerides, and blood pressure. In a different feeding study with 80 overweight or obese adults (18–45 years old), consuming a low GL diet for four weeks resulted in lower C-reactive protein concentrations by approximately 0.24 mg/L relative to the high GL diet phase but only among obese individuals [89]. No effects were reported for other inflammatory cytokines, and lipids were not reported. The only crossover study in which participants were not provided with all meals was a 21-day intervention in which 21 overweight or obese adults were given breakfast meals with different GI [18]. No differences in fasting lipids were reported.

Some of the parallel design studies reporting the effects of GI of the diet on cardiovascular disease risk factors were designed as weight loss interventions ranging from 12 to 24 weeks in duration for overweight and obese adults [38,39,90,91]. In the only controlled feeding intervention in which all meals were provided to study participants, 40 obese adults with at least two components of the metabolic syndrome were assigned to low or high GI hypocaloric diets for 12 weeks [38]. Weight loss was comparable in both groups, and was accompanied by reductions in waist circumference, fasting glucose and HOMA index, total- and LDL-cholesterol, triglycerides, and systolic blood pressure, all of which were not different between groups. The only differential response observed was on endothelial function assessed by flow mediated dilation (FMD), a method that measures the changes in arterial wall dilation after a stimulus. Relative to baseline values, FMD increased 2.3% in the low GI diet group, but decreased 1.0% with the high GI diet, suggesting an improvement in endothelial response with the low GI diet. In the other two parallel design interventions, participants (35–65 years old; 27–35 kg/m^2) were randomized to low or high GL diets and were given advice on energy restriction, weight loss, and how to follow the assigned diet [39,90]. No meals were provided to the participants.

In the 12-week study conducted with 13 healthy adults, the greater weight loss observed with the low GL diet was not accompanied by significant changes in total-, LDL- or HDL-cholesterol or triglycerides [39]. In contrast, a 6-month intervention with 38 men with increased cardiovascular risk resulted in lower total cholesterol and ambulatory 24-h blood pressure among participants in the low GL diet than those following the high GL diet. No differences between groups were observed for other lipids. Finally, a 6-month intervention in which 773 overweight or obese adults (18–65 years) were assigned to LGI or HGI diets (either low or high in protein) reported that consumption of the low GI diets resulted in a reduction in hsCRP concentrations [91]. No other cardiovascular disease risk factors were reported.

Table 10. Intervention studies assessing the effects of diets with different GI on cardiovascular disease risk factors [1].

Study	Sample	Design	Duration	Intervention	Treatment Effects (Low vs. High GI)	Greater Fiber (Low GI)
Botero et al. [62]	12 overweight and obese males 18–35 years 27–45 kg/m²	R; X	10 days/phase	LGL HGL	↓ Glucose, insulin ↔ BP, Total-C, HDL-C, TG, CRP	No
Neuhouser et al. [89]	80 overweight or obese adults 18–45 years 27.5 ± 5.9 kg/m²	R; X	4 weeks/phase	LGL HGL	↓ CRP (if high body fat mass) ↔ Leptin, adiponectin	Yes
Sacks et al. [63]	163 overweight adults 53 ± 11 years 32 ± 6 kg/m²	R; X	5 weeks/phase	HGI-HCHO HGI-LCHO LGI-HCHO LGI-LCHO	With HCHO: ↓ Glucose, insulin sensitivity ↑ LDL-C ↔ HDL-C, TG, BP With LCHO: ↔ Glucose, insulin, LDL-C, HCL-C, TG, BP	Yes
Shikany et al. [64]	24 overweight and obese men 34.5 ± 8.1 years 27.8 ± 3.5 kg/m²	R; X	4 weeks/phase	LGI/GL HGI/GL	↔ Weight, BMI ↔ Glucose, insulin ↔ CRP, IL-6, TNF-a, TNF-RII, PAI-1, Fibrinogen ↑ Total-C, LDL-C, HDL-C	No
Pal et al. [18]	21 overweight and obese adults 25–65 years	R; X	21 days/phase	LGI breakfast replacement HGI breakfast replacement	↓ Glucose ↔ Insulin, HOMA ↔ TG, LDL-C, HDL-C	Yes
Buscemi et al. [38]	40 obese adults 20–60 years 25–49.9 kg/m²	R; =	3 months	LGI diet, hypocaloric HGI diet, hypocaloric	↔ Weight loss, WC, BMI ↔ HbA1c, Glucose, HOMA	No
Philippou et al. [39]	13 adults 35–65 years 27–35 kg/m²	R; =	12 weeks	LGL HGL	↑ Weight loss ↓ Glucose AUC ↔ Total-C, LDL-C, HDL-C, TG, Glucose ↔ WC, Body Fat %	No
Philippou et al. [90]	38 men with high CHD risk 35–65 years 27–35 kg/m²	R; =	6 months	LGL HGL	↓ Insulin, HOMA ↓ TC ↔ BP, LDL-C, HDL-C, TG	No
de Rougemont et al. [92]	38 French adults 20–60 years 25–30 kg/m²	R; =	5 weeks	LGI starchy foods HGI starchy foods	↓ Body weight, BMI ↓ TC, LDL-C	Yes
McMillan-Price et al. [93]	129 overweight and obese young adults 18–40 years 25–30 kg/m²	R; =	12 weeks	HGI/HCHO LGI/HCHO HGI/HProt LGI/HProt (All LFat, HF)	↑ LDL-C w/HighGI-Hprot ↔ weight, HDL-C, TG, FFA, Glucose, Insulin, HOMA, CRP	No
Gogebakan et al. [91]	773 overweight or obese adults 18–65 years 27–45 kg/m²	R; =	6 months (after initial weight loss phase)	LGI/LProt HGI/HProt LGI/HProt HGI/Lprot	↔ Glucose ↓ hsCRP	No

[1] Abbreviations: AUC: area under the curve; BMI: body mass index; BP: blood pressure; CRP: C-reactive protein; CHD: coronary heart disease; FFA: free fatty acids; GI: glycemic index; HbA1c: glycosylated hemoglobin; HCHO: high carbohydrate; HDL-C: high density lipoprotein cholesterol; HF: high fiber; HGI: high GI; HGL: high glycemic load; HOMA: homeostasis model assessment for insulin resistance; HProt: high protein; IL: interleukin; LCHO: low carbohydrate; LDL-C: low density lipoprotein cholesterol; LFat: low fat; LGI: low GI; LGL: low glycemic load; LProt: low protein; PAI: plasminogen activator inhibitor; R: randomized; Total-C: total cholesterol; TG: triglycerides; TNF: tumor necrosis factor; WC: waist circumference; X: crossover design; =: parallel design; ↑: higher; ↓ lower; ↔ no difference.

Two parallel design interventions that assessed cardiovascular disease risk factors, and in which test diets were prescribed without energy restriction to study participants, were identified [92,93]. In a 5-week intervention with 38 adults (20–60 years old; 25–30 kg/m²), participants were randomized to receiving low or high GI starchy foods to incorporate ad libitum with the rest of their diets [92]. At the end of the intervention, participants in the low GI foods group had a significantly greater decrease in weight and body fat mass accompanied by greater, albeit not significantly different, reductions in total and LDL-cholesterol concentrations. In a 12-week intervention, 129 overweight or obese young adults (18–40 years old; 25–30 kg/m^2) were randomized to one of four low-fat diets: high GI/high carbohydrate, low GI/high carbohydrate, high GI/high protein, or low GI/high protein [93]. Participants received sample menus to be used as guide to follow the assigned diets. Relative to baseline, all groups lost weight, with no differences among groups. No differences in lipids were reported, with the exception of LDL-cholesterol, which was significantly greater by about 10 mg/dL at the end of the study for participants consuming the high GI/high protein diet.

In summary, intervention studies that assessed cardiovascular disease risk factors in response to diets with different GI have also provided conflicting results. In two well-controlled crossover feeding trials of at least four weeks in duration, consumption of low GI or GL diets was associated with less favorable LDL/HDL profiles than their high GI or GL counterparts in the context of high carbohydrate diets. In parallel design studies, most of the findings point to the lack of effect of dietary GI or GL on cardiovascular disease risk factors.

6. Conclusions

As outlined in this review of the literature, findings reported over the past decade regarding the clinical utility of the GI for these outcomes are equivocal, consistent with earlier reviews [94,95]. The variety in findings probably depend on a complex interplay between different factors associated with issues related to dietary factors influencing carbohydrate digestion and metabolism (e.g., dietary fiber or amount of carbohydrate in the diet), diversity in study design and study populations, and limitations associated with different study designs. Moreover, outcome measures reported in the studies included herein could have been influenced by other factors not assessed by these studies. For example, studies that controlled for fiber only took total amounts into consideration but not individual food sources such as whole grains, fruit/vegetables, etc. Moreover, the possibility that different GI foods/diets may impact gut microbiome composition, and therefore have distinct downstream metabolic effects related to the outcomes reported in this report, cannot be ruled out.

A particular issue noted is the fact that most data regarding the clinical implications of dietary GI have been derived from observational studies. Given the limitations of dietary assessment in those studies (mostly self-reported data from questionnaires that were not designed and have not been validated to test for GI and GL), there is a need for more highly controlled feeding interventions to test whether diets with different types of carbohydrates indeed elicit different metabolic effects. It is noteworthy that in intervention studies the observed effects of lower GI diets on body weight and markers of glucose homeostasis and CVD risk, when present, are generally of small magnitude. Although this may be beneficial at the public health level, the clinical impact at the individual level is questionable. Moreover, future research regarding the effects of different foods on satiety should focus more on the physiological responses rather than subjective measures.

The use of the GI for clinical guidance also warrants further consideration. At the public level, the concepts of GI and GL are generally misunderstood [96]. Moreover, the large intra- and interindividual variability in glycemic responses to a food [97], coupled with the diversity of GI values reported for some comparable foods [98], suggests that making dietary recommendations based on GI may be misleading, especially since low GI does not always mean high nutritional value, and high GI foods, such as potato, may have other healthful qualities including low energy density and a high satiety rating [99]. Thus, focusing on overall dietary quality and promoting the healthful aspects of the diet (e.g., dietary fiber and fruit and vegetable intake) may be a better approach to help reduce chronic disease risk.

Author Contributions: Conceptualization, S.V.-L., B.J.V., and J.L.S.; Methodology, S.V.-L.; Writing-Original Draft Preparation, S.V.-L.; Writing-Review and Editing, B.J.V. and J.L.S.

Funding: Data gathering for this manuscript was funded by Mars Inc. as part of a larger scope literature review into the science of the glycemic index. Mars Inc. had no input into the design, interpretation of the data, or manuscript preparation.

Acknowledgments: Authors would like to acknowledge Mayra Arias Gastélum for her assistance retrieving manuscripts during the initial phase of reviewing the literature.

Conflicts of Interest: The authors declare no conflicts of interest.

References

1. Triplitt, C.L. Examining the mechanisms of glucose regulation. *Am. J. Manag. Care* **2012**, *18*, S4–S10. [PubMed]
2. Jenkins, D.; Wolever, T.; Barker, H.; Fielden, H.; Baldwin, J.; Bowling, A.; Newman, H.; Jenkins, A.; Goff, D. Glycemic index of foods: A physiological basis for carbohydrate exchange. *Am. J. Clin. Nutr.* **1981**, *34*, 362–366. [CrossRef] [PubMed]
3. Salmerón, J.; Manson, J.E.; Stampfer, M.J.; Colditz, G.A.; Wing, A.L.; Willett, W.C. Dietary fiber, glycemic load, and risk of non-insulin-dependent diabetes mellitus in women. *JAMA* **1997**, *227*, 472–477. [CrossRef]
4. Jenkins, D.J.A.; Ghafari, H.; Wolever, T.M.S.; Taylor, R.H.; Jenkins, A.L.; Barker, H.M.; Fielden, H.; Bowling, A.C. Relationship between rate of digestion of foods and post-prandial glycaemia. *Diabetologia* **1982**, *22*, 450–455. [CrossRef] [PubMed]
5. Choudhury, S.M.; Tan, T.M.; Bloom, S.R. Gastrointestinal hormones and their role in obesity. *Curr. Opin. Endocrinol. Diabetes Obes.* **2016**, *23*, 18–22. [CrossRef] [PubMed]
6. Strader, A.D.; Woods, S.C. Gastrointestinal hormones and food intake. *Gastroenterology* **2005**, *128*, 175–191. [CrossRef] [PubMed]
7. Torrance, G.W.; Feeny, D.; Furlong, W. Visual analog scales: Do they have a role in the measurement of preferences for health states? *Med. Decis. Mak.* **2001**, *21*, 329–334. [CrossRef] [PubMed]
8. Wolever, T.M.S.; Jenkins, D.J.A.; Jenkins, A.L.; Josse, R.G. The glycemic index: Methodology and clinical implications. *Am. J. Clin. Nutr.* **1991**, *54*, 846–854. [CrossRef] [PubMed]
9. Louie, J.C.; Markovic, T.P.; Ross, G.P.; Foote, D.; Brand-Miller, J.C. Timing of peak blood glucose after breakfast meals of different glycemic index in women with gestational diabetes. *Nutrients* **2013**, *5*, 1–9. [CrossRef] [PubMed]
10. Makris, A.P.; Borradaile, K.E.; Oliver, T.L.; Cassim, N.G.; Rosenbaum, D.L.; Boden, G.H.; Homko, C.J.; Foster, G.D. The individual and combined effects of glycemic index and protein on glycemic response, hunger, and energy intake. *Obesity* **2011**, *19*, 2365–2373. [CrossRef] [PubMed]
11. Silva, F.M.; Kramer, C.K.; Crispim, D.; Azevedo, M.J. A high-glycemic index, low-fiber breakfast affects the postprandial plasma glucose, insulin, and ghrelin responses of patients with type 2 diabetes in a randomized clinical trial. *J. Nutr.* **2015**, *145*, 736–741. [CrossRef] [PubMed]
12. Lobos, D.R.; Vicuna, I.A.; Novik, V.; Vega, C.A. Effect of high and low glycemic index breakfast on postprandial metabolic parameters and satiety in subjects with type 2 diabetes mellitus under intensive insulin therapy: Controlled clinical trial. *Clin. Nutr. ESPEN* **2017**, *20*, 12–16. [CrossRef] [PubMed]
13. Png, W.; Bhaskaran, K.; Sinclair, A.J.; Aziz, A.R. Effects of ingesting low glycemic index carbohydrate food for the sahur meal on subjective, metabolic and physiological responses, and endurance performance in ramadan fasted men. *Int. J. Food Sci. Nutr.* **2014**, *65*, 629–636. [CrossRef] [PubMed]
14. Campbell, M.D.; Gonzalez, J.T.; Rumbold, P.L.; Walker, M.; Shaw, J.A.; Stevenson, E.J.; West, D.J. Comparison of appetite responses to high- and low-glycemic index postexercise meals under matched insulinemia and fiber in type 1 diabetes. *Am. J. Clin. Nutr.* **2015**, *101*, 478–486. [CrossRef] [PubMed]
15. Reynolds, R.C.; Stockmann, K.S.; Atkinson, F.S.; Denyer, G.S.; Brand-Miller, J.C. Effect of the glycemic index of carbohydrates on day-long (10 h) profiles of plasma glucose, insulin, cholecystokinin and ghrelin. *Eur. J. Clin. Nutr.* **2009**, *63*, 872–878. [CrossRef] [PubMed]
16. Liu, A.G.; Most, M.M.; Brashear, M.M.; Johnson, W.D.; Cefalu, W.T.; Greenway, F.L. Reducing the glycemic index or carbohydrate content of mixed meals reduces postprandial glycemia and insulinemia over the entire day but does not affect satiety. *Diabetes Care* **2012**, *35*, 1633–1637. [CrossRef] [PubMed]
17. Holt, S.H.; Miller, J.C.; Petocz, P.; Farmakalidis, E. A satiety index of common foods. *Eur. J. Clin. Nutr.* **1995**, *49*, 675–690. [PubMed]
18. Pal, S.; Lim, S.; Egger, G. The effect of a low glycaemic index breakfast on blood glucose, insulin, lipid profiles, blood pressure, body weight, body composition and satiety in obese and overweight individuals: A pilot study. *J. Am. Coll. Nutr.* **2008**, *27*, 387–393. [CrossRef] [PubMed]

19. Chang, K.T.; Lampe, J.W.; Schwarz, Y.; Breymeyer, K.L.; Noar, K.A.; Song, X.; Neuhouser, M.L. Low glycemic load experimental diet more satiating than high glycemic load diet. *Nutr. Cancer* **2012**, *64*, 666–673. [CrossRef] [PubMed]

20. Brownley, K.A.; Heymen, S.; Hinderliter, A.L.; Galanko, J.; Macintosh, B. Low-glycemic load decreases postprandial insulin and glucose and increases postprandial ghrelin in white but not black women. *J. Nutr.* **2012**, *142*, 1240–1245. [CrossRef] [PubMed]

21. Krog-Mikkelsen, I.; Sloth, B.; Dimitrov, D.; Tetens, I.; Bjorck, I.; Flint, A.; Holst, J.J.; Astrup, A.; Elmstahl, H.; Raben, A. A low glycemic index diet does not affect postprandial energy metabolism but decreases postprandial insulinemia and increases fullness ratings in healthy women. *J. Nutr.* **2011**, *141*, 1679–1684. [CrossRef] [PubMed]

22. Aston, L.M.; Stokes, C.S.; Jebb, S.A. No effect of a diet with a reduced glycaemic index on satiety, energy intake and body weight in overweight and obese women. *Int. J. Obes.* **2008**, *32*, 160–165. [CrossRef] [PubMed]

23. Das, S.K.; Gilhooly, C.H.; Golden, J.K.; Pittas, A.G.; Fuss, P.J.; Cheatham, R.A.; Tyler, S.; Tsay, M.; McCrory, M.A.; Lichtenstein, A.H.; et al. Long-term effects of 2 energy-restricted diets differing in glycemic load on dietary adherence, body composition, and metabolism in calerie: A 1-y randomized controlled trial. *Am. J. Clin. Nutr.* **2007**, *85*, 1023–1030. [CrossRef] [PubMed]

24. Juanola-Falgarona, M.; Salas-Salvado, J.; Ibarrola-Jurado, N.; Rabassa-Soler, A.; Diaz-Lopez, A.; Guasch-Ferre, M.; Hernandez-Alonso, P.; Balanza, R.; Bullo, M. Effect of the glycemic index of the diet on weight loss, modulation of satiety, inflammation, and other metabolic risk factors: A randomized controlled trial. *Am. J. Clin. Nutr.* **2014**, *100*, 27–35. [CrossRef] [PubMed]

25. Sluijs, I.; Beulens, J.W.; van der Schouw, Y.T.; van der, A.D.; Buckland, G.; Kuijsten, A.; Schulze, M.B.; Amiano, P.; Ardanaz, E.; Balkau, B.; et al. Dietary glycemic index, glycemic load, and digestible carbohydrate intake are not associated with risk of type 2 diabetes in eight European countries. *J. Nutr.* **2013**, *143*, 93–99. [PubMed]

26. Krishnan, S.; Rosenberg, L.; Singer, M.; Hu, F.B.; Djousse, L.; Cupples, L.A.; Palmer, J.R. Glycemic index, glycemic load, and cereal fiber intake and risk of type 2 diabetes in us black women. *Arch. Intern. Med.* **2007**, *167*, 2304–2309. [CrossRef] [PubMed]

27. Bhupathiraju, S.N.; Tobias, D.K.; Malik, V.S.; Pan, A.; Hruby, A.; Manson, J.E.; Willett, W.C.; Hu, F.B. Glycemic index, glycemic load, and risk of type 2 diabetes: Results from 3 large us cohorts and an updated meta-analysis. *Am. J. Clin. Nutr.* **2014**, *100*, 218–232. [CrossRef] [PubMed]

28. Villegas, R.; Liu, S.; Gao, Y.T.; Yang, G.; Li, H.; Zheng, W.; Shu, X.O. Prospective study of dietary carbohydrates, glycemic index, glycemic load, and incidence of type 2 diabetes mellitus in middle-aged Chinese women. *Arch. Intern. Med.* **2007**, *167*, 2310–2316. [CrossRef] [PubMed]

29. Mendez, M.A.; Covas, M.I.; Marrugat, J.; Vila, J.; Schroder, H. Glycemic load, glycemic index, and body mass index in spanish adults. *Am. J. Clin. Nutr.* **2009**, *89*, 316–322. [PubMed]

30. Hosseinpour-Niazi, S.; Sohrab, G.; Asghari, G.; Mirmiran, P.; Moslehi, N.; Azizi, F. Dietary glycemic index, glycemic load, and cardiovascular disease risk factors: Tehran lipid and glucose study. *Arch. Iran. Med.* **2013**, *16*, 401–407. [PubMed]

31. McKeown, N.M.; Meigs, J.B.; Liu, S.; Rogers, G.; Yoshida, M.; Saltzman, E.; Jacques, P.F. Dietary carbohydrates and cardiovascular disease risk factors in the framingham offspring cohort. *J. Am. Coll. Nutr.* **2009**, *28*, 150–158. [CrossRef] [PubMed]

32. Murakami, K.; Sasaki, S.; Okubo, H.; Takahashi, Y.; Hosoi, Y.; Itabashi, M. Dietary fiber intake, dietary glycemic index and load, and body mass index: A cross-sectional study of 3931 Japanese women aged 18–20 years. *Eur. J. Clin. Nutr.* **2007**, *61*, 986–995. [CrossRef] [PubMed]

33. Wang, M.L.; Gellar, L.; Nathanson, B.H.; Pbert, L.; Ma, Y.; Ockene, I.; Rosal, M.C. Decrease in glycemic index associated with improved glycemic control among latinos with type 2 diabetes. *J. Acad. Nutr. Diet.* **2015**, *115*, 898–906. [CrossRef] [PubMed]

34. Silva, F.M.; Steemburgo, T.; de Mello, V.D.F.; Tonding, S.F.; Gross, J.L.; Azevedo, M.J. High dietary glycemic index and low fiber content are associated with metabolic syndrome in patients with type 2 diabetes. *J. Am. Coll. Nutr.* **2011**, *30*, 141–148. [CrossRef] [PubMed]

35. Farvid, M.S.; Homayouni, F.; Shokoohi, M.; Fallah, A.; Farvid, M.S. Glycemic index, glycemic load and their association with glycemic control among patients with type 2 diabetes. *Eur. J. Clin. Nutr.* **2014**, *68*, 459–463. [CrossRef] [PubMed]

36. Milton, J.E.; Briche, B.; Brown, I.J.; Hickson, M.; Robertson, C.E.; Frost, G.S. Relationship of glycaemic index with cardiovascular risk factors: Analysis of the national diet and nutrition survey for people aged 65 and older. *Public Health Nutr.* **2007**, *10*, 1321–1335. [CrossRef] [PubMed]

37. Castro-Quezada, I.; Artacho, R.; Molina-Montes, E.; Serrano, F.A.; Ruiz-Lopez, M.D. Dietary glycaemic index and glycaemic load in a rural elderly population (60–74 years of age) and their relationship with cardiovascular risk factors. *Eur. J. Nutr.* **2015**, *54*, 523–534. [CrossRef] [PubMed]

38. Buscemi, S.; Cosentino, L.; Rosafio, G.; Morgana, M.; Mattina, A.; Sprini, D.; Verga, S.; Rini, G.B. Effects of hypocaloric diets with different glycemic indexes on endothelial function and glycemic variability in overweight and in obese adult patients at increased cardiovascular risk. *Clin. Nutr.* **2013**, *32*, 346–352. [CrossRef] [PubMed]

39. Philippou, E.; McGowan, B.M.; Brynes, A.E.; Dornhorst, A.; Leeds, A.R.; Frost, G.S. The effect of a 12-week low glycaemic index diet on heart disease risk factors and 24 h glycaemic response in healthy middle-aged volunteers at risk of heart disease: A pilot study. *Eur. J. Clin. Nutr.* **2008**, *62*, 145–149. [CrossRef] [PubMed]

40. Abete, I.; Parra, D.; Martinez, J.A. Energy-restricted diets based on a distinct food selection affecting the glycemic index induce different weight loss and oxidative response. *Clin. Nutr.* **2008**, *27*, 545–551. [CrossRef] [PubMed]

41. Sichieri, R.; Moura, A.S.; Genelhu, V.; Hu, F.; Willett, W.C. An 18-mo randomized trial of a low-glycemic-index diet and weight change in Brazilian women. *Am. J. Clin. Nutr.* **2007**, *86*, 707–713. [CrossRef] [PubMed]

42. Karl, J.P.; Cheatham, R.A.; Das, S.K.; Hyatt, R.R.; Gilhooly, C.H.; Pittas, A.G.; Lieberman, H.R.; Lerner, D.; Roberts, S.B.; Saltzman, E. Effect of glycemic load on eating behavior self-efficacy during weight loss. *Appetite* **2014**, *80*, 204–211. [CrossRef] [PubMed]

43. Karl, J.P.; Roberts, S.B.; Schaefer, E.J.; Gleason, J.A.; Fuss, P.; Rasmussen, H.; Saltzman, E.; Das, S.K. Effects of carbohydrate quantity and glycemic index on resting metabolic rate and body composition during weight loss. *Obesity* **2015**, *23*, 2190–2198. [CrossRef] [PubMed]

44. Juanola-Falgarona, M.; Ibarrola-Jurado, N.; Salas-Salvado, J.; Rabassa-Soler, A.; Bullo, M. Design and methods of the glyndiet study; assessing the role of glycemic index on weight loss and metabolic risk markers. *Nutr. Hosp.* **2013**, *28*, 382–390. [PubMed]

45. Van Aerde, M.A.; Witte, D.R.; Jeppesen, C.; Soedamah-Muthu, S.S.; Bjerregaard, P.; Jorgensen, M.E. Glycemic index and glycemic load in relation to glucose intolerance among greenland's inuit population. *Diabetes Res. Clin. Pract.* **2012**, *97*, 298–305. [CrossRef] [PubMed]

46. Murakami, K.; Sasaki, S.; Takahashi, Y.; Okubo, H.; Hosoi, Y.; Horiguchi, H.; Oguma, E.; Kayama, F. Dietary glycemic index and load in relation to metabolic risk factors in Japanese female farmers with traditional dietary habits. *Am. J. Clin. Nutr.* **2006**, *83*, 1161–1169. [CrossRef] [PubMed]

47. Dominguez Coello, S.; Cabrera de Leon, A.; Rodriguez Perez, M.C.; Borges Alamo, C.; Carrillo Fernandez, L.; Almeida Gonzalez, D.; Garcia Yanes, J.; Gonzalez Hernandez, A.; Brito Diaz, B.; Aguirre-Jaime, A. Association between glycemic index, glycemic load, and fructose with insulin resistance: The CDC of the canary islands study. *Eur. J. Nutr.* **2010**, *49*, 505–512. [CrossRef] [PubMed]

48. Shikany, J.M.; Tinker, L.F.; Neuhouser, M.L.; Ma, Y.; Patterson, R.E.; Phillips, L.S.; Liu, S.; Redden, D.T. Association of glycemic load with cardiovascular disease risk factors: The women's health initiative observational study. *Nutrition* **2010**, *26*, 641–647. [CrossRef] [PubMed]

49. Mayer-Davis, E.J.; Dhawan, A.; Liese, A.D.; Teff, K.; Schulz, M. Towards understanding of glycaemic index and glycaemic load in habitual diet: Associations with measures of glycaemia in the insulin resistance atherosclerosis study. *Br. J. Nutr.* **2006**, *95*, 397–405. [CrossRef] [PubMed]

50. Hodge, A.M.; English, D.R.; O'Dea, K.; Giles, G.G. Glycemic index and dietary fiber and the risk of type 2 diabetes. *Diabetes Care* **2004**, *27*, 2701–2706. [CrossRef] [PubMed]

51. Salmerón, J.; Ascherio, A.; Rimm, E.B.; Colditz, G.A.; Spiegelman, D.; Jenkins, D.J.A.; Stampfer, M.J.; Wing, A.L.; Willett, W.C. Dietary fiber, glycemic load, and risk of NIDDM in men. *Diabetes Care* **1997**, *20*, 545–550. [CrossRef] [PubMed]

52. Schulze, M.B.; Liu, S.; Rimm, E.B.; Manson, J.E.; Willett, W.C.; Hu, F.B. Glycemic index, glycemic load, and dietary fiber intake and incidence of type 2 diabetes in younger and middle-aged women. *Am. J. Clin. Nutr.* **2004**, *80*, 348–356. [CrossRef] [PubMed]

53. Stevens, J.; Ahn, K.; Juhaeri; Houston, D.; Steffan, L.; Couper, D. Dietary fiber intake and glycemic index and incidence of diabetes in African-American and white adults. *Diabetes Care* **2002**, *25*, 1715–1721. [CrossRef] [PubMed]

54. Halton, T.L.; Liu, S.; Manson, J.E.; Hu, F.B. Low-carbohydrate-diet score and risk of type 2 diabetes in women. *Am. J. Clin. Nutr.* **2008**, *87*, 339–346. [CrossRef] [PubMed]

55. Sakurai, M.; Nakamura, K.; Miura, K.; Takamura, T.; Yoshita, K.; Morikawa, Y.; Ishizaki, M.; Kido, T.; Naruse, Y.; Suwazono, Y.; et al. Dietary glycemic index and risk of type 2 diabetes mellitus in middle-aged Japanese men. *Metabolism* **2012**, *61*, 47–55. [CrossRef] [PubMed]

56. Simila, M.E.; Kontto, J.P.; Valsta, L.M.; Mannisto, S.; Albanes, D.; Virtamo, J. Carbohydrate substitution for fat or protein and risk of type 2 diabetes in male smokers. *Eur. J. Clin. Nutr.* **2012**, *66*, 716–721. [CrossRef] [PubMed]

57. Barclay, A.W.; Flood, V.M.; Rochtchina, E.; Mitchell, P.; Brand-Miller, J.C. Glycemic index, dietary fiber, and risk of type 2 diabetes in a cohort of older Australians. *Diabetes Care* **2007**, *30*, 2811–2813. [CrossRef] [PubMed]

58. Mosdol, A.; Witte, D.R.; Frost, G.; Marmot, M.G.; Brunner, E.J. Dietary glycemic index and glycemic load are associated with high-density-lipoprotein cholesterol at baseline but not with increased risk of diabetes in the whitehall ii study. *Am. J. Clin. Nutr.* **2007**, *86*, 988–994. [CrossRef] [PubMed]

59. Sluijs, I.; van der Schouw, Y.T.; van der, A.D.; Spijkerman, A.M.; Hu, F.B.; Grobbee, D.E.; Beulens, J.W. Carbohydrate quantity and quality and risk of type 2 diabetes in the European prospective investigation into cancer and nutrition-Netherlands (EPIC-NL) study. *Am. J. Clin. Nutr.* **2010**, *92*, 905–911. [CrossRef] [PubMed]

60. Van Woudenbergh, G.J.; Kuijsten, A.; Sijbrands, E.J.; Hofman, A.; Witteman, J.C.; Feskens, E.J. Glycemic index and glycemic load and their association with C-reactive protein and incident type 2 diabetes. *J. Nutr. Metab.* **2011**, *2011*, 623076. [CrossRef] [PubMed]

61. Sahyoun, N.R.; Anderson, A.L.; Tylavsky, F.A.; Lee, J.S.; Sellmeyer, D.E.; Harris, T.B. Dietary glycemic index and glycemic load and the risk of type 2 diabetes in older adults. *Am. J. Clin. Nutr.* **2008**, *87*, 126–131. [CrossRef] [PubMed]

62. Botero, D.; Ebbeling, C.B.; Blumberg, J.B.; Ribaya-Mercado, J.D.; Creager, M.A.; Swain, J.F.; Feldman, H.A.; Ludwig, D.S. Acute effects of dietary glycemic index on antioxidant capacity in a nutrient-controlled feeding study. *Obesity* **2009**, *17*, 1664–1670. [CrossRef] [PubMed]

63. Sacks, F.M.; Carey, V.J.; Anderson, C.A.; Miller, E.R., 3rd; Copeland, T.; Charleston, J.; Harshfield, B.J.; Laranjo, N.; McCarron, P.; Swain, J.; et al. Effects of high vs low glycemic index of dietary carbohydrate on cardiovascular disease risk factors and insulin sensitivity: The OmniCarb randomized clinical trial. *JAMA* **2014**, *312*, 2531–2541. [CrossRef] [PubMed]

64. Shikany, J.M.; Phadke, R.P.; Redden, D.T.; Gower, B.A. Effects of low- and high-glycemic index/glycemic load diets on coronary heart disease risk factors in overweight/obese men. *Metabolism* **2009**, *58*, 1793–1801. [CrossRef] [PubMed]

65. Runchey, S.S.; Pollak, M.N.; Valsta, L.M.; Coronado, G.D.; Schwarz, Y.; Breymeyer, K.L.; Wang, C.; Wang, C.Y.; Lampe, J.W.; Neuhouser, M.L. Glycemic load effect on fasting and post-prandial serum glucose, insulin, IGF-1 and IGFBP-3 in a randomized, controlled feeding study. *Eur. J. Clin. Nutr.* **2012**, *66*, 1146–1152. [CrossRef] [PubMed]

66. Jenkins, D.J.; Kendall, C.W.; McKeown-Eyssen, G.; Josse, R.G.; Silverberg, J.; Booth, G.L.; Vidgen, E.; Josse, A.R.; Nguyen, T.H.; Corrigan, S.; et al. Effect of a low-glycemic index or a high-cereal fiber diet on type 2 diabetes: A randomized trial. *JAMA* **2008**, *300*, 2742–2753. [CrossRef] [PubMed]

67. Wolever, T.; Mehling, C.; Chiasson, J.L.; Josse, R.; Leiter, L.; Maheux, P.; Rabasa-Lhoret, R.; Rodger, N.; Ryan, E. Low glycaemic index diet and disposition index in type 2 diabetes (the Canadian trial of carbohydrates in diabetes): A randomised controlled trial. *Diabetologia* **2008**, *51*, 1607–1615. [CrossRef] [PubMed]

68. Wolever, T.M.; Gibbs, A.L.; Mehling, C.; Chiasson, J.L.; Connelly, P.W.; Josse, R.G.; Leiter, L.A.; Maheux, P.; Rabasa-Lhoret, R.; Rodger, N.W.; et al. The Canadian trial of carbohydrates in diabetes (CCD), a 1-y controlled trial of low-glycemic-index dietary carbohydrate in type 2 diabetes: No effect on glycated hemoglobin but reduction in C-reactive protein. *Am. J. Clin. Nutr.* **2008**, *87*, 114–125. [CrossRef] [PubMed]

69. Pereira, E.V.; Costa Jde, A.; Alfenas Rde, C. Effect of glycemic index on obesity control. *Arch. Endocrinol. MeTable* **2015**, *59*, 245–251. [CrossRef] [PubMed]

70. Gomes, J.M.G.; Fabrini, S.P.; Alfenas, R.C.G. Low glycemic index diet reduces body fat and attenuates inflammatory and metabolic responses in patients with type 2 diabetes. *Arch. Endocrinol. Metab.* **2017**, *61*, 137–144. [CrossRef] [PubMed]

71. American Diabetes Association. 3. Foundations of care and comprehensive medical evaluation. *Diabetes Care* **2016**, *39*, S23–S35. [CrossRef] [PubMed]

72. Ojo, O.; Ojo, O.O.; Adebowale, F.; Wang, X.H. The effect of dietary glycaemic index on glycaemia in patients with type 2 diabetes: A systematic review and meta-analysis of randomized controlled trials. *Nutrients* **2018**, *10*, 373. [CrossRef] [PubMed]

73. Jenkins, D.J.; Kendall, C.W.; Augustin, L.S.; Mitchell, S.; Sahye-Pudaruth, S.; Blanco Mejia, S.; Chiavaroli, L.; Mirrahimi, A.; Ireland, C.; Bashyam, B.; et al. Effect of legumes as part of a low glycemic index diet on glycemic control and cardiovascular risk factors in type 2 diabetes mellitus: A randomized controlled trial. *Arch. Intern. Med.* **2012**, *172*, 1653–1660. [CrossRef] [PubMed]

74. Levitan, E.B.; Cook, N.R.; Stampfer, M.J.; Ridker, P.M.; Rexrode, K.M.; Buring, J.E.; Manson, J.E.; Liu, S. Dietary glycemic index, dietary glycemic load, blood lipids, and c-reactive protein. *Metabolism* **2008**, *57*, 437–443. [CrossRef] [PubMed]

75. Liese, A.D.; Gilliard, T.; Schulz, M.; D'Agostino, R.B., Jr.; Wolever, T.M. Carbohydrate nutrition, glycaemic load, and plasma lipids: The insulin resistance atherosclerosis study. *Eur. Heart J.* **2007**, *28*, 80–87. [CrossRef] [PubMed]

76. Juanola-Falgarona, M.; Salas-Salvado, J.; Buil-Cosiales, P.; Corella, D.; Estruch, R.; Ros, E.; Fito, M.; Recondo, J.; Gomez-Gracia, E.; Fiol, M.; et al. Dietary glycemic index and glycemic load are positively associated with risk of developing metabolic syndrome in middle-aged and elderly adults. *J. Am. Geriatr. Soc.* **2015**, *63*, 1991–2000. [CrossRef] [PubMed]

77. Nagata, C.; Wada, K.; Tsuji, M.; Kawachi, T.; Nakamura, K. Dietary glycaemic index and glycaemic load in relation to all-cause and cause-specific mortality in a Japanese community: The takayama study. *Br. J. Nutr.* **2014**, *112*, 2010–2017. [CrossRef] [PubMed]

78. Burger, K.N.; Beulens, J.W.; van der Schouw, Y.T.; Sluijs, I.; Spijkerman, A.M.; Sluik, D.; Boeing, H.; Kaaks, R.; Teucher, B.; Dethlefsen, C.; et al. Dietary fiber, carbohydrate quality and quantity, and mortality risk of individuals with diabetes mellitus. *PLoS ONE* **2012**, *7*, e43127. [CrossRef] [PubMed]

79. Levitan, E.B.; Mittleman, M.A.; Wolk, A. Dietary glycemic index, dietary glycemic load and mortality among men with established cardiovascular disease. *Eur. J. Clin. Nutr.* **2009**, *63*, 552–557. [CrossRef] [PubMed]

80. Levitan, E.B.; Mittleman, M.A.; Hakansson, N.; Wolk, A. Dietary glycemic index, dietary glycemic load, and cardiovascular disease in middle-aged and older Swedish men. *Am. J. Clin. Nutr.* **2007**, *85*, 1521–1526. [CrossRef] [PubMed]

81. Yu, D.; Shu, X.O.; Li, H.; Xiang, Y.B.; Yang, G.; Gao, Y.T.; Zheng, W.; Zhang, X. Dietary carbohydrates, refined grains, glycemic load, and risk of coronary heart disease in Chinese adults. *Am. J. Epidemiol.* **2013**, *178*, 1542–1549. [CrossRef] [PubMed]

82. Burger, K.N.; Beulens, J.W.; Boer, J.M.; Spijkerman, A.M.; van der, A.D. Dietary glycemic load and glycemic index and risk of coronary heart disease and stroke in Dutch men and women: The EPIC-MORGEN study. *PLoS ONE* **2011**, *6*, e25955. [CrossRef] [PubMed]

83. Hardy, D.S.; Hoelscher, D.M.; Aragaki, C.; Stevens, J.; Steffen, L.M.; Pankow, J.S.; Boerwinkle, E. Association of glycemic index and glycemic load with risk of incident coronary heart disease among whites and African Americans with and without type 2 diabetes: The atherosclerosis risk in communities study. *Ann. Epidemiol.* **2010**, *20*, 610–616. [CrossRef] [PubMed]

84. Sieri, S.; Krogh, V.; Berrino, F.; Evangelista, A.; Agnoli, C.; Brighenti, F.; Pellegrini, N.; Palli, D.; Masala, G.; Sacerdote, C.; et al. Dietary glycemic load and index and risk of coronary heart disease in a large Italian cohort: The EPICOR study. *Arch. Intern. Med.* **2010**, *170*, 640–647. [CrossRef] [PubMed]

85. Beulens, J.W.; de Bruijne, L.M.; Stolk, R.P.; Peeters, P.H.; Bots, M.L.; Grobbee, D.E.; van der Schouw, Y.T. High dietary glycemic load and glycemic index increase risk of cardiovascular disease among middle-aged women: A population-based follow-up study. *J. Am. Coll. Cardiol.* **2007**, *50*, 14–21. [CrossRef] [PubMed]

86. Levitan, E.B.; Mittleman, M.A.; Wolk, A. Dietary glycaemic index, dietary glycaemic load and incidence of myocardial infarction in women. *Br. J. Nutr.* **2010**, *103*, 1049–1055. [CrossRef] [PubMed]

87. Levitan, E.B.; Mittleman, M.A.; Wolk, A. Dietary glycemic index, dietary glycemic load, and incidence of heart failure events: A prospective study of middle-aged and elderly women. *J. Am. Coll. Nutr.* **2010**, *29*, 65–71. [CrossRef] [PubMed]

88. Ma, X.Y.; Liu, J.P.; Song, Z.Y. Glycemic load, glycemic index and risk of cardiovascular diseases: Meta-analyses of prospective studies. *Atherosclerosis* **2012**, *223*, 491–496. [CrossRef] [PubMed]

89. Neuhouser, M.L.; Schwarz, Y.; Wang, C.; Breymeyer, K.; Coronado, G.; Wang, C.-Y.; Noar, K.; Song, X.; Lampe, J.W. A low-glycemic load diet reduces serum C-reactive protein and modestly increases adiponectin in overweight and obese adults. *J. Nutr.* **2012**, *142*, 369–374. [CrossRef] [PubMed]

90. Philippou, E.; Bovill-Taylor, C.; Rajkumar, C.; Vampa, M.L.; Ntatsaki, E.; Brynes, A.E.; Hickson, M.; Frost, G.S. Preliminary report: The effect of a 6-month dietary glycemic index manipulation in addition to healthy eating advice and weight loss on arterial compliance and 24-hour ambulatory blood pressure in men: A pilot study. *Metabolism* **2009**, *58*, 1703–1708. [CrossRef] [PubMed]

91. Gogebakan, O.; Kohl, A.; Osterhoff, M.A.; van Baak, M.A.; Jebb, S.A.; Papadaki, A.; Martinez, J.A.; Handjieva-Darlenska, T.; Hlavaty, P.; Weickert, M.O.; et al. Effects of weight loss and long-term weight maintenance with diets varying in protein and glycemic index on cardiovascular risk factors: The diet, obesity, and genes (diogenes) study: A randomized, controlled trial. *Circulation* **2011**, *124*, 2829–2838. [CrossRef] [PubMed]

92. De Rougemont, A.; Normand, S.; Nazare, J.A.; Skilton, M.R.; Sothier, M.; Vinoy, S.; Laville, M. Beneficial effects of a 5-week low-glycaemic index regimen on weight control and cardiovascular risk factors in overweight non-diabetic subjects. *Br. J. Nutr.* **2007**, *98*, 1288–1298. [CrossRef] [PubMed]

93. McMillan-Price, J.; Petocz, P.; Atkinson, F.; O'Neill, K.; Samman, S.; Steinbeck, K.; Caterson, I.; Brand-Miller, J. Comparison of 4 diets of varying glycemic load on weight loss and cardiovascular risk reduction in overweight and obese young adults: A randomized controlled trial. *Arch. Intern. Med.* **2006**, *166*, 1466–1475. [CrossRef] [PubMed]

94. Vega-López, S.; Mayol-Kreiser, S. Use of the glycemic index for weight loss and glycemic control: A review of recent evidence. *Curr. Diab. Rep.* **2009**, *9*, 379–388. [CrossRef]

95. Kristo, A.S.; Matthan, N.R.; Lichtenstein, A.H. Effect of diets differing in glycemic index and glycemic load on cardiovascular risk factors: Review of randomized controlled-feeding trials. *Nutrients* **2013**, *5*, 1071–1080. [CrossRef] [PubMed]

96. Pi-Sunyer, X. Do glycemic index, glycemic load, and fiber play a role in insulin sensitivity, disposition index, and type 2 diabetes? *Diabetes Care* **2005**, *28*, 2978–2979. [CrossRef] [PubMed]

97. Vega-López, S.; Ausman, L.M.; Griffith, J.L.; Lichtenstein, A.H. Interindividual variability and intra-individual reproducibility of glycemic index values for commercial white bread. *Diabetes Care* **2007**, *30*, 1412–1417. [CrossRef] [PubMed]

98. Foster-Powell, K.; Holt, S.H.; Brand-Miller, J.C. International table of glycemic index and glycemic load values: 2002. *Am. J. Clin. Nutr.* **2002**, *76*, 5–56. [CrossRef] [PubMed]

99. Anderson, G.H.; Soeandy, C.D.; Smith, C.E. White vegetables: Glycemia and satiety. *Adv. Nutr.* **2013**, *4*, 356S–367S. [CrossRef] [PubMed]

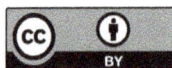

nutrients

MDPI

Article

The Comparative Effect on Satiety and Subsequent Energy Intake of Ingesting Sucrose or Isomaltulose Sweetened Trifle: A Randomized Crossover Trial

Fiona E. Kendall, Olivia Marchand, Jillian J. Haszard and Bernard J. Venn *

Department of Human Nutrition, University of Otago, P.O. Box 56, Dunedin 9054, New Zealand;
fkendall831@gmail.com (F.E.K.); liv.marchand@gmail.com (O.M.); jill.haszard@otago.ac.nz (J.J.H.)
* Correspondence: bernard.venn@otago.ac.nz; Tel.: +64-3-479-5068

Received: 25 September 2018; Accepted: 13 October 2018; Published: 15 October 2018

check for updates

Abstract: The effect that blood glucose concentration has on feelings of satiety is unclear. Our aims were to assess satiety and subsequent energy intake following the ingestion of trifle sweetened with sucrose or isomaltulose whilst measuring plasma glucose concentration to confirm glycemic differences between trifles. Seventy-seven healthy adults participated in a double-blind crossover trial where trifle sweetened with sucrose or isomaltulose was consumed on separate days with a two-week washout. Blood was sampled at the baseline, 1 and 2 h postprandially, and satiety assessed using visual analogue scales (VAS). Weighed diet records were taken on test days. A statistically significant difference in blood glucose concentration between trifles was found at 60 min following consumption, with the isomaltulose trifle having a 0.69 mmol/L (95% confidence interval (CI): −1.07, −0.31) lower concentration when compared with the sucrose trifle. Mean satiety response by area-under-the-curve (AUC) was not significantly different between trifles. Mean (SD) appetite scores for the sucrose and isomaltulose trifles were 4493 (2393) and 4527 (2590) mm·min, respectively, with a between trifle difference of −9 (95% CI: −589, 572) mm·min. Mean (SD) energy intake for the remainder of the day following trifle consumption was 3894 kJ (1950 kJ) and 3530 kJ (1926 kJ) after the sucrose and isomaltulose trifles, respectively, and was not significantly different ($p = 0.133$). The differing glycemic response to trifle was not related to satiety or to subsequent energy intake.

Keywords: satiety; sugars; sucrose; isomaltulose; glycemia

---

1. Introduction

Overweight and obesity occur on a global scale and efforts are needed to counteract the problems of obesity-related diseases [1]. The World Health Organization estimated that 1.9 billion adults were overweight in 2016 [2]. A contributing factor to weight gain is likely to be the satiating property of foods [3]. Several factors have been variably associated with the satiating properties of food including protein content [4], fat content [5], fiber [6], and food volume [7]. Another factor suggested to regulate food intake is circulating blood glucose where it has been hypothesized that raised blood glucose concentrations promote satiety and low concentrations signal hunger [8]. A possible link between circulating blood glucose concentration and satiety has persisted with suggestions that diets producing low glycemic responses enhance weight control by promoting satiety [9,10]. A suggested mechanism is that slowly absorbed glucose interacts with nutrient receptors in the gut over an extended period, signaling prolonged satiety stimulus in the brain [11].

However, any effects of circulating blood glucose on satiety are unclear, as findings have been inconsistent [12]. Part of this inconsistency may be due to factors other than glycemic response that differ between test foods, for example, foods chosen on the basis of glycemic index (GI). Practical advice from the Glycemic Index Foundation is to exchange high for low GI foods [13]. If this advice is followed, there may be factors other than the glycemic response that differ between foods, for example, macronutrients [7] or fiber content [14].

The problem of attributing satiogenic effects to the glycemic response properties of foods selected on the basis of GI, independent of other properties of the food, has been reviewed [11]. The authors of the review found 14 studies by which to assess the effect of GI on satiety; in six of the studies, the fiber content of the lower GI foods was greater than that of the higher GI food; in another three studies, the low GI property of the test foods was achieved by adding extrinsic fiber; thus, the independent effect of the glycemic response per se on satiety has been difficult to assess [11]. It is possible to control for these food factors and in one such study, postprandial glycemia and satiety were found to differ in men consuming lunches containing different proportions of amylose to amylopectin in the starch fraction of otherwise comparable meals [15]. In a subsequent follow-up study by the same authors, despite lower glycemia after high were compared with the low amylose lunches, no differences in satiety were found [16].

Another strategy to manipulate glycemic responses by exchanging food ingredients is to use sugars with different GI. Isomaltulose (Palatinose™) is a non-cariogenic sugar found in trace amounts in honey [17] and in Japan, it has been commercially produced from sucrose and added to processed foods since the 1980s [18]. Isomaltulose is a structural isomer of sucrose, both disaccharides comprise one glucose and one fructose moiety but the glycosidic bond between the monosaccharides differs [19]. The different bonds result in isomaltulose being fully digested but at a slower rate than sucrose, creating a flattened blood glucose response curve following isomaltulose when compared with sucrose ingestion [20]. When groups of rats were sustained with these disaccharides over 24 h, it was found that food and energy intakes were lower in the animals fed isomaltulose when compared with the sucrose-fed group [21]. The effect on satiety of providing humans with foods containing these sugars has not been tested.

The objective of this experiment was to compare the acute effect on satiety by incorporating a higher and a lower GI sugar as an ingredient into a solid food that could be consumed in practice. In order to test the hypothesis that feelings of satiety would be increased following the consumption of a food containing a lower GI ingredient, it was necessary to identify a food with a relatively high sugar content so that it would generate a difference in glycemic response between test foods. Trifle was chosen because each of its components (jelly, sponge, and custard) contain a considerable proportion of sugar. Hence, the current study was designed to measure glycemic responses and to test for short-term effects on satiety and subsequent energy intake by providing participants with trifle sweetened with either isomaltulose or sucrose. The main outcomes were satiety and subsequent energy intake, with plasma glucose concentration measured as confirmation of the effectiveness in generating glycemic differences between trifles.

2. Materials and Methods

Participants were a convenience sample of students from the University of Otago. Inclusion criteria were students enrolled in a third year human nutrition course older than 18 years of age. Students were invited to participate in the study providing they had no food allergies to any of the trifle ingredients. Students were not obliged to take part and were given an information sheet and the opportunity to seek clarification of what the study involved. The University of Otago Human Ethics Committee approved the study (reference H17/011) and students signed a consent form. The study has been registered with the Australian and New Zealand Clinical Trials Registry ACTRN12618001137280.

2.1. Study Design

Seventy-seven young adults received a sucrose- or isomaltulose-sweetened trifle at lunchtime in a cross-over design randomized to the order in which they received the trifle. Participants attended two testing days on Fridays starting at 12 p.m. with a 2-week washout. Participants were stratified by the weeks when they could attend the test sessions to ensure equal distribution at each clinic for the order in which the trifles were consumed.

The day before the first test day, each participant indicated to the investigators the type and amount of cereal that he or she wished to consume at breakfast the following morning and this was weighed and packaged in a sealable plastic bag for the participant to take home. Participants were instructed to eat all of the cereal on the morning of the test day at his or her usual breakfast time and then not to eat or drink (apart from water) until 12 p.m. Participants were provided with the same breakfast and asked to eat the breakfast at the same time on each of those days to ensure that appetite and energy intake prior to the lunchtime test sessions were consistent.

At 12 p.m., participants were seated in the testing facility and asked to consume the trifle within 20 min. No other food was consumed for the following 150 min. A staff member independent of the study used the random number generator in Excel (Microsoft, Redmond, Washington, WA, USA) to allocate the order in which each student received the sucrose- or isomaltulose-sweetened trifle. This staff member placed a colored sticker (red or green) onto the lid of the trifle container corresponding to sucrose or isomaltulose. The students, study investigators, and the biostatistician were blinded to trifle type with the colored code revealed after the completion of the statistical analysis. On the morning of the first test day, the participants' heights were recorded to the nearest mm using a stadiometer (Holtain, Crymych, UK); and weight was measured to the nearest gram using calibrated electronic scales (Seca Deutschland, Hamburg, Germany). Body mass index was calculated as weight divided by height squared. Participants filled out a questionnaire regarding sex, age, and ethnicity.

2.2. Test Foods

The trifles were made in the metabolic kitchen of the Department of Human Nutrition at the University of Otago. The ingredients were: eggs, sugar (isomaltulose or sucrose in the form of castor sugar), plain flour, cornflour, baking powder, water, lemon juice, gelatin, full fat milk, and cream. Each serving weighed 446 g and contained 2600 kJ. The nutritional composition of the two trifles on a fresh weight basis were identical: protein 15.8 g; fat 18.6 g; available carbohydrate 98.2 g; total sugars 80.5 g (of which sucrose or isomaltulose 73.2 g); dietary fiber 0.6 g, and ash 2.1 g; with a moisture content of 70%.

2.3. Blood Testing

A 500 µL capillary blood sample was collected into a microcontainer containing potassium ethylenediaminetetraacetic acid (EDTA) (Becton, Dickinson and Company, Franklin Lakes, NJ, USA) using a contact-activated disposable lancet at the baseline and at 1 and 2 h following consumption of the trifles. The tubes were centrifuged for 10 min at $2000 \times g$ within 20 min of blood collection and the plasma was extracted and stored at $-80\,^{\circ}\text{C}$ until analysis. Plasma glucose concentration was measured using the glucose hexokinase method on a Cobas c311 auto analyzer (Roche Diagnostics, Indianapolis, IN, USA). Coefficients of variation for Roche control sera Precinorm U plus (nominal 4 mmol/L) and Precipath U plus (nominal 13 mmol/L) were 1.25% and 0.67%, respectively.

2.4. Satiety and Dietary Recording

Feelings of satiety were assessed using 100 mm Visual Analogue Scales (VAS) using methodology validated by Flint and colleagues [22]. Four questions were asked with anchoring statements as given in parentheses "How hungry do you feel?" (I am not hungry at all/I have never been more hungry); "How satisfied do you feel?" (I am completely empty/I cannot eat another bite); "How full do you feel?" (Not at all full/Totally full); and "How much do you think you can eat?" (Nothing at all/A lot). The set of four questions were asked at the baseline and at 30, 60, 90, 120, and 150 min after eating the trifles. Responses to each question at each timepoint were marked on a 100 mm line and the sheets removed. Each of the four satiety questions were analyzed for each person using area under the curve over 150 min (AUC). In addition, a composite appetite score was generated by taking the average AUC of the four questions at each time point. Cronbach's alphas were calculated for the overall appetite scale at each time point.

Training was given to participants in the use of the Model 3010 Salter electronic kitchen scales reading to 1 g (Salter Housewares, Tonbridge, UK). Participants took the scales home and weighed and recorded all food and beverages consumed throughout the day from waking on the morning of each test day through to midnight. The dietary data were entered into a University of Otago dietary analysis program that uses the New Zealand Food Composition database as the source of nutrient information [23].

2.5. Statistical Analysis

A sample of 60 was required to detect a difference of 0.5 standard deviations for all outcomes in standardized form with 90% power and $\alpha = 0.01$. Seventy-seven participants were recruited as a convenience sample, which allowed for some dropout. Random effects regression analysis was used to test for between-treatment differences in plasma glucose at the 60 and 120 min timepoints and for AUC satiety responses with participant id as a random effect and adjusted for randomized order and baseline satiety. Analysis was also undertaken for standardized AUC and to estimate differences in subsequent energy intake. A p-value < 0.05 was considered statistically significant. Stata 15.1 (StataCorp, College Station, TX, USA) was used to analyze the VAS satiety data.

3. Results

Seventy-seven participants were randomized to order and complete blood and satiety data were available for 66 people. A diagram of participant flow through the study is given in Figure 1.

Anthropometric and demographic characteristics of the sample are given in Table 1.

Participants were mainly young female adults of European descent, with Asian and Māori ethnicities combined constituting 30% of the sample.

Table 1. Baseline demographics and characteristics ($n = 77$).

Characteristic	Mean (SD) or n (%)
Height (m)	1.7 (0.1)
Weight (kg)	66.4 (13.5)
Body Mass Index (kg/m^2)	23.7 (3.6)
Sex n (Female/Male)	59 F/18 M
Age (year)	21.9 (5.6)
Ethnicity n (%)	
New Zealand European	49 (65%)
Asian	17 (23%)
Māori	5 (7%)
Other	4 (5%)

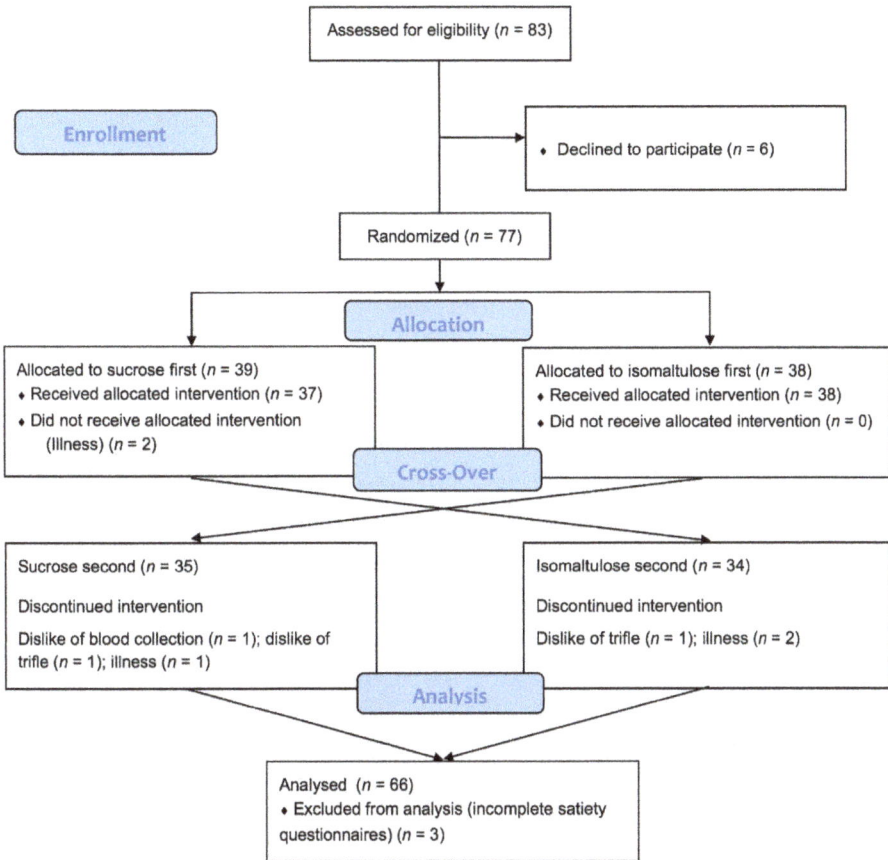

Figure 1. CONSORT diagram showing the flow of participants through the study.

3.1. Blood Glucose

The mean (SD) plasma glucose concentrations at the baseline were 5.2 (0.7) and 5.1 (0.7) mmol/L for the sucrose and isomaltulose-sweetened trifles, respectively, and these concentrations were not different (p = 0.253). The mean blood glucose concentration data sampled at 60 and 120 min and comparisons between treatments at 60 and 120 min are given in Table 2.

Table 2. Blood glucose concentrations (mmol/L) and difference between trifles (*n* = 66).

Time (min)	Sucrose Mean (SD)	Isomaltulose Mean (SD)	Isomaltulose-Sucrose Mean Difference (95% Confidence Interval) [1]	p
60	7.3 (1.7)	6.6 (1.1)	−0.69 (−1.07, −0.31)	<0.001
120	5.9 (0.9)	6.1 (0.9)	0.18 (−0.10, 0.45)	0.215

[1] Random effects regression analysis adjusted for baseline and order of treatment.

Blood glucose rose at 60 min then declined at 120 min, though remained above the baseline for both trifles. A statistically significant difference between trifles was observed at 60 min following consumption.

3.2. Satiety

AUC was used to measure appetite response across the testing time period on both days, spanning the baseline (prior to trifle ingestion) to 150 min postprandial. This enabled six VAS questionnaires to be completed by each participant on a given testing day. There were no significant differences for mean difference between the isomaltulose- and sucrose-sweetened trifle or in mean AUC for each satiety question across all time points following the consumption of the trifles (Table 3).

Table 3. Subjective satiety area under the curve (AUC) using visual analogue scales over 150 min (*n* = 66).

VAS Question	Sucrose Mean (SD) mm·min	Isomaltulose Mean (SD) mm·min	Mean Difference (95% CI) mm·min	Mean Standardized Difference (95% CI)
How hungry do you feel?	3628 (2457)	3697 (2454)	37 (−616, −691)	0.02 (−0.25, 0.28)
How satisfied do you feel?	4928 (2506)	4886 (2667)	−97 (−717, −523)	0.04 (−0.28, 0.20)
How full do you feel?	4768 (2668)	4899 (2859)	23 (−673, −718)	0.01 (−0.24, 0.26)
How much do you think you can eat?	4718 (2777)	4729 (2979)	9 (−600, −617)	0.00 (−0.21, 0.22)
Overall appetite score [a]	4493 (2393)	4527 (2590)	−9 (−589, −572)	0.00 (−0.24, 0.23)

[a] The overall appetite score was an average of the AUC values of the four satiety questions. The questions were highly correlated with internal reliability (Cronbach's alpha) of 0.86–0.94 at each time point. There were no significance between-trifle differences for any of the questions. VAS: visual analogue scales.

A meaningful effect was ruled out as the mean difference and 95% CI were all under 0.3 standard deviations. Therefore, it is unlikely that there is a real difference in satiety between the trifles. Sixty-six participants recorded subsequent energy intake for the rest of the day after the trial; mean (SD) energy intake after the sucrose trifle was 3894 kJ (1950 kJ), and after the isomaltulose trifle it was 3530 kJ (1926 kJ). Energy intake for the remainder of the day after consuming the trifle did not differ significantly between treatments with a mean difference (sucrose arm-isomaltulose arm) of 364 kJ (95% CI: −110 kJ, 838 kJ), *p* = 0.133.

4. Discussion

In the present study, differences in postprandial glycemia were found between trifles, but there were no significant differences in the participants feelings of satiety or in their subsequent energy intake. These findings are consistent with other work. When comparing satiety among 38 foods, food volume or energy density were found to be the strongest predictors of satiety index scores, with satiety index defined as area under the 120 min satiety curve (AUC) of the test food divided by the AUC of white bread [24]. Using the same index, the portion sizes of seven isocaloric breads were predictors of satiety and subsequent energy intake with no significant relationship found between glycemic response and satiety [7]. We controlled for both volume and energy density as the trifles were identical in these factors. Thus, there is consistency that volume or energy density of foods are predictive of satiety, whereas differences in glycemia, at least of the magnitude attained in these studies, is not.

In contrast, differences in some appetite measures have been found from studies where comparison treatments have been designed using food choices based on GI. In one such study, food was requested approximately three-quarters of an hour earlier after the high GI meal when compared with the low GI meals, although there was no difference in subsequent energy intake [25]. In a study in which shepherd's pie contained either low GI beans or high GI potato puree, feelings of hunger were delayed and stomach fullness was greater four hours after eating the bean when compared with the potato meal [26]. The authors of that study were unable to exclude the possibility that factors other than glycemic responses were influential over satiety, as the nutrient compositions of the meals differed [26]. In a longer-term crossover study conducted over 28 days using low and high GI foods, the mean hunger rating of 80 participants over the study period was not different between diets, but people reported feeling fuller while eating the low GI diet [14].

The outcomes of these studies are variable both within and among studies, but in each study there was some indication that low, as opposed to high GI foods, resulted in some greater measure of satiety. However, whether any of the differences found were due to glycemic responses is uncertain. The fiber content of foods has been found in some studies to affect satiety [6]. In the study by Chang et al., the low GI diets contained 55 g/day fiber, considerably more than the 28 g/day in the high GI diets [14]. In the study by Leathwood and colleagues, the shepherd's pie containing bean puree had more protein, less carbohydrate, and more fiber (13 vs. 6 g) than the potato meal [26]. The fiber content was not reported by Ball et al., but the low GI foods were products designed to contain relatively high fiber contents (USANA, Salt Lake City, UT, USA) while the high GI products comprising a maltodextrin based beverage and an Ensure bar (Ross Products Division, Abbott Laboratories, Columbus, OH, USA) were likely to have contained less fiber [25]. Thus, because different foods were used to generate glycemic differences between treatment arms, it is possible that factors other than glycemic responses may have contributed to, or have been the cause of, differences in satiety.

Controlling for factors such as fiber, energy, and macronutrient content is possible with the use of beverages sweetened with sugars with different glycemic-inducing characteristics. Beverages sweetened with glucose (G) and fructose (F) mixtures of G80:F20 (high glycemic) and G20:F80 (low glycemic) ratios were given to 12 and 19 people (two experiments), resulting in no difference in the ratings of appetite but a lower subsequent energy intake 80 min after drinking the high-compared with the low-glycemic beverage [27]. In another trial involving 15 adolescents, subsequent food intake was lower after a glucose beverage compared with a sucralose control; and appetite ratings were higher after ingesting a glucose beverage compared with a high-fructose corn syrup beverage [28]. These data are suggestive that glucose has a satiating effect, potentially via its glycemic-raising capacity in accordance with the glucostatic theory where an elevated blood glucose concentration is hypothesized to induce appetite dampening [8]. However, fructose undergoes different metabolic processes to glucose and therefore it is possible that differences in satiety may result from differences in the metabolism of the two sugars, for example, via cerebral blood flow acting on appetite signals [29].

A means of isolating the glycemic effects of sugars on satiety is the use of isomaltulose and sucrose as the comparison treatments as these two sugars have identical monosaccharide constituents. It has been found that rats provided with sucrose or isomaltulose ingested more energy over 24 h when exposed to sucrose compared with isomaltulose [21]. However, these were extreme diets in that the intakes were 100% of either sugar in an animal model. In humans, using a practical approach, the trifles our participants consumed generated differences in glycemia, but resulted in no difference in the immediate ratings of satiety or in subsequent energy intake throughout the day. A limitation of our work was the infrequent sampling of blood glucose, at the baseline, one and two hours later. The infrequency was to avoid participant anxiety at having multiple fingerpricks taken during the time when subjective feelings of satiety were being collected. Nevertheless, we were able to confirm a significant difference in glycemic response at the one-hour timepoint. Generalizability may also be limiting as our participants were young, healthy, and predominantly female. A difference in feelings of fullness over time following ad libitum consumption of yogurt between adolescent and elderly participants has been found [30],however, it is unknown how age would effect change in satiety when comparing between two test foods.

A major strength of the study was the use of isomaltulose and sucrose as the sweeteners that allowed for double-blinding and for the control of many factors associated with satiety including volume of food, macronutrients, fiber, and energy content. The study also had a strong design, being a crossover, participants were randomized to treatment order, and it was adequately powered with a relatively large sample. A limitation was the inclusion of these sugars into trifle that limited the glycemic difference between treatments. A maximum difference of around 1.5 mmol/L in blood glucose concentration between sucrose and isomaltulose has been found when participants ingested

50 g solutions of these beverages [20] whereas the difference between trifles was 0.69 mmol/L using 73 g of the sugars. The reason for the diminished glycemic difference could be that the infrequency of sampling missed the time of maximum separation, or could be due to the inclusion of fat and protein in the trifles. Co-ingestion of fat and carbohydrate lessens the glycemic response when compared with carbohydrate alone [31] and protein stimulates insulin, thereby encouraging glucose disposal out of circulation [32]. It is possible that greater differences in glycemia could be related to satiety and this could be tested by feeding sucrose or isomaltulose beverages without the addition of fat and protein; or by increasing still further the amount of these sugars incorporated into test foods. Generalizability is also limiting as our sample was predominantly young, healthy females. Testing for the effects of these sugars on the satiety of other age groups and in people with impaired glucose tolerance would be informative.

5. Conclusions

In conclusion, sucrose and isomaltulose contain identical glucose and fructose molecules but differ in the glycosidic bond joining the monosaccharides, resulting in the slower digestion of isomaltulose when compared with sucrose. The slower rate of digestion of isomaltulose compared with sucrose generated a glycemic difference between the two trifles at lunchtime, but this glycemic difference did not result in differences in feelings of satiety or in subsequent food intake over the remainder of the day. These data are novel and will hopefully lead to other investigators testing the satiating properties of these sugars amongst a wider demographic.

Author Contributions: Conceptualization, B.J.V.; Methodology, F.E.K., O.M., J.J.H. and B.J.V.; Formal analysis, J.J.H.; Investigation, F.E.K. and O.M.; Resources, B.J.V.; Data curation, J.J.H.; Writing—original draft preparation, F.E.K. and B.J.V.; Writing—review and editing, F.E.K., O.M., J.J.H. and B.J.V.; Supervision, B.J.V.; Project administration, B.J.V.

Funding: This research was funded by University of Otago.

Acknowledgments: The authors thank Kieran Columb and Ivy Salih for their laboratory assistance.

Conflicts of Interest: The authors declare no conflict of interest.

References

1. Must, A.; McKeown, N.M. The Disease Burden Associated with Overweight and Obesity. Available online: https://www.ncbi.nlm.nih.gov/books/NBK279095/ (accessed on 12 June 2018).
2. World Health Organization. Obesity and Overweight. Available online: http://www.who.int/news-room/fact-sheets/detail/obesity-and-overweight (accessed on 29 June 2018).
3. Blundell, J.; De Graaf, C.; Hulshof, T.; Jebb, S.; Livingstone, B.; Lluch, A.; Mela, D.; Salah, S.; Schuring, E.; van der Knaap, H.; et al. Appetite control: Methodological aspects of the evaluation of foods. *Obes. Rev.* **2010**, *11*, 251–270. [CrossRef] [PubMed]
4. Anderson, G.H.; Moore, S.E. Dietary proteins in the regulation of food intake and body weight in humans. *J. Nutr.* **2004**, *134*, 974S–979S. [CrossRef] [PubMed]
5. Robinson, T.M.; Gray, R.W.; Yeomans, M.R.; French, S.J. Test-meal palatability alters the effects of intragastric fat but not carbohydrate preloads on intake and rated appetite in healthy volunteers. *Physiol. Behav.* **2005**, *84*, 193–203. [CrossRef] [PubMed]
6. Clark, M.J.; Slavin, J.L. The effect of fiber on satiety and food intake: A systematic review. *J. Am. Coll. Nutr.* **2013**, *32*, 200–211. [CrossRef] [PubMed]
7. Holt, S.H.; Brand-Miller, J.C.; Stitt, P.A. The effects of equal-energy portions of different breads on blood glucose levels, feelings of fullness and subsequent food intake. *J. Am. Diet. Assoc.* **2001**, *101*, 767–773. [CrossRef]
8. Mayer, J. Glucostatic mechanism of regulation of food intake. *N. Engl. J. Med.* **1953**, *249*, 13–16. [CrossRef] [PubMed]
9. Brand-Miller, J.; Holt, S.; Pawlak, D.; McMillan, J. Glycaemic Index and Obesity. *Am. J. Clin. Nutr.* **2002**, *76*, 281S–285S. [CrossRef] [PubMed]

10. Brand-Miller, J.; McMillan-Price, J.; Steinbeck, K.; Caterson, I. Dietary glycemic index: Health implications. *J. Am. Coll. Nutr.* **2009**, *28*, 446S–449S. [CrossRef] [PubMed]

11. Bornet, F.R.; Jardy-Gennetier, A.E.; Jacquet, N.; Stowell, J. Glycaemic response to foods: Impact on satiety and long-term weight regulation. *Appetite* **2007**, *49*, 535–553. [CrossRef] [PubMed]

12. Anderson, G.H.; Woodend, D. Effect of glycemic carbohydrates on short-term satiety and food intake. *Nutr. Rev.* **2003**, *61*, 172S–176S. [CrossRef]

13. Brand-Miller, J. GI Update with Prof Jennie Brand-Miller 2013. Available online: http://ginews.blogspot. com/2013/06/gi-update-with-prof-jennie-brand-miller.html (accessed on 21 September 2018).

14. Chang, K.T.; Lampe, J.W.; Schwarz, Y.; Breymeyer, K.L.; Noar, K.A.; Song, X.; Neuhouser, M.L. Low glycemic load experimental diet more satiating than high glycemic load diet. *Nutr. Cancer* **2012**, *64*, 666–673. [CrossRef] [PubMed]

15. Van Amelsvoort, J.M.; Weststrate, J.A. Amylose-amylopectin ratio in a meal affects postprandial variables in male volunteers. *Am. J. Clin. Nutr.* **1992**, *55*, 712–718. [CrossRef] [PubMed]

16. Weststrate, J.A.; van Amelsvoort, J.M. Effects of the amylose content of breakfast and lunch on postprandial variables in male volunteers. *Am. J. Clin. Nutr.* **1993**, *58*, 180–186. [CrossRef] [PubMed]

17. Siddiqui, I.; Furgala, B. Isolation and Characterization of Oligosaccharides from Honey. Part I. Disaccharides. *J. Apic. Res.* **1967**, *6*, 139–145. [CrossRef]

18. Nakajima, Y. Manufacture and Utilization of Palatinose. *J. Jpn. Soc. Starch Sci.* **1988**, *35*, 131–139. (In Japanese) [CrossRef]

19. Park, J.Y.; Jung, J.H.; Seo, D.H.; Ha, S.J.; Yoon, J.W.; Kim, Y.C.; Shim, J.H.; Park, C.S. Microbial production of palatinose through extracellular expression of a sucrose isomerase from *Enterobacter* sp. FMB-1 in *Lactococcus lactis* MG1363. *Bioresour. Technol.* **2010**, *101*, 8828–8833. [CrossRef] [PubMed]

20. Holub, I.; Gostner, A.; Theis, S.; Nosek, L.; Kudlich, T.; Melcher, R.; Scheppach, W. Novel findings on the metabolic effects of the low glycaemic carbohydrate isomaltulose (Palatinose). *Br. J. Nutr.* **2010**, *103*, 1730–1737. [CrossRef] [PubMed]

21. Sasagawa, K.; Mineo, S.; Hirayama, M.; Sata, S. Sustained effect of isomaltulose on satiety in rats. *J. Jpn. Soc. Nutr. Food Sci.* **2013**, *66*, 301–307. (In Japanese) [CrossRef]

22. Flint, A.; Raben, A.; Blundell, J.; Astrup, A. Reproducibility, power and validity of visual analogue scales in assessment of appetite sensations in single test meal studies. *Int. J. Obes.* **2000**, *24*, 38–48. [CrossRef]

23. The New Zealand Institute for Plant & Food Research Limited and the Ministry of Health (New Zealand). New Zealand Food Files. 2016. Available online: https://www.foodcomposition.co.nz/foodfiles/ (accessed on 12 June 2018).

24. Holt, S.; Brand-Miller, J. Increased insulin responses to ingested foods are associated with lessened satiety. *Appetite* **1995**, *24*, 43–54. [CrossRef]

25. Ball, S.D.; Keller, K.R.; Moyer-Mileur, L.J.; Ding, Y.W.; Donaldson, D.; Jackson, W.D. Prolongation of satiety after low versus moderately high glycemic index meals in obese adolescents. *Pediatrics* **2003**, *111*, 488–494. [CrossRef] [PubMed]

26. Leathwood, P.; Pollet, P. Effects of slow release carbohydrates in the form of bean flakes on the evolution of hunger and satiety in man. *Appetite* **1988**, *10*, 1–11. [CrossRef]

27. Akhavan, T.; Anderson, G.H. Effects of glucose-to-fructose ratios in solutions on subjective satiety, food intake, and satiety hormones in young men. *Am. J. Clin. Nutr.* **2007**, *86*, 1354–1363. [CrossRef] [PubMed]

28. Van Engelen, M.; Khodabandeh, S.; Akhavan, T.; Agarwal, J.; Gladanac, B.; Bellissimo, N. Effect of sugars in solutions on subjective appetite and short-term food intake in 9- to 14-year-old normal weight boys. *Eur. J. Clin. Nutr.* **2014**, *68*, 773–777. [CrossRef] [PubMed]

29. Page, K.A.; Chan, O.; Arora, J.; Belfort-Deaguiar, R.; Dzuira, J.; Roehmholdt, B.; Cline, G.W.; Naik, S.; Sinha, R.; Constable, R.T.; et al. Effects of fructose vs glucose on regional cerebral blood flow in brain regions involved with appetite and reward pathways. *JAMA* **2013**, *309*, 63–70. [CrossRef] [PubMed]

30. Rolls, B.J.; McDerrmott, T.M. Effects of age on sensory-specific satiety. *Am. J. Clin. Nutr.* **1991**, *54*, 988–996. [CrossRef] [PubMed]

31. Collier, G.; O'Dea, K. The effect of coingestion of fat on the glucose, insulin, and gastric inhibitory polypeptide responses to carbohydrate and protein. *Am. J. Clin. Nutr.* **1983**, *37*, 941–944. [CrossRef] [PubMed]
32. Nuttall, F.Q.; Mooradian, A.D.; Gannon, M.C.; Billington, C.; Krezowski, P. Effect of protein ingestion on the glucose and insulin response to a standardized oral glucose load. *Diabetes Care* **1984**, *7*, 465–470. [CrossRef] [PubMed]

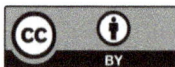

nutrients

Article

Kiwifruit Exchanges for Increased Nutrient Richness with Little Effect on Carbohydrate Intake, Glycaemic Impact, or Insulin Response

John Monro [1,2,*], Kerry Bentley-Hewitt [1] and Suman Mishra [1]

1 New Zealand Institute for Plant & Food Research, Private Bag 11600, Palmerston North 4442, New Zealand; kerry.bentley-hewitt@plantandfood.co.nz (K.B.-H.); suman.mishra@plantandfood.co.nz (S.M.)
2 Riddet Institute, Massey University, Palmerston North 4442, New Zealand
* Correspondence: john.monro@plantandfood.co.nz; Tel.: +64-6355-6137

Received: 22 October 2018; Accepted: 5 November 2018; Published: 8 November 2018

Abstract: Background: Kiwifruit are nutrient-rich and have properties which indicate a low glycaemic impact compared with many cooked cereal foods, suggesting that they may be used for dietary enrichment of vitamin C without glycaemic cost. Aim: To develop tables for equi-carbohydrate and equi-glycaemic partial exchange of kiwifruit for glycaemic carbohydrate foods. Method: The available carbohydrate content of Zespri® Green and Zespri® SunGold kiwifruit was determined as sugars released during in vitro digestive analysis. Glycaemic potency was determined as grams of glucose equivalents (GGEs) in a clinical trial using 200 g (a two-kiwifruit edible portion) of each cultivar, non-diabetic subjects ($n = 20$), and a glucose reference. GGE values were also estimated for a range of carbohydrate foods in the New Zealand Food Composition Database for which available carbohydrate and glycaemic index values were available. The values allowed exchange tables to be constructed for either equi-carbohydrate or equi-glycaemic partial exchange of kiwifruit for the foods. Results: GGE values of both kiwifruit cultivars were low ("Hayward", 6.6 glucose equivalents/100 g; "Zesy002", 6.7 glucose equivalents/100 g). Partial equi-carbohydrate substitution of foods in most carbohydrate food categories substantially increased vitamin C with little change in glycaemic impact, while equi-glycaemic partial substitution by kiwifruit could be achieved with little change in carbohydrate intake. Conclusion: Equi-carbohydrate partial exchange of kiwifruit for starchy staple foods is a means of greatly increasing nutrient richness in a diet without the physiological costs of increased glycaemia and insulin responses or carbohydrate intake.

Keywords: kiwifruit; carbohydrate exchanges; glycaemic response; glycaemic glucose equivalents; vitamin C

---

1. Introduction

Kiwifruit is one of the most nutrient-rich of readily available fruits, and can make a valuable contribution to dietary intakes of micronutrients and phytochemicals that foster good health through a variety of protective mechanisms. So much so that it has recently been recommended that kiwifruit should be considered as part of a natural and effective dietary strategy to address some of the major global health and wellness concerns [1]. One kiwifruit per day has been shown to be sufficient to achieve "healthy" plasma levels of vitamin C [2] and to saturate muscle tissue vitamin C concentrations [3].

Fruits are also generally rich in available carbohydrate in the form of approximately equal proportions of glucose and fructose. In kiwifruit, for instance, sugars make up about 12% of the edible portion of the fresh fruit, consisting of glucose, fructose, and sucrose (about 2:2:1), and represent a major proportion of the skin-free dry matter (New Zealand Food Composition Database, 2015). Consequently, with an increasing global incidence of diabetes and obesity, the high content of sugars is often seen as reason to avoid fruit, ignoring the fact that fruit phytochemicals, including vitamin C, may have a valuable role in counteracting body states and processes such as glycaemia-induced oxidative stress and inflammation [4], which are implicated in the development of diabetic complications [5]. It is therefore important that the need to control intakes of glycaemic carbohydrate should not be misconstrued as a need to decrease intakes of fruits, particularly as fruit structure, fruit sugar (fructose), and other fruit constituents that retard glycaemic response, such as cell wall debris (dietary fibre), organic acids, and phenolics acting in the gut, may lead to a relatively low glycaemic response to sugars in fruit. We have shown that in kiwifruit, both the available carbohydrates and other components, contribute to an improved glycaemic response upon equal-carbohydrate partial substitution of kiwifruit for starchy breakfast cereal [6].

One of the strategies for glycaemia management that has been used in dietetic practice is to substitute highly glycaemic carbohydrates in the diet with less glycaemic carbohydrates using the "carbohydrate exchange" system [7]. Carbohydrate exchanges are generally carried out by substituting low glycaemic impact carbohydrate for higher glycaemic impact carbohydrate sources, while maintaining a more or less constant nutrient composition. However, rather than simply substituting one carbohydrate source for another, carbohydrate exchanges provide an opportunity to improve the nutrient richness of the diet by partially substituting nutrient-rich carbohydrate products, such as fresh kiwifruit, for less nutrient-rich foods such as starch-based staples and refined cereal products.

To facilitate the more general use of kiwifruit in food exchange for nutrient enrichment or glycaemic control we determined the available carbohydrate content of two cultivars of kiwifruit (*Actinidia chinensis* var. *deliciosa* "Hayward" marketed as Zespri® Green kiwifruit, and *Actinidia chinensis* var. *chinensis* "Zesy002", marketed as Zespri® SunGold kiwifruit) by in vitro digestive analysis, and their glycaemic potencies relative to a glucose reference in a human intervention study. The results allowed quantities to be calculated for either equi-carbohydrate or equi-glycaemic substitution of a range of foods, and construction of tables of kiwifruit exchanges to show:

(1) How much of a range of carbohydrate foods could be substituted by one kiwifruit while keeping available carbohydrate content constant.
(2) Approximately how much glycaemic impact would be altered by equal carbohydrate partial substitution of one kiwifruit for a food.
(3) Approximately how much of a number of foods could be substituted by one kiwifruit while keeping glycaemic impact constant.

The aim of the study was to demonstrate the feasibility and glycaemic safety of using kiwifruit exchanges to increase intake of nutrients such as vitamin C within the diet with little effect on its glycaemic impact or carbohydrate load.

2. Methods

2.1. Test Components

"Hayward" (GR) and "Zesy002" (SG) kiwifruit were provided by Zespri Group Ltd., Tauranga, New Zealand, in a ready-to-eat state of ripeness, and processed within a few days of receipt. They were peeled and the hard apical core removed from the green kiwifruit, then halved and frozen ($-20\,^{\circ}$C). The frozen fruit were allowed to thaw partially and were then crushed to a coarse pulp by briefly (10 s) chopping in a Halde food processor. The pulp was then divided accurately into individual 200-g portions, each stored frozen within a plastic, capped, freezer-proof sundae container until required.

The glucose used was dextrose monohydrate (Davis Food Ingredients, Palmerston North, New Zealand), which contains 91% glucose. It is henceforth referred to as glucose, and an allowance was made for its water content in all calculations and weight measurements.

2.2. Carbohydrate Analysis of Kiwifruit

The available carbohydrate contents of the fruit (GR and SG) were determined by a standard digestive analysis, involving simulated gastric (pepsin pH 2.5, 30 min) and small intestinal digestion (pancreatin/amyloglucosidase, pH 6.2, 120 min), with the available carbohydrate content of the digested pulp measured after invertase digestion using a reduced scale modification of the dinitrosalicylic acid method [8]. The fructose content was measured by the thiobarbituric acid procedure [9].

2.3. Formulation of Meals

The subjects consumed three materials:

(1)   40 g of glucose (reference).
(2)   200 g of "Hayward" kiwifruit alone
(3)   200 g of "Zesy002" kiwifruit alone.

2.4. Human Intervention Study

This study was conducted according to the guidelines laid down in the Declaration of Helsinki and all procedures involving human subjects were approved by the Human and Disabilities Ethics Committee of the New Zealand Ministry of Health (ethics approval number 14/CEN/207). Written informed consent was obtained from all subjects. The trial was registered with the Australia New Zealand Clinical Trials Registry (Trial ID: ACTRN12615000222549) (URL: http://www.anzctr.org.au). The participant flow chart shows ethical approval, recruitment, and intervention processes for the trial (Figure 1).

The trial was run as a non-blinded randomised repeated measures study. It was not possible to blind the subjects to the meals they were consuming. However, the data and statistical analysis were performed by an analyst who was blinded to the treatments. Meal order was randomised for each subject using a computerised random number generator.

Participants: Twenty participants, eight male and 12 female, were recruited by flyer and email. Respondents were interviewed and given an information pack including a description of the study and a consent form. Prospective participants were asked to complete a health questionnaire and provide a capillary blood glucose sample for glucose and glycated haemoglobin analysis. Exclusion criteria included known intolerance of kiwifruit, glucose intolerance as indicated by the fasting blood glucose and HbA1c, and recent ill health. The characteristics (mean $\pm$ SD) of the study group were as follows: age 36.7 $\pm$ 8.1 years, BMI 24.5 $\pm$ 5.2 kg.m^{-2}, fasting glucose 4.6 $\pm$ 0.4 mmol.L^{-1}, HbA1c 33.9 $\pm$ 4 mmol.mol^{-1}).

Ingestion: The kiwifruit were thawed in a microwave with care to avoid heating, immediately before being consumed. The glucose and kiwifruit were consumed with enough water to give an equal intake volume (300 mL) in all meals.

Glycaemic response: Subjects were asked to eat moderately the evening before and to fast overnight and present themselves at 0830 h for the dietary intervention. They were asked to consume the meals within a 10-min period and avoid physical exertion for three hours afterward, during which time blood glucose determinations were made. Blood glucose concentrations were measured by finger-prick analysis of capillary blood using a HemoCue (Ängelholm, Sweden) blood glucose analyser. Blood samplings were made immediately before consuming the diets (duplicate, baseline), and at 15, 30, 45, 60, 90, 120, and 180 min after the start of food consumption.

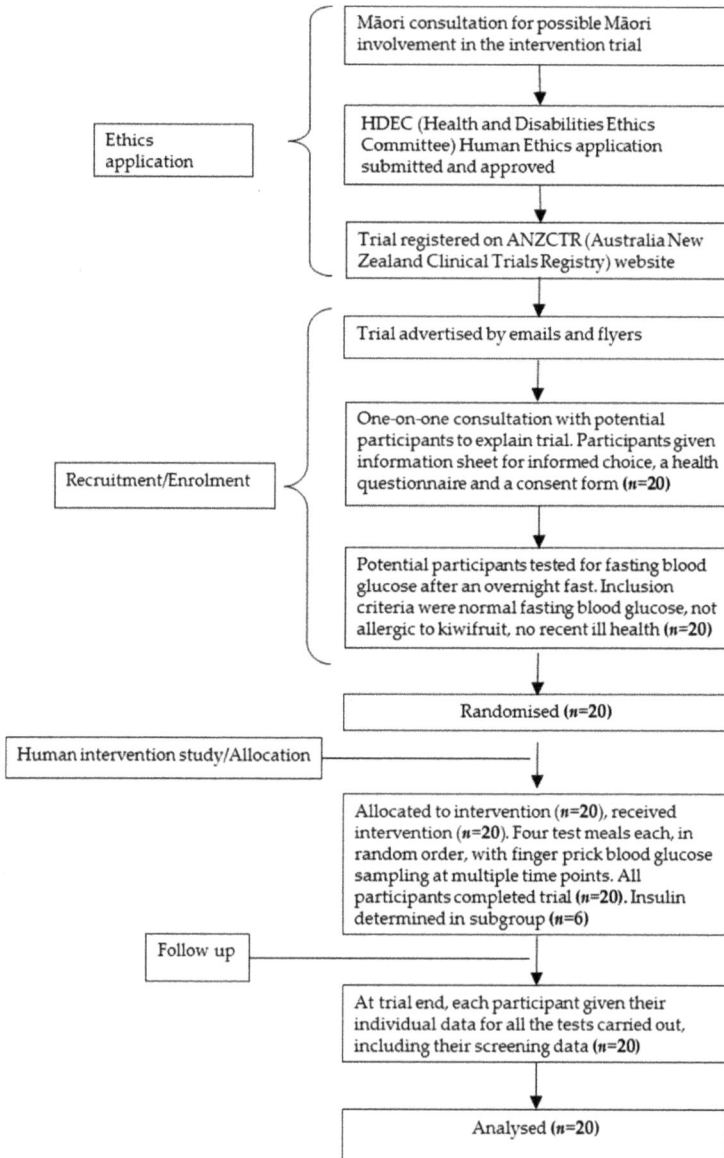

Figure 1. Participant flow chart for clinical determination of the relative glycaemic potency of kiwifruit.

Plasma insulin: Plasma insulin was determined with a Human Insulin Elisa kit (Millipore Hertfordshire, UK) using 0.8-mL capillary blood glucose samples collected at the same time as capillary blood glucose measurements of the glucose reference and SG kiwifruit. A subset of six subjects was used for insulin determination, with their response to SG compared with response to the glucose reference. The aim was to show that kiwifruit exchange did not induce a disproportionately high insulin response. An obvious outlier was removed from the glucose and kiwifruit groups because of technical problems with the glucose analysis, so the analysis involved five subjects. Removal of the outlier did not affect conclusions drawn from the results.

2.5. Data Analysis

Glycaemic potency of kiwifruit carbohydrate: Incremental blood glucose responses were calculated by subtracting each individual's average baseline value from their subsequent measurements and were then used to determine the incremental area under the curve (IAUC) for each individual by trapezoid summation of positive increments [10]. Data were entered into a Microsoft® Excel spreadsheet for preliminary analysis. For statistical comparison of means (ANOVA), GenStat software was used (version 11.1, VSNi Ltd., Hemel Hempstead, UK). Data were analysed using unbalanced analysis of variance (ANOVA), testing differences between meals after adjusting for participant and order effects.

Relative glycaemic potency of the carbohydrate (CHO) in kiwifruit (grams of glucose equivalents (GGEs)/100 g CHO) was used as an estimate of glycaemic index and calculated from the areas under the blood glucose response curves for the kiwifruit ($IAUC_{200\,g\,KF}$) relative to the glucose reference ($IAUC_{40\,g\,Glucose}$), with adjustment for weights of carbohydrate involved (Table 1):

$$\text{Relative glycaemic potency (RGP)} = \frac{(IAUC_{KF}/IAUC_{glucose}) \times (\text{Wt. glucose/Wt. KF}) \times 100}{GGE/100\ g\ CHO} \quad (1)$$

$$RGP = (IAUC_{200\,g\,KF}/IAUC_{40\,g\,Glucose}) \times (40/200) \times 100 \quad GGE/100\ g\ CHO \quad (2)$$

GGE expresses the effects of foods on blood glucose on a whole-food basis relative to glucose, as grams of glucose equivalents (GGEs) [11]. The GGE has weight (g) units, so it can be expressed per serving or per reference amount customarily consumed, or per 100 g of food. Thus, it behaves like a nutrient value, and has been termed a virtual food component [12]. It allows direct comparison of foods, and indicates how much glucose a food quantity would be equivalent to in its glycaemic effect. A food composition table containing GGE values allows one to see not only what a food is, but also what it does in terms of its relative glycaemic effect.

Kiwifruit equivalents and kiwifruit exchanges: From a knowledge of the available carbohydrate and GGE content of various foods, including kiwifruit, it was possible to construct tables as guides to incorporating kiwifruit into diets while managing postprandial glycaemia as follows. Because the glycaemic potencies of the two kiwifruit cultivars were similar, the exchange tables have been based on the SunGold values for carbohydrate (12.3 g/100 g) and GGE (6.7 g/100 g) content.

(1) Equi-carbohydrate exchanges (Table 2)

The amount of a food that could be exchanged for (substituted by) one kiwifruit without altering carbohydrate intake was calculated from the available carbohydrate content (%) of kiwifruit and the substituted food.

Where $\%CHO_f$ is the percentage of available carbohydrate in the food (New Zealand Food Composition Database), and $\%CHO_k$ is the percentage of carbohydrate in the kiwifruit, 100 g kiwifruit (one kiwifruit) would exchange: $(\%CHO_k/\%CHO_f) \times 100$ g of the food, or $((\%CHO_k/\%CHO_f) \times 100)/Sf$ servings of the food, where Sf is the serving size (g) of the food.

(2) Glycaemic impact of carbohydrate-based kiwifruit exchange

From the glycaemic potencies (GGE contents) of kiwifruit and foods, and their carbohydrate contents, one may estimate the reduction in relative glycaemic impact that could be expected by equi-carbohydrate partial substitution of kiwifruit for a food. This would allow estimation of possible changes in glycaemic response, for the purposes of blood glucose management.

The proportional reduction in glycaemic impact as a result of substitution by kiwifruit is the relative glycaemic potency of the food (GGE/serving) after substituting plus the GGE added in the substituting kiwifruit, as a proportion of the relative glycaemic potency of the unsubstituted food. The relative glycaemic potency of the food (RGP_f) may be estimated as glycaemic load from its carbohydrate content and glycaemic index (Table 1).

The glycaemic potency of the food before substituting (GGE_B) is:

$$(GGE_B) = Wt\ food \times RGP_f/100 \tag{3}$$

After substituting (GGE_A), it is:

$$GGE_A = ((Wt\ food \times \%\ CHO) - CHO_{KF}) \times RGP_f/\%\ CHO \tag{4}$$

where CHO_{KF} is the carbohydrate in the substituting kiwifruit. Including the GGE contribution from the substituting kiwifruit (6.7 GGE), the proportional (%) decrease as a result of substitution would be:

$$\%\ decrease\ in\ GGE = (GGE_A + 6.7) \times 100/GGE_B \tag{5}$$

(3) Equi-glycaemic partial substitution (Table 3)

From the relative glycaemic potencies of kiwifruit and a food (GGE/100 g = RGP) one can estimate the amount of the food that should be removed from a meal to include a kiwifruit without increasing postprandial glycaemia. This approach may be useful where the aim is to include fruits in the diet while maintaining a constant blood glucose response.

If the RGP of a food is RGP_f, and the RGP of kiwifruit is RGP_{KF}, the weight of food (W_f) equivalent to 100 g of kiwifruit is given by:

$$W_f = RGP_f/RGP_{KF} \times 100 \tag{6}$$

Similarly, the weight of kiwifruit (W_{KF}) that is the glycaemic equivalent of any given food quantity (W_f), such as a serving, is easily calculated from the relationship between the relative glycaemic potencies of the kiwifruit (RGP_{KF}) and the food (RGP_f):

$$W_{KF} = W_f \times RGP_{KF}/RGP_f \tag{7}$$

This information may be useful where it is desired to replace a complete item with kiwifruit without altering glycaemic response.

Table 1. Estimation of relative glycaemic potency (RGP) of foods as glycaemic load for a selection of foods with available glycaemic index (GI) and available carbohydrate (% CHO avail.) values.

Description	Portion Size [1] (CSM)	Weight [2] (g)	GI [3] (%)	CHO Avail. (%)	RGP [4] (GGE/100 g)	GGEs/CSM [5]
Bakery Products						
Bread, white	1 medium slice	26	70	43.4	30.4	7.9
Crispbread	1 biscuit	6	65	64.4	41.9	2.5
Mixed grain bread "heavy"	1 medium slice	28	45	36.7	16.5	4.6
Bread, wholemeal	1 medium slice	28	69	37.1	25.6	7.2
Muffin, bran	1 muffin	80	60	32.5	19.5	15.6
Breakfast Cereal						
Bran cereal	1 cup	45	42	37.4	15.7	7.1
Corn flakes	1 cup	31	80	84.8	67.8	21.0
Porridge, prepared	1 cup	260	61	10.5	6.4	16.7
Cereal Grain						
Rice, brown, boiled	1 cup	206	55	29.2	16.1	33.1
Rice, white, boiled	1 cup	144	56	17.5	9.8	14.1
Dairy						
Yoghurt, fat red, unsweetened	1 pottle	150	20	14.8	3.0	4.4
Fruit						
Apple, dessert, flesh, raw	1 apple	130	36	10.7	3.9	5.0
Apricot, dried	10 halves	35	31	48.8	15.1	5.3
Banana, raw	1 banana	128	53	24.1	12.8	16.3
Cherries	10 cherries	67	22	14.0	3.1	2.1
Grapefruit	1 grapefruit	236	25	10.1	2.5	6.0
Grapes, black and white	10 grapes	54	43	15.8	6.8	3.7
Kiwifruit	1 kiwi fruit	100	52	10.0	5.2	5.2
Mango	1 cup slices	176	55	14.6	8.0	14.1

Table 1. *Cont.*

Description	Portion Size [1] (CSM)	Weight [2] (g)	GI [3] (%)	CHO Avail. (%)	RGP [4] (GGE/100 g)	GGEs/CSM [5]
Orange, raw	1 orange	128	43	7.7	3.3	4.2
Pawpaw	1 slice	140	58	6.9	4.0	5.6
Pineapple, raw	1 cup chopped	164	66	11.4	7.5	12.3
Peaches, canned in juice	1 cup slices	264	30	22.2	6.7	17.6
Pear, raw	1 pear	148	33	12.8	4.2	6.3
Plum, raw	1 plum	49	24	13.9	3.3	1.6
Rock melon	1 cup sliced	168	65	6.4	4.1	7.0
Raisins	1 cup	154	64	71.3	45.6	70.3
Watermelon	1 cup flesh	169	72	5.1	3.7	6.2
Legumes						
Chickpeas, cooked	1 cup	173	33	8.6	2.8	4.9
Haricot beans, boiled	1 cup	180	31	15.2	4.7	8.5
Kidney beans, red, boiled	1 cup	187	27	15.9	4.3	8.0
Lentils, red, cooked	1 cup	209	26	10.4	2.7	5.7
Pasta						
Spaghetti, boiled	1 cup	148	40	23.9	9.6	14.1
Macaroni, boiled	1 cup	149	45	16.8	7.6	11.3
Noodles, instant, chicken	1 packet	200	47	5.8	2.7	6.0
Treats						
Jelly beans	10 jelly beans	20	80	91.8	73.4	14.7
Potato crisps	1 small packet	50	54	47.6	25.7	12.9
Honey	1 tablespoon	21	73	79.6	58.1	12.2
Vegetables						
Beetroot, boiled	1 cup slices	180	64	9.8	6.3	11.3
Broad beans, boiled	1 cup	170	79	8.6	6.8	11.5
Carrot, boiled	1 carrot	49	71	5.5	3.9	1.9
Corn-sweet, boiled	1 cob	128	55	20.9	11.5	14.7
Kumara, baked	1 kumara	114	44	23.3	10.3	11.7
Parsnip, boiled	1 parsnip	160	97	12.3	11.9	19.1
Peas, green	1 cup	164	48	7.1	3.4	5.6
Potato, rua, boiled	1 potato	114	56	18.2	10.2	11.6
Potato, mashed	1 cup	209	70	14.5	10.2	21.2
Pumpkin, boiled	1 cup	220	75	4.0	3.0	6.6
Swede	1 cup chopped	150	72	3.7	2.7	4.0
Taro corms, cooked	1 cup sliced	142	54	27.4	14.8	21.0
Yams, boiled	1 cup cubes	144	51	27.1	13.8	19.9

[1] Portion size used was a "Common Standard Measure" (CSM); [2] Weight of a portion (g); [3] From the international tables of glycaemic index and glycaemic load a [13]; [4] GI·% available carbohydrate (CHO avail (%)); [5] Relative glycaemic impact per portion expressed as glucose equivalents.

Table 2. Kiwifruit exchanges that would maintain a constant carbohydrate intake, based on the available carbohydrate content of selected carbohydrate foods.

Description	Portion Size	Weight (g)	SG Equivalents per 100 g [1]	SG Equivalents per Portion [2]	1 Zespri® SunGold Kiwifruit (SG) Replaces (g) [3]	1 Zespri® SunGold Kiwifruit (SG) Replaces Portions [4]	GGE (g) [5]
Bakery Products							
Bread, white	1 medium slice	26	3.53	0.9	28	1.09	−1.9
Crispbread	1 biscuit	6	5.24	0.3	19	3.18	−1.3
Mixed grain bread	1 medium slice	28	2.98	0.8	34	1.20	1.2
Bread, wholemeal	1 medium slice	28	3.02	0.8	33	1.18	−1.8
Muffin, bran	1 muffin	80	2.64	2.1	38	0.47	−0.7
Breakfast Cereal							
Bran cereal	1 cup	45	3.04	1.4	33	0.73	1.5
Corn flakes	1 cup	31	6.89	2.1	15	0.47	−3.1
Porridge, prepared	1 cup	260	0.85	2.2	117	0.45	−0.8
Cereal Grain							
Rice, brown, boiled	1 cup	206	2.37	4.9	42	0.20	−0.1
Rice, white, boiled	1 cup	144	1.42	2.0	70	0.49	−0.2
Dairy							
Yoghurt, fat red, unsweetened	1 pottle	150	1.20	1.8	83	0.55	4.2
Fruit							
Apple, dessert, raw	1 apple	130	0.87	1.1	115	0.88	2.3
Apricot, dried	10 halves	35	3.97	1.4	25	0.72	2.9
Banana, raw	1 banana	128	1.96	2.5	51	0.40	0.2

Table 2. *Cont.*

Description	Portion Size	Weight (g)	SG Equivalents per 100 g [1]	SG Equivalents per Portion [2]	1 Zespri® SunGold Kiwifruit (SG) Replaces (g) [3]	1 Zespri® SunGold Kiwifruit (SG) Replaces Portions [4]	GGE (g) [5]
Cherries	10 cherries	67	1.14	0.8	88	1.31	4.0
Grapefruit	1 grapefruit	236	0.82	1.9	122	0.52	3.6
Grapes	10 grapes	54	1.28	0.7	78	1.44	1.4
Kiwifruit	1 kiwi fruit	100	1.00	1.0	100	1.00	0
Mango	1 cup slices	176	1.19	2.1	84	0.48	−0.1
Orange, raw	1 orange	128	0.63	0.8	160	1.25	1.4
Pawpaw	1 slice	140	0.56	0.8	178	1.27	−0.4
Pineapple, raw	1 cup	164	0.93	1.5	108	0.66	−1.4
Peaches, canned	1 cup slices	264	1.80	4.8	55	0.21	3.0
Pear, raw	1 pear	148	1.04	1.5	96	0.65	2.6
Plum, raw	1 plum	49	1.13	0.6	88	1.81	3.7
Rock Melon	1 cup sliced	168	0.52	0.9	193	1.15	−1.3
Raisins	1 cup	154	5.80	8.9	17	0.11	−1.2
Watermelon	1 cup flesh	169	0.41	0.7	241	1.43	−2.2
Legumes							
Chickpeas, cooked	1 cup	173	0.70	1.2	143	0.83	2.6
Haricot beans, boiled	1 cup	180	1.24	2.2	81	0.45	2.9
Kidney beans, boiled	1 cup	187	1.29	2.4	77	0.41	3.4
Lentils, red, cooked	1 cup	209	0.85	1.8	118	0.57	3.5
Pasta							
Spaghetti, boiled	1 cup	148	1.94	2.9	51	0.35	1.8
Macaroni, boiled	1 cup	149	1.37	2.0	73	0.49	1.2
Noodles, instant	1 packet	200	0.47	0.9	212	1.06	0.9
Treats							
Jelly beans	10 jelly beans	20	7.46	1.5	13	0.67	−3.1
Potato crisps	1 small packet	50	3.87	1.9	26	0.52	0.1
Honey	1 tablespoon	21	6.47	1.4	15	0.74	−2.3
Vegetables							
Beetroot, boiled	1 cup slices	180	0.80	1.4	126	0.70	−1.2
Broad beans, boiled	1 cup	170	0.70	1.2	143	0.84	−3.0
Carrot, boiled	1 carrot	49	0.45	0.2	224	4.56	−2.0
Corn, sweet, boiled	1 cob	128	1.70	2.2	59	0.46	−0.1
Kumara, baked	1 kumara	114	1.89	2.2	53	0.46	1.3
Parsnip, boiled	1 parsnip	160	1.00	1.6	100	0.63	−5.2
Peas, green	1 cup	164	0.58	0.9	173	1.06	0.8
Potato, rua, boiled	1 potato	114	1.48	1.7	68	0.59	−0.2
Potato, mashed	1 cup	209	1.18	2.5	85	0.41	−1.9
Pumpkin, boiled	1 cup	220	0.33	0.7	308	1.40	−2.5
Swede	1 cup	150	0.30	0.5	332	2.22	−2.2
Taro corms, cooked	1 cup sliced	142	2.23	3.2	45	0.32	0.1
Yams, boiled	1 cup cubes	144	2.20	3.2	45	0.32	0.4

[1] % carbohydrate in food/12.3 (12.3 = % available carbohydrate in kiwifruit); [2] (Portion weight × % carbohydrate in food/100)/12.3; [3] (12.3 × 100)/% available carbohydrate in food; [4] ((12.3 × 100)/% available carbohydrate in food)/portion weight; [5] 6.7—(12.3 × GI of food/100). GGEs = grams of glucose equivalents.

Table 3. Equi-glycemic kiwifruit exchanges based on the relative glycaemic potency of Zespri® SunGold Kiwifruit (SG) and a selection of carbohydrate foods for which relative glycaemic potency (RGP) could be estimated from GI and available carbohydrate as grams of glucose equivalents (GGEs)/100 g, to maintain a constant glycaemic response.

Description	Portion Size	Weight (g)	SG Equivalents (per 100 g) [1]	SG Equivalents (per Portion) [2]	1 SG Replaces (g) [3]	1 SG Replaces (Portions) [4]
Bakery Products						
Bread, white	1 medium slice	26	4.5	1.2	22	0.8
Crispbread	1 biscuit	6	6.2	0.4	16	2.7
Mixed grain bread "heavy"	1 medium slice	28	2.5	0.7	41	1.4
Bread, wholemeal	1 medium slice	28	3.8	1.1	26	0.9
Muffin, bran	1 muffin	80	2.9	2.3	34	0.4
Breakfast Cereal						
Bran cereal	1 cup	45	2.3	1.1	43	0.9
Corn flakes	1 cup	31	10.1	3.1	10	0.3
Porridge, prepared	1 cup	260	1.0	2.5	105	0.4
Cereal Grain						
Rice, brown, boiled	1 cup	206	2.4	4.9	42	0.2
Rice, white, boiled	1 cup	144	1.5	2.1	68	0.5

Table 3. *Cont.*

Description	Portion Size	Weight (g)	SG Equivalents (per 100 g) [1]	(per Portion) [2]	1 SG Replaces (g) [3]	(Portions) [4]
Dairy						
Yoghurt, fat red, unsweetened	1 pottle	150	0.4	0.7	226	1.5
Fruit						
Apple, dessert, flesh, raw	1 apple	130	0.6	0.7	174	1.3
Apricot, dried	10 halves	35	2.3	0.8	44	1.3
Banana, raw	1 banana	128	1.9	2.4	52	0.4
Cherries	10 cherries	67	0.5	0.3	218	3.2
Grapefruit	1 grapefruit	236	0.4	0.9	265	1.1
Grapes, black and white	10 grapes	54	1.0	0.5	99	1.8
Kiwifruit	1 kiwifruit	100	1.0	1.0	97	1.0
Mango	1 cup slices	176	1.2	2.1	83	0.5
Orange, raw	1 orange	128	0.5	0.6	202	1.6
Pawpaw	1 slice	140	0.6	0.8	167	1.2
Pineapple, raw	1 cup chopped	164	1.1	1.8	89	0.5
Peaches, canned in juice	1 cup slices	264	1.0	2.6	101	0.4
Pear, raw	1 pear	148	0.6	0.9	159	1.1
Plum, raw	1 plum	49	0.5	0.2	201	4.1
Rock melon	1 cup sliced	168	0.6	1.0	162	1.0
Raisins	1 cup	154	6.8	10.5	15	0.1
Watermelon	1 cup flesh	169	0.5	0.9	182	1.1
Legumes						
Chickpeas, cooked	1 cup	173	0.4	0.7	236	1.4
Haricot beans, boiled	1 cup	180	0.7	1.3	142	0.8
Kidney beans, red, boiled	1 cup	187	0.6	1.2	156	0.8
Lentils, red, cooked	1 cup	209	0.4	0.8	248	1.2
Pasta						
Spaghetti, boiled	1 cup	148	1.4	2.1	70	0.5
Macaroni, boiled	1 cup	149	1.1	1.7	89	0.6
Noodles, instant, chicken	1 packet	200	0.4	0.9	246	1.1
Treats						
Jelly beans	10 jelly beans	20	11.0	2.2	9	0.5
Potato crisps	1 small packet	50	3.8	1.9	26	0.5
Honey	1 tablespoon	21	8.7	1.8	12	0.5
Vegetables						
Beetroot, boiled	1 cup slices	180	0.9	1.7	107	0.6
Broad beans, boiled	1 cup	170	1.0	1.7	99	0.6
Carrot, boiled	1 carrot	49	0.6	0.3	172	3.5
Corn, sweet, boiled	1 cob	128	1.7	2.2	58	0.5
Kumara, baked	1 kumara	114	1.5	1.7	65	0.6
Parsnip, boiled	1 parsnip	160	1.8	2.8	56	0.4
Peas, green	1 cup	164	0.5	0.8	197	1.2
Potato, rua, boiled	1 potato	114	1.5	1.7	66	0.6
Potato, mashed	1 cup	209	1.5	3.2	66	0.3
Pumpkin, boiled	1 cup	220	0.4	1.0	223	1.0
Swede	1 cup chopped	150	0.4	0.6	252	1.7
Taro corms, cooked	1 cup sliced	142	2.2	3.1	45	0.3
Yams, boiled	1 cup cubes	144	2.1	3.0	48	0.3

[1] RGP (Table 1)/6.7; [2] GGE per CSM (Table 1)/6.7; [3] 6.7 × 100/RGP; [4] 6.7/(GGE per CSM (Table 1)).

3. Results

Analysis of kiwifruit: Digestive analysis showed the available carbohydrate contents of the kiwifruit to be as follows: "Hayward" green kiwifruit, 11.2% *w/w*; "Zesy002" gold kiwifruit, 12.3% *w/w*.

The figures were close to values from previous analyses of six cultivars of kiwifruit (New Zealand Food Composition Database). The sugars consisted of approximately equal proportions of glucose and fructose, with a lesser sucrose component, in the approximate ratio 2:2:1.

Blood glucose responses: All 20 subjects completed the trial and the results from all of them were used in the data analysis. The between-subject variations were large, as is typical of such studies, but no outliers were removed. The different diets induced blood glucose responses that were clearly distinctive (Figure 2). The responses to the two kiwifruit cultivars were very similar and less than for the glucose reference.

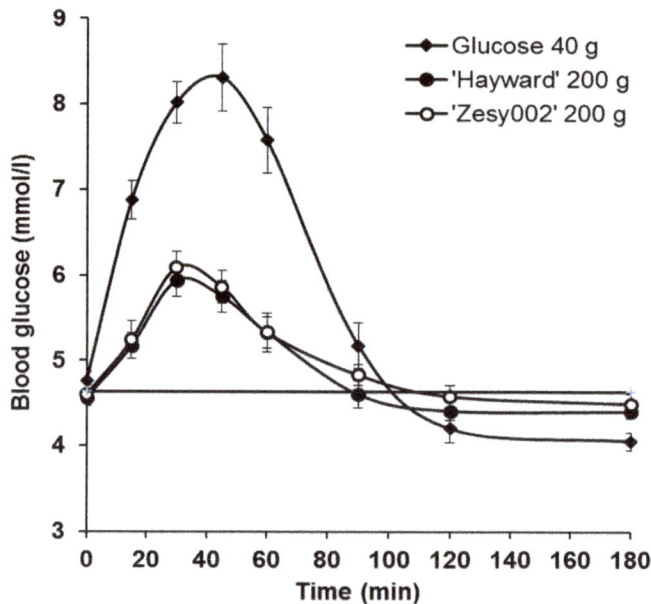

Figure 2. Mean (± SEM) blood glucose responses used to determine the relative glycaemic potency of "Hayward" (GR) and "Zesy002" (SunGold, SG) kiwifruit.

Relative glycaemic potency: The relative glycaemic potency (RGP; grams of glucose equivalents (GGE)) of the whole fruit, calculated from the glycaemic response to 200 g kiwifruit compared with the response to 40 g of glucose reference (Figure 2), and based on the area under the blood glucose response curve, showed that in terms of blood glucose-raising potential, one 100-g piece of "Hayward" kiwifruit would have a blood glucose-raising (glycaemic) potency equivalent to that of 6.6 g of glucose, and one 100-g piece of "Zesy002" kiwifruit would have a glycaemic potency equivalent to 6.7 g glucose (Table 4).

Table 4. Relative glycaemic potency (RGP) expressed as grams of glucose equivalents (GGEs) per 100 g of kiwifruit, determined from the relative areas under the blood glucose response curves (incremental area under the curve, IAUC) shown in Figure 2.

	IAUC		GGE/200 g		RRGP (GGEs/100 g) (GGEs/100 g)	
	Mean	SEM	Mean	SEM	Mean	SEM
Glucose (40 g)	234.7	18.8				-
"Hayward" kiwifruit (200 g)	75.1	7.3	13.2	1.25	6.6	0.8
"Zesy002" kiwifruit (200 g)	76.2	8.5	13.4	1.44	6.7	0.4

The RGP of the available carbohydrate alone in "Hayward", its approximate glycaemic index, was 59 ± 7.03 GGE/100 g carbohydrate (mean ± SEM) and that of "Zesy002" was 54 ± 3.05 GGE/100 g carbohydrate (mean ± SEM), with the difference between the values non-significant.

Insulin responses: On an equal carbohydrate basis, insulin response was lower for kiwifruit carbohydrate than for than for glucose (Table 5), consistent with the lower insulinaemic potential of fructose compared with glucose [14]. A lower insulin response to kiwifruit than to rice in equal carbohydrate meals has similarly been measured recently [15]. When expressed per GGE the insulin responses were very similar (Table 5), indicating that it is physiologically valid to express glycaemic potency of mixed sugars in fruit as glucose equivalents, as indicated in previous studies of the relative effects of glucose and fructose on the insulin response [14].

With the one removed outlier subject included in the analysis the median insulin response (μU mL^{-1}.min^{-1}) per gram of carbohydrate was: glucose 39.7, SunGold 24.1; and the insulin response per GGE was: glucose 39.7, SunGold 42.1.

Table 5. Insulin response to glucose and to glycaemic glucose equivalents (GGEs) in kiwifruit.

	Insulin Response (μU mL^{-1}.min^{-1}) per g Carbohydrate		Insulin Response (μU mL^{-1}.min^{-1}) per GGE	
	Mean	SEM	Mean	SEM
Glucose	40.9	2.2	40.9	2.2
Kiwifruit	28.8	5.3	39.6	4.5

4. Discussion

The tables of equi-carbohydrate (Table 2) and equi-glycaemic (Table 3) exchanges of kiwifruit show that kiwifruit exchanges over a range of food categories will result in very small changes in glycaemic impact, based purely on the glycaemic potency of the sugars involved. The change in GGE intake using one kiwifruit exchange is within the range ± 5 GGE for most of the foods considered (Figure 3). Because the exchange is on a carbohydrate basis, whether kiwifruit exchange increases or decreases glycaemic impact will depend on the glycaemic index (GI) of the food being substituted relative to the GI of kiwifruit. Substitution of any foods with a GI less than that of kiwifruit (GI = 54) will increase glycaemic impact, and substitution of foods with a GI greater than 54 will reduce glycaemic impact. However, because the substitution involves quite small amounts of carbohydrate, due to the high water content of kiwifruit and the fact that kiwifruit has a low GI, the change in GGE intake will be small. Food groups in which kiwifruit substitution would slightly increase glycaemic impact include pasta, pulses, and some fruits. Kiwifruit substitution of cereal-based starchy foods such as bakery products and breakfast cereals would reduce glycaemic impact most.

The exchange tables indicate the change in relative glycaemic impact that may be attributed to carbohydrate exchange (Table 2, Figure 3). However, kiwifruit substitution is likely to cause a greater reduction in glycaemic impact than would be predicted from carbohydrate substitution alone because of the presence of organic acids, dietary fibre, and other fruit components such as phenolics. Thus, where kiwifruit exchange indicates an increase in relative glycaemic impact, as in the case of pulses and pasta, the increase is likely to be smaller than indicated in Figure 3. Furthermore, the pattern of food intake can have a sizeable effect on glycaemic response: if the kiwifruit portion of the substituted meal is consumed 30 min before the rest of the meal, the overall glycaemic response can be substantially suppressed [15], by as much as 30%.

The results of insulin analysis in a subset of participants (Table 5) showed that the insulin response per kiwifruit GGE was almost identical to the response per gram of glucose. Therefore, substitution of kiwifruit carbohydrate for food carbohydrate would not lead to a disproportionately large increase in insulin response compared with glucose. Because the exchange involves no more than 6–7 GGEs per kiwifruit, any disproportionate increase in insulin per GGE from kiwifruit would in any case give a small net change in insulin for the meal. Kiwifruit exchanges will not, therefore, appreciably increase insulin demand.

The vitamin C content of the kiwifruit was not determined for the present study because it has been previously well established as consistently higher than in most other fruits [1], with a concentration of about 150 mg per 100 g SunGold fruit—enough for a single fruit to raise vitamin C intake to the recommended daily allowance. The present analysis of the effects of kiwifruit exchanges has shown that using kiwifruit to improve intakes of vitamin C or other fruit components would have very little effect on glycaemic impact over a range of food categories, and is therefore glycaemically safe.

With the aid of exchange tables, kiwifruit may be used to improve vitamin C intakes while maintaining either a constant carbohydrate intake, or a more or less constant glycaemic impact and insulin demand.

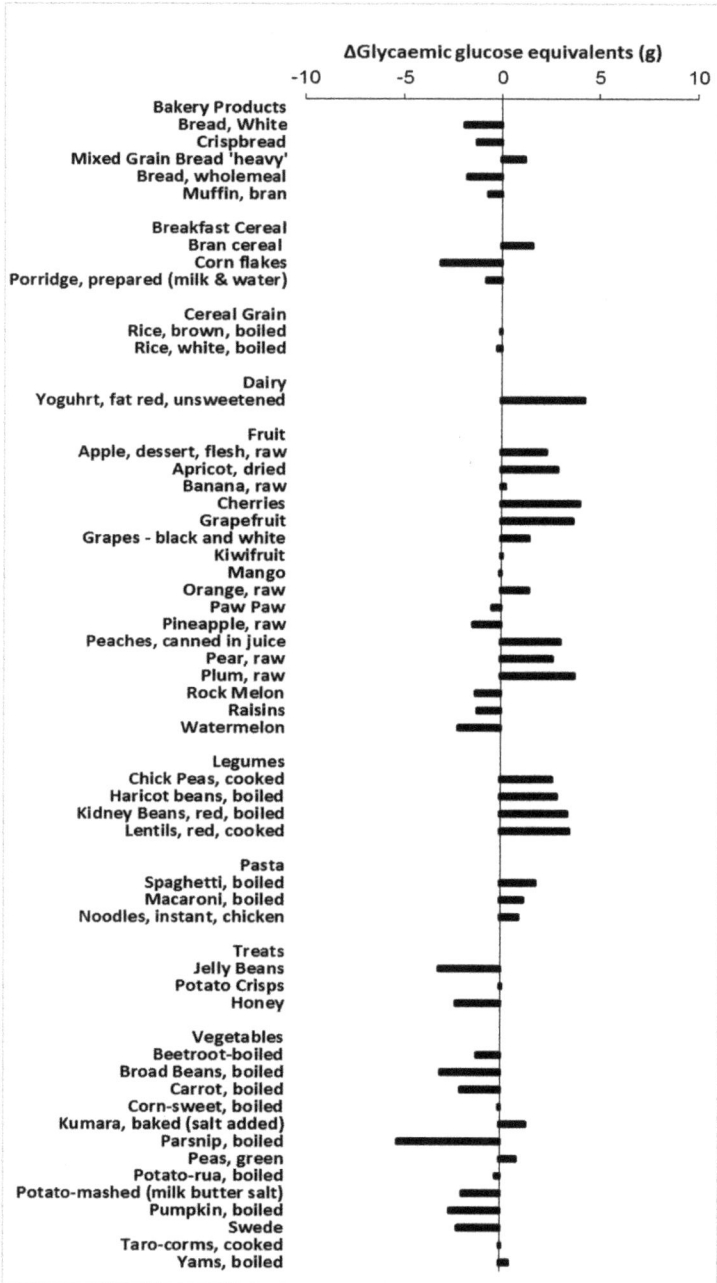

Figure 3. Change in glycaemic potential (GGE (g)) upon equi-carbohydrate substitution of one SunGold kiwifruit for various foods.

Although the focus has been on vitamin C in this paper, it is noteworthy that kiwifruit have a high content of potassium, 315 mg per 100 g (about one fruit) [1]. When kiwifruit exchange involves substitution of refined cereal products, including many breakfast cereals, a substantial increase in potassium may result. For instance, one cup of cornflakes containing 24.4 g of available carbohydrate provides 27 mg of potassium. Exchange for two SunGold kiwifruit providing 24.6 g of available carbohydrate, according to the analysis in this paper, would provide 630 mg of potassium, a 24-fold increase. Similarly, substitution of highly refined cereal products by kiwifruit on an equal carbohydrate basis may help to address the shortfall in dietary fibre in many modern diets.

The utility of the exchange tables in dietary management of glycaemia, and how accurately they achieve this purpose, requires further validation, particularly for the equi-glycaemic exchanges which are based on glycaemic response. The equal carbohydrate exchanges can be conducted accurately, because the measurements on which they are based are purely chemical analyses of available carbohydrate content of foods. If measured directly, available carbohydrate is accurate, although it is often measured indirectly "by difference", which is not as accurate. However, measures involving glycaemic responses such as GGEs, RGP, and GI involve intrinsically larger errors [16], arising from individual differences and variations in physiological response to foods.

Calculating the glucose equivalent of 200 g kiwifruit with a 40-g glucose reference involves a small error because of the non-linearity of the glucose dose–blood glucose response curve [11]. The present study was about the glycaemic impact of foods, not about GI per se, so there was no need to use a 50-g glucose reference as specified for GI determination. Instead, the reference glucose dose of 40 g was closer to the carbohydrate dose of 23 g ingested in the realistic 200 g intake of kiwifruit, which is the edible portion of two fresh kiwifruit, used in the clinical trial of the present study. Therefore, no adjustment for non-linearity was required when calculating the glucose equivalence (GGE content) of the kiwifruit [17]. We have also shown that the difference between GGE estimated as glycaemic load from GI and carbohydrate content, and GGE measured directly, is small [18]. Thus, glycaemic load values may be used as estimates of RGP with little loss of accuracy in guiding food choices for glycaemia management [19].

The present study has shown the glycaemic potencies of "Hayward" and "Zesy002" in comparison to a glucose reference (their relative glycaemic potencies) to be very low. Both kiwifruit cultivars had an RGP of 6–7 GGEs per 100 g. That is, 100 g (one kiwifruit edible portion) would have the same glycaemic effect as 6–7 g of glucose. Converting the GGE content to a per 100-g carbohydrate basis gave estimates of GI for "Hayward" and "Zesy002" of 59 and 54, respectively. The values were slightly higher than previously published [20] perhaps because the fruit were consumed after disintegration and freezing. However, with the very low relative glycaemic potency and low available carbohydrate content of kiwifruit, a difference of 10 GI units would translate to a difference of about 1 g of glucose equivalents per kiwifruit. With a carbohydrate content of about 10%, a difference of 10 GI units would make a difference of only about 1 GGEs (the effect equivalent to 1 g glucose) in a 100 g edible portion of kiwifruit. This underlines the irrelevance of GI to management of intakes of kiwifruit and other fresh fruits for postprandial glycaemic control, and the need to use more realistic means of expressing glycaemic potency, such as RGP. So even if consumed on an equal carbohydrate basis as a partial replacement of low GI foods there would be little glycaemic cost compared with the benefit of a greatly increased intake of vitamin C.

Similarly, when kiwifruit is used in an exchange format to partially substitute other carbohydrate foods, the net effect on GGE intake of removing carbohydrate in the substituted food and adding it in the substituting kiwifruit is only a few GGE units (Figure 3). Furthermore, partially substituting fresh kiwifruit, with a vitamin C content of about 100 mg per fruit, for starch-based foods such as breakfast cereals and cereal-based cooked staples, has the potential to enormously improve vitamin C status. As vitamin C is heat-labile and most cereal products and other starchy staples are cooked and therefore contain very low amounts of vitamin C, partial substitution by one or two kiwifruit would be a useful strategy for naturally improving vitamin C intakes.

Substituting kiwifruit for unsweetened starchy products would increase fructose intakes slightly, but by an amount that would not produce the metabolic changes that are associated with high fructose intakes in sweetened processed foods [21]. In fact, a modest intake of fructose has the benefit of enhancing glucose metabolism and facilitating glucose disposal [22]. We have found that consuming two kiwifruit per day for 12 weeks did not cause any of the metabolic changes that have been reported for high intakes of fructose (paper in preparation).

The present paper has illustrated the concept of kiwifruit exchange tables, but the practicality of using the exchange tables, and the range of foods they contain also needs further development. While the tables in their present form would be easily understood by nutritionists and dieticians, how the information could be best used in a user-friendly format for public use, could be the subject of consumer research. Further research in long-term trials should also be conducted to determine whether or not sustained use of kiwifruit exchanges leads to improvements, or delays decline, in key biomarkers of health outcomes.

The exchange tables are based on a value for ready-to-eat ripe fruit, but such a value is likely to depend on the stage of ripeness of the fruit when consumed, so it is also important to determine the stability of the GGE values determined in the present study. In that respect, the values are likely to be similar to any other values in a food composition database that are guides, but do not pretend to be exact predictors of effects of any given food ingestion event.

Overall, the results indicate that including kiwifruit or other fruits in diets by equi-carbohydrate substitution of highly digestible and therefore high GI starch components will generally lead to glycaemic benefits, while also enriching the diets functionally and nutritionally. At the very least, despite the perception of fruits as sweet-flavoured and therefore high in glycaemic sugars, the glycaemic change associated with consuming fresh fruits in a carbohydrate exchange format is small. Including fresh fruit in the diet need not have a negative glycaemic impact when its introduction is guided by tables of exchanges based on carbohydrate or glycaemic equivalents, as presented here for kiwifruit.

Author Contributions: Conceptualisation: J.M. Funding acquisition: J.M. Ethics application: S.M., J.M. Clinical trial management and sampling: S.M. In vitro digestive analysis: S.M. Insulin analysis: K.B.-H. Data curation and analysis: S.M., J.M. Preparation of manuscript: J.M.

Funding: This research was funded by The New Zealand National Science Challenge (subcontract UOAX1421) and The New Zealand Institute for Plant & Food Research Limited (Contract no.33115).

Acknowledgments: The research was funded as part of the "Kiwi, fruity and friendly" research programme in the High Value Nutrition theme of the New Zealand National Science Challenge (subcontract UOAX1421), and by the New Zealand Institute for Plant & Food Research (Contract no. 33115). Technical help from Sue Middlemiss-Kraak is gratefully acknowledged.

Conflicts of Interest: The authors declare no conflict of interest.

References

1. Richardson, D.P.; Ansell, J.; Drummond, L.N. The nutritional and health attributes of kiwifruit: A review. *Eur. J. Nutr.* **2018**. [CrossRef] [PubMed]
2. Carr, A.C.; Pullar, J.M.; Moran, S.; Vissers, M.C.M. Bioavailability of vitamin C from kiwifruit in non-smoking males: Determination of 'healthy' and 'optimal' intakes. *J. Nutr. Sci.* **2012**, *1*, e14. [CrossRef] [PubMed]
3. Carr, A.C.; Bozonet, S.M.; Pullar, J.M.; Simcock, J.M.; Vissers, M.C.M. Human skeletal muscle ascorbate is highly responsive to changes in vitamin C intake and plasma concentrations. *Am. J. Clin. Nutr.* **2013**, *97*, 800–807. [CrossRef] [PubMed]
4. Frei, B.; England, L.; Ames, B.N. Ascorbate is an outstanding antioxidant in human-blood plasma. *Proc. Natl. Acad. Sci. USA* **1989**, *86*, 6377–6381. [CrossRef] [PubMed]
5. Brownlee, M. Biochemistry and molecular cell biology of diabetic complications. *Nature* **2001**, *414*, 813–820. [CrossRef] [PubMed]
6. Mishra, S.; Edwards, H.; Hedderley, D.; Podd, J.; Monro, J. Kiwifruit Non-Sugar Components Reduce Glycaemic Response to Co-Ingested Cereal in Humans. *Nutrients* **2017**, *9*, 1195. [CrossRef] [PubMed]

Nutrients **2018**, *10*, 1710

7. Wheeler, M.L.; Franz, M.; Barrier, P.; Holler, H.; Cronmiller, N.; Delahanty, L.M. Macronutrient and energy database for the 1995 Exchange Lists for Meal Planning: A rationale for clinical practice decisions. *J. Am. Diet. Assoc.* **1996**, *96*, 1167–1171. [CrossRef]

8. Monro, J.A.; Mishra, S.; Venn, B. Baselines representing blood glucose clearance improve in vitro prediction of the glycemic impact of customarily consumed food quantities. *Br. J. Nutr.* **2010**, *103*, 295–305. [CrossRef] [PubMed]

9. Blakeney, A.; Mutton, L. A simple colourimetric method for determination of sugars in fruit and vegetables. *J. Sci. Food Agric.* **1980**, *31*, 889–897. [CrossRef]

10. Brouns, F.; Bjorck, I.; Frayn, K.; Gibbs, A.; Lang, V.; Slama, G.; Wolever, T. Glycaemic index methodology. *Nutr. Res. Rev.* **2005**, *18*, 1–28. [CrossRef] [PubMed]

11. Monro, J.A.; Shaw, M. Glycemic impact, glycemic glucose equivalents, glycemic index, and glycemic load: Definitions, distinctions and implications. *Am. J. Clin. Nutr.* **2008**, *87*, S237–S243. [CrossRef] [PubMed]

12. Monro, J.A. Virtual food components: Functional food effects expressed as food components. *Eur. J. Clin. Nutr.* **2004**, *58*, 219–230. [CrossRef] [PubMed]

13. Foster-Powell, K.; Holt, S.H.A.; Brand-Miller, J.C. International table of glycemic index and glycemic load values: 2002. *Am. J. Clin. Nutr.* **2002**, *76*, 5–56. [CrossRef] [PubMed]

14. Lee, B.M.; Wolever, T.M.S. Effect of glucose, sucrose and fructose on plasma glucose and insulin responses in normal humans: Comparison with white bread. *Eur. J. Clin. Nutr.* **1998**, *52*, 924–928. [CrossRef] [PubMed]

15. Lubransky, A.; Monro, J.; Mishra, S.; Yu, H.; Haszard, J.J.; Venn, B.J. Postprandial Glycaemic, Hormonal and Satiety Responses to Rice and Kiwifruit Preloads in Chinese Adults: A Randomised Controlled Crossover Trial. *Nutrients* **2018**, *10*, 1110. [CrossRef] [PubMed]

16. Venn, B.J.; Green, T.J. Glycemic index and glycemic load: Measurement issues and their effect on diet-disease relationships. *Eur. J. Clin. Nutr.* **2007**, *61*, S1221–S1231. [CrossRef] [PubMed]

17. Wallace, A.; Monro, J.; Brown, R.; Frampton, C. A glucose reference curve is the optimum method to determine the Glycemic Glucose Equivalent values of foods in humans. *Nutr. Res.* **2008**, *28*, 753–759. [CrossRef] [PubMed]

18. Venn, B.J.; Wallace, A.J.; Monro, J.A.; Perry, T.; Brown, R.; Frampton, C.; Green, T.J. The glycemic load estimated from the glycemic index does not differ greatly from that measured using a standard curve in healthy volunteers. *J. Nutr.* **2006**, *136*, 1377–1381. [CrossRef] [PubMed]

19. Monro, J.A.; Mishra, S. Database values for food-based dietary control of glycaemia. *J. Food Compos. Anal.* **2010**, *23*, 406–410. [CrossRef]

20. Monro, J.A. Kiwifruit, carbohydrate availability, and the glycemic response. *Adv. Food Nutr. Res.* **2013**, *68*, 257–271. [PubMed]

21. Stanhope, K.L. Role of Fructose-Containing Sugars in the Epidemics of Obesity and Metabolic Syndrome. *Ann. Rev. Med.* **2012**, *63*, 329–343. [CrossRef] [PubMed]

22. Laughlin, M.R. Normal Roles for Dietary Fructose in Carbohydrate Metabolism. *Nutrients* **2014**, *6*, 3117–3129. [CrossRef] [PubMed]

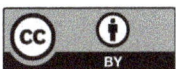

nutrients

MDPI

Article

Subjective Satiety Following Meals Incorporating Rice, Pasta and Potato

Zhuoshi Zhang [1], Bernard J. Venn [1], John Monro [2] and Suman Mishra [2,*]

[1] Department of Human Nutrition, University of Otago, P.O. Box 56, Dunedin 9054, New Zealand;
     zhuoshi.zhang@gmail.com (Z.Z.); bernard.venn@otago.ac.nz (B.J.V.)
[2] New Zealand Institute for Plant & Food Research, Private Bag 11600, Palmerston North 4442, New Zealand;
     John.Monro@plantandfood.co.nz
*   Correspondence: Suman.Mishra@plantandfood.co.nz; Tel.: +64-6-355-6146

Received: 24 October 2018; Accepted: 9 November 2018; Published: 12 November 2018

check for updates

Abstract: The satiating capacity of carbohydrate staples eaten alone is dependent upon the energy density of the food but relative satiety when starchy staples are incorporated into mixed meals is uncertain. Our aim was to assess the satiating effects of three carbohydrate staples; jasmine rice, penne pasta, and Agria potato, each consumed within a standard mixed meal. Cooked portions of each staple containing 45 g carbohydrate were combined with 200 g of meat sauce and 200 g of mixed vegetables in three mixed meals. The quantities of staple providing 45 g carbohydrate were: Rice, 142 g; pasta, 138 g and potato 337 g. Participants ($n = 14$) consumed each of the mixed meals in random order on separate days. Satiety was assessed with using visual analogue scales at baseline and for 3 h post meal. In an area-under-the-curve comparison, participants felt less hungry (mean (SD)) following potato 263 (230) than following rice 374 (237) or pasta 444 (254) mm·min, and felt fuller, more satisfied, and wanted to eat less following the potato compared with the rice and pasta meals (p for all <0.01). The superior satiating effect of potato compared with rice and pasta in a mixed meal was consistent with its lower energy density.

Keywords: carbohydrate; satiety; mixed meal; potato; pasta; rice

1. Introduction

The World Health Organization estimates that more than half of the world's adults are overweight or obese and warns of dramatic rises in overweight and obesity in low- and middle-income countries [1]. Overweight and obesity statuses are multifactorial in aetiology with such factors as the food environment, decreased physical activity, inadequate sleep and medication being involved [2,3]. Highly palatable foods that are hard to resist eating are said to be 'hyperpalatable' and are characterized as being inexpensive, highly caloric, fat-laden, potentially addictive and a major contributor to chronic weight gain [4,5]. The involvement of high calorie foods as a contributing factor to overweight and obesity has some credibility as food energy density has been associated with body weight change [6]. A strategy used to reduce dietary energy density has been to add pureed (hidden) vegetables into meals, resulting in a reduction in energy intake [7]. However, the effectiveness of adding fruit and vegetables into diets as a means of reducing overall dietary energy density is questionable as a meta-analysis of the body of literature indicated no long-term effect on weight loss [8]. This may be due to foods such as non-starchy vegetables having a low impact on feelings of satiety when eaten in typical amounts [9]. The authors of the meta-analysis concluded that increasing the fruit and vegetable intake of a diet is unlikely to be a successful weight control strategy because people tend not to decrease their overall dietary energy intake, suggesting that mechanisms underlying participant perceptions of hunger and satiety need to be better understood [8].

At a population level, low energy dense diets of good nutritional quality in Irish children and teenagers have been characterized as having higher intakes of fruits, vegetables, grains, rice, pasta and potato (boiled, baked, mashed); and lower intakes of carbonated beverages and chipped, fried and roasted potatoes [10]. The consumption of low energy dense foods must be accompanied with a concomitant reduction in the intake of high energy dense foods in order for an effect on body weight to be observed [8]. Indeed, the energy density of diets, characterized by a combination of lower fat and higher fruit and vegetable intake, have been associated with long-term weight loss [11]. In an ad libitum dietary intervention in which fat was replaced with either starch- or sugar-rich foods, spontaneous weight loss was achieved with the starchy diet over 2 weeks with the authors suggesting that the starch-based diet was more satiating than the higher fat or sugar diets [12]. Satiety is an important aspect to consider when changing the energy density of meals. When foods were consumed in servings containing 1000 kJ, satiety was inversely related to the energy density of the food, with a strong positive correlation found between the satiety index of food and the serving weight ($r = 0.66$, $p < 0.001$) [13]. The least satiating foods were energy-dense snacks, confectionary and high-fat bakery products; among the starchy foods, white rice and pasta had satiety indices 1.19 and 1.38 times higher than white bread, respectively, with potato having a satiety index over three times (3.23) that of white bread [13].

This evidence is indicative that potato may be of research interest in relation to satiety. In a comparison of instant mashed potato and barley containing 49.5 g and 46.6 g carbohydrate, respectively, there was no difference in satiety between foods although half of the 10 test participants could not finish all of the food [14]. However, people seldom eat single foods so the incorporation of starchy foods into test meals may have more practical relevance. In one such study, 12 participants consumed breakfast meals that included 50–52 g available carbohydrate in the form of baked potato, instant potato, brown rice, white bread and pasta [15]. There was no difference in area-under-the-curve (AUC) hunger or fullness ratings among the meals, with a possible explanation being that a cup of water of variable volume accompanied the food such that the overall water content of the meals plus drink was standardized to 400 mL [15]. This would have evened out differences in energy density among the meals and may have obscured the previously observed effect of energy density on satiety [13]. Therefore, although previous studies are suggestive of a differential effect of starchy foods on satiety, the data are inconsistent, possibly as a consequence of study design. We hypothesized that preserving differences in energy density among meals would maintain differences in feelings of satiety.

Thus, we provided cooked meals for lunch, a usual time for such food to be served, accompanied with a fixed volume of water to drink in order to preserve differences in energy density among meals. Our aims were to assess, in a realistic and normal lunchtime setting, the immediate effect on satiety following meals containing the starchy staple foods; rice, pasta and potato, as part of a mixed meal.

2. Materials and Methods

2.1. Experimental Design

A randomized crossover design was used. On three different days, participants consumed a lunchtime meal comprising minced beef in a Bolognese sauce, mixed vegetables, and a serving of either whole boiled potato, white rice or penne pasta. The order in which participants received the meals was randomized and there was a minimum two-day washout between meals. Participants were asked to keep breakfast consistent on each of the three test days, to avoid consuming any food between breakfast and lunch, and to avoid any food intake for three hours after finishing the test meal, the period during which satiety was measured.

2.2. Recruitment

Volunteers were recruited using a flyer that briefly described the study. In advance of the study each respondent was presented with an information sheet and an informed consent form.

Fourteen healthy volunteers (nine females and five males) were recruited using the following inclusion/exclusion criteria.

2.3. Inclusion Criteria

Age: Aged between 18 and 70.

Sex: Male or female.

Gastrointestinal function: No history of gastrointestinal dysfunction that could have an impact on appetite in the three hours after consuming the meal.

Health: Healthy as gauged by self-assessment and results on the General Health Questionnaire.

Activity: Not involved in prolonged strenuous activity on the day of the trial

Agreement: Subject having given written informed consent to comply with the conditions of the trial.

2.4. Exclusion Criteria

Self-reported intolerance to any of the meal components.

Having a gastrointestinal disorder.

Being involved in a physically demanding work on the day of the trial.

Eligible volunteers who were willing to participate were invited to attend the study at the Plant & Food premises.

Ethical approval was obtained from the New Zealand Health and Disabilities Ethics Committee (HDEC 15/CEN/71). This study was registered on the Australian New Zealand Clinical Trials Registry (www.anzctr.org), registration number ACTRN12615000721505. All participants signed a consent form.

2.5. Test Meal Preparation and Composition

All meals were prepared in advance, frozen as individual meals and reheated before consumption. The carbohydrate foods were cooked and served in equal carbohydrate and calorie portions, and consumed with the standardized meat and vegetable sauce, and 250 mL of water. The meat sauce contained fried beef mince, bacon, onions, chopped celery, thyme, bay leaves and chopped black olives. A commercial pasta sauce (Dairymaid foods, Christchurch, New Zealand) was added and the whole mixture stirred and simmered for 90 min. The mixed vegetables were a commercial frozen mixture consisting of peas, chopped carrots and corn (Heinz Wattie's Ltd., Hastings, New Zealand) and were boiled for 5 min. The pasta (penne; Diamond brand, Wilson Consumer Products, Auckland, New Zealand), rice (Jasmine; SunRice, New South Wales, Australia) and whole potatoes (Agria; Morgan Laurenson Ltd., Palmerston North, New Zealand) were weighed, cooked according to package instructions, and reweighed after cooking. The meals were assembled by placing 200 g vegetables, 200 g Bolognese sauce, and the weight of the rice, penne pasta or whole potato containing 45 g of carbohydrate (Table 1) into aluminum containers which were sealed and frozen until required. Before consumption, the meals were thawed overnight in a refrigerator and heated in a convection oven.

Table 1. Test meal composition.

Meal	Meal Components			Total CHO (g)	Total Energy (kJ)	Energy Density (kJ/g)
	Mince + Sauce (g)	Vegetables (g)	Starchy Staple (g)			
Rice	200	200	142	112	3010	5.55
Pasta	200	200	138	112	3010	5.59
Whole potato	200	200	337	112	3010	4.08

On test days each participant was asked to consume his or her normal breakfast and to refrain from eating between 8 a.m. and 12.00 p.m. (lunch time). Participants were asked to consume a similar breakfast on each of the 3 test days. At lunch time the participants were provided with the test meal and asked to consume it within 20 min.

2.6. Satiety

Satiety was measured using a 100 mm visual analogue scale (VAS) consisting of four questions anchored at either end with the following statements:

- How hungry do you feel? (Not at all hungry–Extremely hungry)
- How full do you feel? (Not at all full–Totally full)
- How strong is your desire to eat? (Not at all strong–Extremely strong)
- How much food do you think you can eat? (Nothing at all–A large amount)

These scales have been recommended in a methodological review of the evaluation of foods for their validity and reliability [16]. The length of the scale was measured from the start to the point that was marked. Participants were asked to rate their hunger/appetite using the VAS immediately before lunch, immediately after lunch and at 1, 2 and 3 h after lunch. The VAS rating for each time was on a separate sheet and participants were instructed not to refer back to ratings of earlier times.

2.7. Sample Size Calculation

In a study on the validity of appetite visual analogue scales, a Table was presented in which sample sizes were given in relation to detectable differences and power [17]. Using this information, 18 subjects would be sufficient to detect a 10% difference in satiety, with 80% power at the 0.05 significance level for a paired design.

2.8. Statistical Analysis

All appetite ratings were recorded in a spreadsheet using the Microsoft Excel for Macintosh (Microsoft® Excel®. Version 15.31. Microsoft Corporation 2017, Redmond, WA, USA). Area under the curve (AUC) was calculated. Results were expressed as means with standard deviation. Random effects regression analysis was used to test for between-treatment differences in AUC satiety responses, with participant id as a random effect and adjusted for randomized order and baseline satiety. Microsoft Stata/MP 14.0 for Macintosh (Stata Corporation, College Station, TX, USA) was used for the regression analysis. p-value of less than 0.05 was set as statistical significance in all analyses.

3. Results

Fourteen adults completed the intervention in a balanced three-arm crossover. The mean (SD) age of the participants was 40.9 (14.6) years with a range of 28–70 years. Eleven participants were of European- and 3 of Asian-descent. The flow of participants through the study is given in Figure 1.

The baseline scores to the satiety questions are given in Table 2. People were randomized to the order in which they received the meals.

At baseline, there was no difference in mean scores of hunger and fullness before eating. There was a lesser desire to eat and people indicated they could eat less on the potato and rice days compared with the pasta day. The main outcomes arising from the visual analogue scale data are given in Table 3. The outcomes are total postprandial AUC over three hours; the difference (mm) between the pre- and post-meal scores (0–15 min); and a rate of return to hunger (15–180 min).

Table 2. Mean (SD) baseline satiety scores of 14 people.

Satiety Measure (mm) *	Pasta	Potato	Rice
Hunger	77.4 (21.9)	77.1 (10.2)	72.9 (19.8)
Fullness	18.9 (16.9)	18.7 (12.1)	19.6 (14.9)
Desire	87.9 (11.1) [a]	77.1 (12.5) [b]	77.3 (19.1) [b]
Quantity	81.9 (11.4) [a]	68.9 (11.2) [b]	68.6 (19.8) [b]

Different superscript letters within a row signify statistically significant. differences. * A high score indicates hunger; fullness, desire to eat; and ability to eat a large quantity.

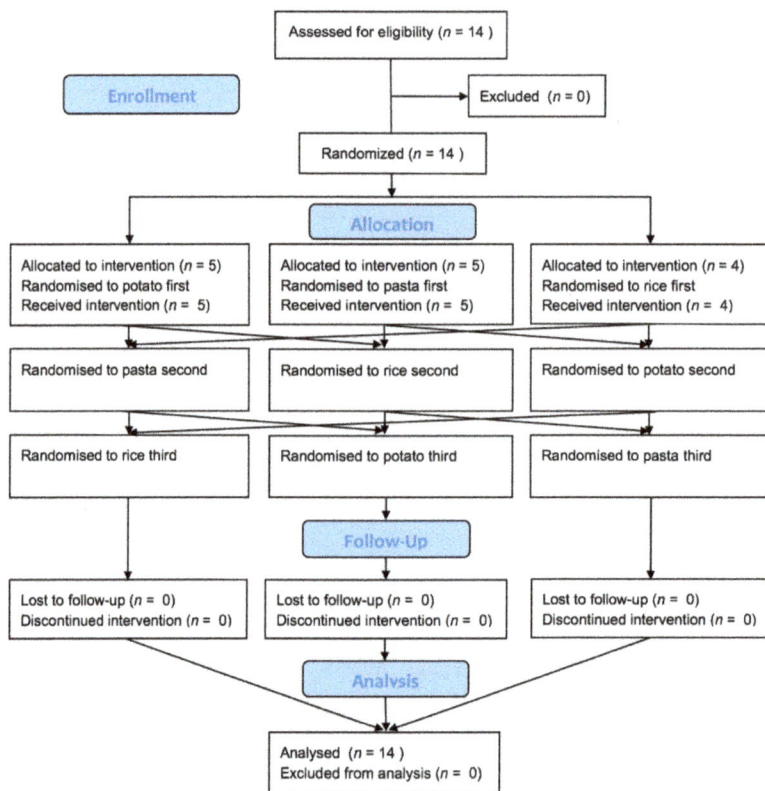

Figure 1. CONSORT diagram showing the flow of participants through the study.

Table 3. Mean visual analogue scale (VAS) outcomes of 14 people in response to four satiety questions.

Satiety Measure [1]	Mean (SD)			Mean Difference (95% Confidence Interval) Comparing between Meals Given in the Column Headings above		
	Pasta	Potato	Rice	Pasta vs. Potato	Pasta vs. Rice	Rice vs. Potato
Hunger AUC	448 (254)	264 (230)	376 (236)	184 (105, 263) $p < 0.001$	−72 (−151, 8) $p = 0.076$	112 (33, 191) $p = 0.006$
Fullness AUC	964 (468)	1120 (345)	954 (423)	−155 (−335, 24) $p = 0.090$	−10 (−189, 170) $p = 0.914$	−165 (−344, 14.3) $p = 0.071$
Desire AUC	427 (220)	210 (190)	361 (218)	217 (147, 287) $p < 0.001$	−66 (−136, 4) $p = 0.064$	151 (87, 214) $p < 0.001$
Quantity AUC	436 (231)	289 (257)	389 (221)	148 (65, 230) $p < 0.001$	−47 (−130, 36) $p = 0.265$	100 (30, 171) $p = 0.005$
	Change (mm) in VAS scores from commencement of eating to finishing the meal					
Hunger drop [2]	76 (18)	72 (15)	71 (16)	3.6 (−2.5, 9.8) $p = 0.249$	−4.6 (−10.9, 1.6) $p = 0.146$	−1.0 (−7.2, 5.2) $p = 0.755$
Fullness rise [2]	70.6 (18.3)	75.7 (13.3)	71.4 (19.7)	−5.1 (−8.0, −2.2) $p = 0.001$	0.7 (−2.1, 3.7) $p = 0.617$	−4.3 (−7.2, −1.4) $p = 0.004$
Desire drop	87.9 (11.1)	77.1 (12.5)	77.3 (19.1)	10.9 (2.3, 19.4) $p = 0.013$	−10.6 (−19.2, −2.1) $p = 0.015$	0.2 (−8.4, 8.8) $p = 0.961$
Quantity drop	81.9 (11.4)	68.9 (11.2)	68.6 (19.8)	13.0 (5.2, 20.8) $p = 0.001$	−13.4 (−21.2, −5.5) $p = 0.001$	−0.4 (−8.1, 7.5) $p = 0.929$
	Rate of return of VAS scores (mm/h) from eating cessation to 3 h post-baseline					
Hunger return [3]	9.8 (6.5)	6.5 (9.0)	10.6 (9.3)	3.2 (−0.1, 6.6) $p = 0.061$	0.9 (−2.5, 4.3) $p = 0.609$	4.1 (0.7, 7.5) $p = 0.017$
Fullness return	−10.6 (7.0)	−6.3 (8.5)	−12.2 (9.4)	−4.2 (−8.3, −0.2) $p = 0.040$	−1.6 (−5.7, 2.4) $p = 0.425$	−5.9 (−9.9, −1.8) $p = 0.004$
Desire return	9.7 (6.1)	5.7 (9.6)	10.2 (8.8)	4.0 (−1.1, 9.1) $p = 0.121$	0.5 (−4.6, 5.6) $p = 0.850$	4.5 (−0.2, 9.2) $p = 0.060$
Quantity return	8.2 (3.9)	3.5 (3.6)	8.6 (6.2)	4.7 (1.5, 7.9) $p = 0.004$	0.4 (-2.8, 3.6) $p = 0.803$	5.1 (2.3, 7.9) $p < 0.001$

[1] AUC Area-Under-the-Curve (cm·min); [2] drop/rise = change in score (mm) from baseline to immediately after finishing the meal; [3] return from a satiated to a less satiated condition over time (mm/h). A positive difference in hunger, desire and quantity represent being hungrier, having greater desire and a feeling of being able to eat more. A negative difference in fullness represents feeling less full. Bolded *p*-values indicate differences between treatments.

The plots of visual analogue scale data over time are shown in Figure 2.

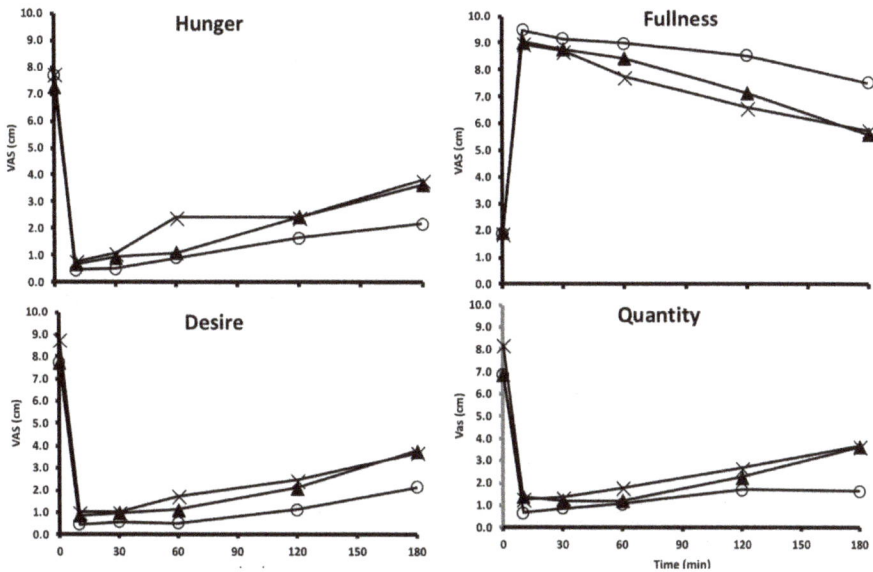

Figure 2. Plots of visual analogue scales (VAS) in response to four questions over time starting at baseline (t = 0) and following the consumption of pasta (×), potato (○) and rice (▲) meals. Data were analyzed by comparing the area-under-the-curve (AUC) among the meals for each of the questions. Interpretation of the data: How hungry do you feel? (Small AUC—Not at all hungry; Large AUC—Extremely hungry). How full do you feel? (Small AUC—Not at all full; Large AUC—Totally full). How strong is your desire to eat? (Small AUC—Not at all strong; Large AUC—Extremely strong). How much do you think you can eat? (Small AUC—Nothing at all; Large AUC—A large amount).

4. Discussion

The study results are indicative that the rice and the pasta meals were equally satiating, whilst participants felt fuller and more satisfied after eating the potato meals compared with the rice and the pasta meals. In this experiment, the comparison among different carbohydrate foods was standardized to an equal carbohydrate content. Similar results have been found when testing foods on an isoenergetic basis in which boiled potatoes eaten alone were more satiating than either rice or pasta eaten alone [13]. The data from the present study in a meal setting, are therefore consistent with differences in satiety found when these foods are eaten alone.

Our findings may be compared with a study in which investigators tested the effects on satiety of consuming meals containing various starchy staples [15]. In that study, desire to eat was lower following baked potato compared with pasta but contrary to our findings, hunger and fullness AUC did not differ among meals containing instant potato, baked potato, brown rice, pasta and white bread [15]. A difference between study designs was that Geleibter et al. standardized the total water content of the meals (food plus water provided as a beverage) whereas we only standardized the volume of water given as an accompanying beverage. Thus, the meals and beverages that Geleibter et al provided presumably tended to be equi-volumetric [15]. This may have obscured a difference in satiety among the meals given that food volume is a determinant of satiety [18]. This is suggestive that if starchy foods are to be exchanged, keeping accompanying drink volume constant may be important when assessing effects on satiety.

With comparable protein, fat, dietary fiber and calorie content, possible explanations for potato being more satiating than rice or pasta are differences in the energy density of the foods. Potatoes have a higher water content and lower energy density than rice or pasta [19]. Therefore, a larger volume of potatoes than rice and pasta needed to be consumed when served in equal carbohydrate portions. A large food volume increases gastric distension and stimulates postprandial satiety [20–22]. When eaten ad libitum, potato, rice and pasta consumed with a pork steak resulted in satiating effects that were not different among the meals despite the total carbohydrate and calorie intake after eating potatoes being significantly less than after eating rice and pasta meals [23]. In a randomized crossover study involving 11 to 13-year-old children, 30–40% less calories ($p < 0.0001$) were consumed after eating ad libitum meals containing boiled and mashed potatoes compared with comparable pasta and rice meals [24]. These observations may have practical and clinical relevance because the amount of carbohydrate consumed directly impacts postprandial glycaemia. If satiety can be maintained whilst consuming a smaller portion of potato compared to other starchy staples, this may offset the potential for a larger glycemic excursion due to potato having a high glycemic index (GI) relative to rice and pasta [25]. A consequence of a smaller portion reduces not only the glycemic load (GI x grams available carbohydrate) but also the energy content of the meal. As suggested, potatoes could be a suitable food option to reduce energy intake whilst maintaining satiety and mitigating postprandial glycaemia as less carbohydrate is consumed [26]. This effect has been observed among an older group consuming an equivalent amount of carbohydrate either as a glucose beverage, instant potato or barley [14]. All 10 participants were able to ingest the beverage but four and five of the participants were unable to eat all of the potato and barley, respectively [14]. Despite the differences in carbohydrate intake of the subset who could not finish their food, as a group mean satiety was greater after potato than after the glucose beverage.

It is interesting to note that the satiating effect of the carbohydrate foods was not clearly related to GI, even though it has been proposed that GI, as an indicator of sustained carbohydrate digestion, is a strong determinant of satiety [27,28]. Potato and jasmine rice are generally considered to be of moderate to high GI, and pasta of low GI, yet the rice and pasta meals did not differ in satiation and the potato meal was more satiating than the pasta meal. The results suggest that the effect of food volume on the proportion of a meal released from the stomach per unit time may have been sufficient to override the effects of differences in digestibility of the carbohydrates. Indeed, the rate of gastric emptying has been found to be affected by food volume and by energy density [29]. There is also a relationship between glycaemia and gastrointestinal motor control indicative that hyperglycemia slows gastric emptying [30]. More research in which blood glucose responses and gastric emptying are measured in conjunction with satiety would be helpful in interpreting the results of the present study.

It has also been found that although the glycemic response to mashed potato was greater compared with rice and pasta when consumed as part of a meal containing vegetables and salmon, the glycemic responses to all three meals were not different [31]. If the same effect has occurred in the present study due to the presence of meat sauce and vegetables, the effects of differences in glycemic response on satiety may have been eliminated leaving food volume as a dominant influence on satiety.

The healthfulness of carbohydrates in the human diet has been examined from a migratory perspective in which carbohydrate-rich staple foods consumed in the country of birth have been replaced by an increased intake of refined carbohydrate, meat and dairy in the adopted country contributing to a higher risk of non-communicable disease [32]. The rice and pasta used in our study were refined and perhaps equivalent whole-grain products would have induced different satiety responses. In previous work there was no difference in satiety found between white and brown rice; brown pasta appeared to be more satiating than white pasta; and boiled potatoes were the most satiating of all of the foods tested [13]. Plant-based starchy and non-starchy foods in general have lower energy density than animal derived foods and foods that are highly possessed with sugar and fat [19]. In practice, a plant-based diet in which starchy foods were recommended to be eaten ad libitum to satiation resulted in a greater reduction in body mass index compared with a usual care control group [33]. Thus, there is evidence to suggest that low energy-dense starchy foods are healthful components of a diet even when eaten ad libitum to satiation.

A potential limitation to our work was the sample size. The study had been powered to detect a difference in satiety among meals and it was sufficient for this purpose. Also, there were no differences at baseline in VAS responses to the questions "How hungry do you feel?" and "How full do you feel?". However, the data were indicative that people had a greater desire to eat; and could eat a larger quantity before the pasta meal compared with the rice and potato meals. We are unsure why this difference occurred as the order in which participants received the meals was randomized and we would not have expected baseline differences to occur. It is unclear whether this is a sample size issue, a chance finding, or whether anticipatory effects could have caused such an outcome. VAS methodology is widely used for assessing satiety [16] but subsequent energy consumption and satiety hormone responses could be informative as objective measurements in future research. A strength of this study was that all test meals were realistic in composition. It provides evidence that reflects real life when meat and vegetables are consumed in combination with starchy staples. A limitation to generalization of this study was that it was not conducted in people who are overweight or obese, a demographic who may have an impaired satiety response [34]. Similar studies undertaken in groups of people who are overweight or obese could provide evidence on which to base dietary recommendations suitable for weight loss.

5. Conclusions

In summary, on an equal carbohydrate basis, potato meals were more satiating than rice or pasta meals. If serving sizes of potato could be reduced such that the satiating properties match that of larger servings of rice or pasta, there would be a caloric intake saving and the potential to bring the glycemic response of high GI potato down to the glycemic responses of the rice and pasta meals, making potatoes an excellent choice of a low energy-dense food with the capacity to satiate.

Author Contributions: Conceptualization, Z.Z. and B.J.V.; Methodology, J.M. and S.M.; Formal Analysis, B.J.V.; Investigation, S.M., J.M., Z.Z. and B.J.V.; Resources, J.M. and S.M.; Data Curation, S.M. and J.M.; Writing-Original Draft Preparation, B.J.V., J.M. and Z.Z.; Writing-Review & Editing, J.M., Z.Z., S.M. and B.J.V.; Supervision, J.M. and B.J.V.; Project Administration, J.M. and S.M.; Funding Acquisition, J.M.

Funding: This research was funded by a New Zealand Ministry of Business Innovation and Employment grant to the New Zealand Institute of Plant & Food Research under the 'Foods for Health' research programme.

Conflicts of Interest: The authors declare no conflict of interest.

References

1. World Health Organization. Available online: http://www.who.int/topics/obesity/en/ (accessed on 24 August 2018).
2. Wright, S.M.; Aronne, L.J. Causes of obesity. *Abdom. Imaging* **2012**, *37*, 730–732. [CrossRef] [PubMed]
3. Wilding, P.H. Causes of obesity. *Pr. Diabetes Int.* **2001**, *18*, 288–292. [CrossRef]
4. Lerma-Cabrera, J.M.; Carvajal, F.; Lopez-Legarrea, P. Food addiction as a new piece of the obesity framework. *Nutr. J.* **2016**, *15*, 5. [CrossRef] [PubMed]
5. Gearhardt, A.N.; Grilo, C.M.; DiLeone, R.J.; Brownell, K.D.; Potenza, M.N. Can food be addictive? Public health and policy implications. *Addiction* **2011**, *106*, 1208–1212. [CrossRef] [PubMed]
6. Stelmach-Mardas, M.; Rodacki, T.; Dobrowolska-Iwanek, J.; Brzozowska, A.; Walkowiak, J.; Wojtanowska-Krosniak, A.; Zagrodzki, P.; Bechthold, A.; Mardas, M.; Boeing, H. Link between food energy density and body weight changes in obese adults. *Nutrients* **2016**, *8*, 229. [CrossRef] [PubMed]
7. Blatt, A.D.; Roe, L.S.; Rolls, B.J. Hidden vegetables: An effective strategy to reduce energy intake and increase vegetable intake in adults. *Am. J. Clin. Nutr.* **2011**, *93*, 756–763. [CrossRef] [PubMed]
8. Kaiser, K.A.; Brown, A.W.; Bohan Brown, M.M.; Shikany, J.M.; Mattes, R.D.; Allison, D.B. Increased fruit and vegetable intake has no discernible effect on weight loss: A systematic review and meta-analysis. *Am. J. Clin. Nutr.* **2014**, *100*, 567–576. [CrossRef] [PubMed]
9. Gustafsson, K.; Asp, N.G.; Hagander, B.; Nyman, M. Effects of different vegetables in mixed meals on glucose homeostasis and satiety. *Eur. J. Clin. Nutr.* **1993**, *47*, 192–200. [PubMed]
10. O'Connor, L.; Walton, J.; Flynn, A. Dietary energy density and its association with the nutritional quality of the diet of children and teenagers. *J. Nutr. Sci.* **2013**, *2*, e10. [CrossRef] [PubMed]

11. Flood, A.; Mitchell, N.; Jaeb, M.; Finch, E.A.; Laqua, P.S.; Welsh, E.M.; Hotop, A.; Langer, S.L.; Levy, R.L.; Jeffery, R.W. Energy density and weight change in a long-term weight-loss trial. *Int. J. Behav. Nutr. Phys. Act.* **2009**, *6*, 57. [CrossRef] [PubMed]

12. Marckmann, P.; Raben, A.; Astrup, A. Ad libitum intake of low-fat diets rich in either starchy foods or sucrose: effects on blood lipids, factor VII coagulant activity, and fibrinogen. *Metabolism* **2000**, *49*, 731–735. [CrossRef] [PubMed]

13. Holt, S.H.; Miller, J.C.; Petocz, P.; Farmakalidis, E. A satiety index of common foods. *Eur. J. Clin. Nutr.* **1995**, *49*, 675–690. [PubMed]

14. Kaplan, R.J.; Greenwood, C.E. Influence of dietary carbohydrates and glycaemic response on subjective appetite and food intake in healthy elderly persons. *Int. J. Food Sci. Nutr.* **2002**, *53*, 305–316. [CrossRef] [PubMed]

15. Geliebter, A.; Lee, M.I.; Abdillahi, M.; Jones, J. Satiety following intake of potatoes and other carbohydrate test meals. *Ann. Nutr. Metab.* **2013**, *62*, 37–43. [CrossRef] [PubMed]

16. Blundell, J.; de Graaf, C.; Hulshof, T.; Jebb, S.; Livingstone, B.; Lluch, A.; Mela, D.; Salah, S.; Schuring, E.; van der Knaap, H.; et al. Appetite control: methodological aspects of the evaluation of foods. *Obes. Rev.* **2010**, *11*, 251–270. [CrossRef] [PubMed]

17. Flint, A.; Raben, A.; Blundell, J.E.; Astrup, A. Reproducibility, power and validity of visual analogue scales in assessment of appetite sensations in single test meal studies. *Int. J. Obes. Relat. Metab. Disord.* **2000**, *24*, 38–48. [CrossRef] [PubMed]

18. Rolls, B.J.; Castellanos, V.H.; Halford, J.C.; Kilara, A.; Panyam, D.; Pelkman, C.L.; Smith, G.P.; Thorwart, M.L. Volume of food consumed affects satiety in men. *Am. J. Clin. Nutr.* **1998**, *67*, 1170–1177. [CrossRef] [PubMed]

19. The New Zealand Institute for Plant & Food Research Limited and the Ministry of Health (New Zealand). New Zealand FOODfiles 2016. Available online: https://www.foodcomposition.co.nz/downloads/foodfiles-2016-manual.pdf (accessed on 12 November 2018).

20. Deutsch, J.A.; Young, W.G.; Kalogeris, T.J. The stomach signals satiety. *Science* **1978**, *201*, 165–167. [CrossRef] [PubMed]

21. Geliebter, A. Gastric distension and gastric capacity in relation to food intake in humans. *Physiol. Behav.* **1988**, *44*, 665–668. [CrossRef]

22. Poppitt, S.D.; Prentice, A.M. Energy density and its role in the control of food intake: Evidence from metabolic and community studies. *Appetite* **1996**, *26*, 153–174. [CrossRef] [PubMed]

23. Erdmann, J.; Hebeisen, Y.; Lippl, F.; Wagenpfeil, S.; Schusdziarra, V. Food intake and plasma ghrelin response during potato-, rice- and pasta-rich test meals. *Eur. J. Nutr.* **2007**, *46*, 196–203. [CrossRef] [PubMed]

24. Akilen, R.; Deljoomanesh, N.; Hunschede, S.; Smith, C.E.; Arshad, M.U.; Kubant, R.; Anderson, G.H. The effects of potatoes and other carbohydrate side dishes consumed with meat on food intake, glycemia and satiety response in children. *Nutr. Diabetes* **2016**, *6*, e195. [CrossRef] [PubMed]

25. Atkinson, F.S.; Foster-Powell, K.; Brand-Miller, J.C. International tables of glycemic index and glycemic load values: 2008. *Diabetes Care* **2008**, *31*, 2281–2283. [CrossRef] [PubMed]

26. Anderson, G.H.; Soeandy, C.D.; Smith, C.E. White vegetables: Glycemia and satiety. *Adv. Nutr.* **2013**, *4*, 356S–367S. [CrossRef] [PubMed]

27. Brand-Miller, J.; McMillan-Price, J.; Steinbeck, K.; Caterson, I. Dietary glycemic index: Health implications. *J. Am. Coll. Nutr.* **2009**, *28*, 446S–449S. [CrossRef] [PubMed]

28. Brand-Miller, J.C.; Holt, S.H.; Pawlak, D.B.; McMillan, J. Glycemic index and obesity. *Am. J. Clin. Nutr.* **2002**, *76*, 281S–285S. [CrossRef] [PubMed]

29. Hunt, J.N.; Smith, J.L.; Jiang, C.L. Effect of meal volume and energy density on the gastric emptying of carbohydrates. *Gastroenterology* **1985**, *89*, 1326–1330. [CrossRef]

30. Rayner, C.K.; Samsom, M.; Jones, K.L.; Horowitz, M. Relationships of upper gastrointestinal motor and sensory function with glycemic control. *Diabetes Care* **2001**, *24*, 371–381. [CrossRef] [PubMed]

31. Ballance, S.; Knutsen, S.H.; Fosvold, O.W.; Fernandez, A.S.; Monro, J. Predicting mixed-meal measured glycaemic index in healthy subjects. *Eur. J. Nutr.* **2018**. [CrossRef] [PubMed]

32. Holmboe-Ottesen, G.; Wandel, M. Changes in dietary habits after migration and consequences for health: A focus on South Asians in Europe. *Food Nutr. Res.* **2012**, *56*. [CrossRef] [PubMed]

Nutrients **2018**, *10*, 1739

33. Wright, N.; Wilson, L.; Smith, M.; Duncan, B.; McHugh, P. The BROAD study: A randomised controlled trial using a whole food plant-based diet in the community for obesity, ischaemic heart disease or diabetes. *Nutr. Diabetes* **2017**, *7*, e256. [CrossRef] [PubMed]

34. Suzuki, K.; Jayasena, C.N.; Bloom, S.R. Obesity and appetite control. *Exp. Diabetes Res.* **2012**, *2012*, 824305. [CrossRef] [PubMed]

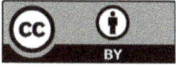

nutrients

MDPI

Article

The Timing of Activity after Eating Affects the Glycaemic Response of Healthy Adults: A Randomised Controlled Trial

Andrew N. Reynolds [1,2] and Bernard J. Venn [1,*]

[1]   Department of Human Nutrition, University of Otago, P.O. Box 56, Dunedin 9054, New Zealand; andrew.reynolds@otago.ac.nz

[2]   Edgar National Centre for Diabetes and Obesity Research, Dunedin School of Medicine, University of Otago, P.O. Box 56, Dunedin 9054, New Zealand

*   Correspondence: bernard.venn@otago.ac.nz; Tel.: +64-3-479-5068

Received: 18 October 2018; Accepted: 12 November 2018; Published: 13 November 2018

check for
updates

Abstract: There is scant information on how a time lag between the cessation of eating and commencement of physical activity affects postprandial glycaemia. Starting at baseline (t = 0), participants ingested white bread containing 50 g of available carbohydrates within 10 min. Using two crossover conditions, we tested the effect over 2 h on postprandial glycaemia of participants undertaking light activity at 15 or 45 min following baseline and compared it with a sedentary control condition. The activity involved cycling on a stationary ergometer for 10 min at 40 revolutions per min with zero resistance. Seventy-eight healthy adults were randomized to the 15 or 45 min activity arm and then randomised to the order in which they undertook the active and sedentary conditions. Cycling 45 min after baseline changed the course of the blood glucose response (likelihood ratio chi square = 31.47, $p < 0.01$) and reduced mean blood glucose by 0.44 mmol/L (95% confidence interval 0.14 to 0.74) at 60 min when compared with the sedentary control. No differences in postprandial blood glucose response were observed when cycling started 15 min after baseline compared with the sedentary control. Undertaking activity after waiting for 30 min following eating might be optimal in modifying the glycaemic response.

Keywords: postprandial; glycaemia; activity; exercise; timing

---

1. Introduction

Poor blood glucose control is a risk factor for the development of type 2 diabetes [1] and cardiovascular disease [2–4], even when at subclinical levels [5,6]. Regular physical activity assists in maintaining blood glucose control [7,8], with activity-mediated skeletal muscle glucose uptake able to reduce circulating levels [9]. This is one reason that regular activity is widely promoted [10,11] to both the general population and subgroups of the population where internal glycaemic regulation may no longer be sufficient.

One aspect central to blood glucose control is the postprandial response. Repeated bouts of postprandial hyperglycaemia occurring over months and years result in accumulated micro- and macro-vascular damage [2,3,12], are the primary determinants of glycaemic variability [13] and are drivers of protein glycation [14]. It has been found that both pre- and postprandial physical activity in adults with normal glucose tolerance has dampened postprandial blood glucose excursions [15–22]. Based on the findings of a review, it has been concluded that activity commenced after eating produces a more favourable post-meal glycaemic response compared with a comparable amount of pre-meal activity [23]. A variable that has received little attention is the timing of commencement of activity following a meal. It has been suggested that the optimum timing for the commencement of post-meal activity is 30 min after finishing a meal using the rationale that this coincides with the greatest influx of dietary-derived glucose into the bloodstream [24]. Given the increase in glucose utilisation at higher concentrations of plasma glucose [25], it is feasible that activity undertaken at the blood glucose peak may be more effective at reducing blood glucose than when activity is taken during carbohydrate absorption.

However, the precision with which the timing of activity needs to be undertaken after eating is unclear. It has been found that light walking commenced immediately following a meal lowered postprandial glycaemia [26], as did activity commenced 30 min after the start of a meal [27]. In contrast, delaying the commencement of activity for one hour following the start of eating resulted in no glycaemic benefit compared with a sedentary condition [28]. However, within each of these studies there was no comparison of glycaemic effectiveness between activity started at different times after eating. Nor was there consistency in the duration or intensity of the activity. In the studies by Lunde et al. [26], Nelson et al. [27], and Borer et al. [28], the activities were slow walking for 20 min, cycle ergometer for 45 min at 55% VO_2 max, and treadmill walking for two hours at 43% VO_2 max respectively.

Effects of low-intensity activity carried out for a short duration after eating had variable effects on postprandial glucose excursions. Among 14 healthy women, slow walking for 15 min started immediately following a meal resulted in a 1.5 mmol/L reduction in blood glucose concentration at the end of the active period compared with a sedentary arm [22]. In contrast, blood glucose concentration was not different among 11 adults when eight minutes of moderate intensity cycling was undertaken immediately following eating compared with control [29] and was higher by ~1 mmol/L 30 min after finishing 15 min bouts of cycling by six healthy volunteers compared with a control arm [30]. There may be a number of reasons for the discrepant findings, including differences in participant demographics and study design, but of note, the sample numbers were small. Given this heterogeneity in findings we were interested in exploring whether low intensity activity over a short duration could influence postprandial glycaemia of a larger group. The duration and intensity of the activity are factors that require consideration if lowering postprandial glycaemia is a long-term goal requiring sustained adherence over years or a lifetime.

Thus, the primary aim of this experiment was to compare the effects on postprandial blood glucose concentration of undertaking activity at two timepoints commenced either 15 min (during glucose absorption) or 45 min (coinciding with peak glucose) after the consumption of a meal in comparison to a sedentary control. The activity chosen was a cycle ergometer set at zero resistance, in order that anyone could undertake the activity regardless of fitness, and for a duration of 10 min to ensure that in practice people would be more likely to have the time to commit to the activity after meals over months and years compared with a longer duration.

2. Materials and Methods

This randomised controlled trial was conducted between February and March of 2014 at the research clinic of the Department of Human Nutrition, University of Otago, Dunedin, New Zealand. This study has University of Otago Human Ethics Committee approval (09/012) and is registered with the Australian New Zealand Clinical Trials Registry (ACTRN12614000264684).

2.1. Study Design

The study was designed as two crossover trials run in parallel (Figure 1). A three-arm crossover would have been another option but, due to resourcing constraints, it was more efficient to undertake the experiment as described.

2.2. Participants

We recruited young adults without a self-reported diagnosis of dysglycaemia. Diagnosed diabetes mellitus, cardiovascular disease, cancer, diseases of the digestive system, food allergies, and pregnancy were exclusion criteria for study participation. The study was designed as a crossover (activity vs. sedentary), but also as a randomised parallel trial in which two groups were studied: Group 1, in which the activity arm was commenced 5 min after eating (15 min from baseline), and Group 2, in which the activity commenced 35 min after eating (45 min from baseline).

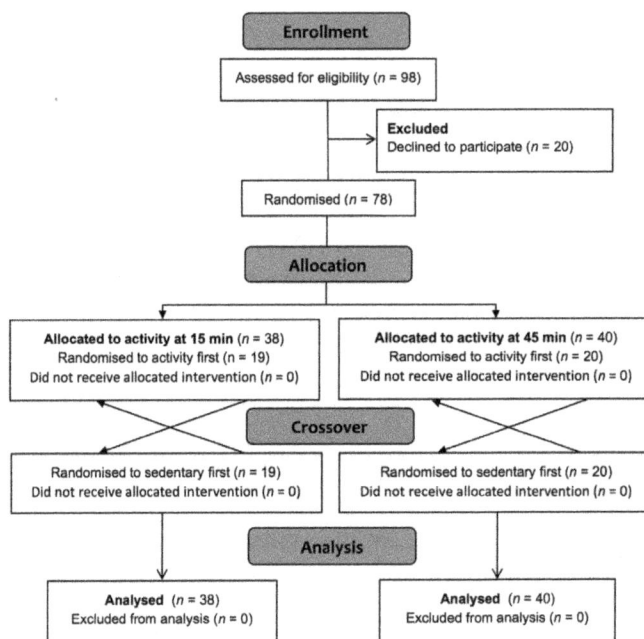

Figure 1. Consolidated Standards of Reporting Trials (CONSORT) diagram showing the flow of participants through the study.

2.3. Randomisation

Allocation to group (15 or 45 min activity start) and allocation to order (active or sedentary) was achieved using a computer-generated randomisation protocol. Randomisation took place at a separate site before study commencement.

2.4. Intervention

Each participant attended two fasted morning tests. Participants were advised to avoid alcohol, caffeine, and be consistent with their physical activity level and diet in the 24 h before each morning test. Participants were advised to walk slowly or drive to the test facility each morning and were seated for a minimum of five minutes before testing commenced. Morning tests were separated by a one-week washout.

Each morning the participants consumed a weighed amount (150 g) of white bread corresponding to just over two slices, containing a nominal 50 g of available carbohydrate according to the manufacturer's nutrition information panel (Nature's Fresh, Goodman Fielder, Auckland, New Zealand). Participants were provided with a 250 mL glass of water. The bread was ingested within ten minutes, with baseline defined as the commencement of eating. Each participant remained sedentary in the two hours following carbohydrate ingestion on one morning and on the alternative morning cycled at very light intensity for 10 min after eating, commencing at either 15 or 45 min after baseline. Cycling was on seated ergocycles maintained at 40 rotations per minute on a setting of zero resistance.

2.5. Measurements

Anthropometric measurements of height and weight were recorded before the first morning test. Each test morning participants sat for a minimum of five minutes before two fasting capillary blood samples were taken. Capillary blood glucose values were then taken at 15, 30, 45, 60, 90, and 120 min after carbohydrate consumption, in line with published guidelines [31]. Capillary blood glucose over the testing period was measured on HemoCue 201+ systems (Radiometer, Copenhagen, Denmark). The coefficient of variation (CV) was 0.11%. The primary outcome was change in the postprandial blood glucose response between sedentary control and physical activity interventions. Incremental area under the blood glucose curve (iAUC) was calculated using the trapezoidal method [32].

2.6. Statistical Analysis

The sample size estimate was based on a power calculation at an alpha of 0.05 and a power of 0.80 to detect within group differences in outcome variables: A 0.5 mmol/L difference in capillary blood glucose at any time point or a 20% difference in iAUC. This estimate required 31 participants to complete both morning tests, however, we over-recruited to allow for dropouts. Data were analysed according to intention to treat. A mixed model was used to examine the difference in postprandial blood glucose response and included terms for both treatment and order. Blood glucose outcomes are presented comparing the physical activity intervention with the sedentary exposure. Comparisons among test conditions were made using a likelihood ratio (LR) chi-square statistic with 14 degrees of freedom comparing static differences between blood glucose at each time point and comparing iAUC among test conditions. Analyses were undertaken in Stata Version 13, (StataCorp, College Station, TX, USA) with the statistician blinded to the intervention type.

3. Results

The characteristics of participants are shown in Table 1. There were no differences in the baseline measurements of participants randomised to physical activity starting at either 15 or 45 min post-baseline.

Table 1. Participant characteristics.

Characteristic	Activity at 15 min (n = 38)	Activity at 45 min (n = 40)	p
Women/Men	32/6	30/10	0.915
BMI (kg/m^2)	23.7 (4.07)	23.9 (3.63)	0.710
Age (year)	21.4 (1.35)	22.3 (5.16)	0.353
Fasting blood glucose (mmol/L)	4.65 (0.51)	4.70 (0.61)	0.384

Values are mean (SD). BMI is Body Mass Index.

Physical activity starting 45 min after the commencement of eating coincided with the observed blood glucose peak. The postprandial blood glucose responses to physical activity are given in Figure 2.

There was no difference in any measured parameter of postprandial blood glucose when a matched bout of cycling began 15 min after carbohydrate ingestion when compared with the sedentary response. In the 15 min post-baseline test, the mean (SD) iAUC in the sedentary and active conditions were 140.5 (85) and 139.8 (91) respectively and were not different (p = 0.938). In the 45 min post-baseline test, the shape of the blood response curve differed when compared to the sedentary exposure (likelihood ratio chi-square = 31.47, p < 0.01). This difference in shape was driven by a reduction in blood glucose immediately following physical activity. The blood glucose concentration over the postprandial periods are given in Table 2.

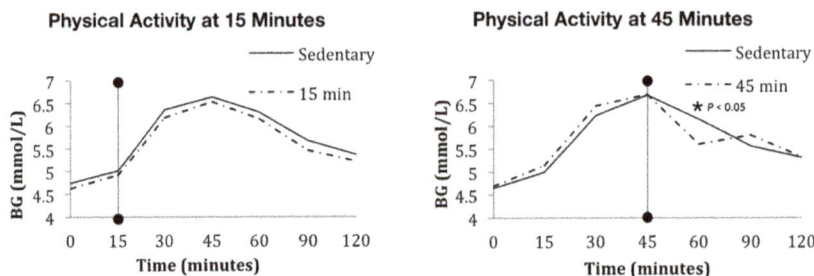

Figure 2. Blood glucose (BG) response to light cycling at 15 or 45 min after meal commencement. The vertical line with the filled circle ends represents the start of 10 min of cycling.

Table 2. Mean (SD) blood glucose concentration (mmol/L) during the sedentary and active arms in the groups assigned to 10 min of cycling starting either 15 or 45 min post-baseline.

Time (min)	Group Assigned to Activity Starting at Time = 15		Group Assigned to Activity Starting at Time = 45	
	Sedentary	Active	Sedentary	Active
0	4.7 (0.43)	4.6 (0.57)	4.7 (0.55)	4.7 (0.69)
15	5.0 (0.66)	4.9 (0.63)	5.1 (0.83)	5.2 (0.73)
30	6.3 (0.99)	6.2 (0.86)	6.3 (0.97)	6.5 (0.71)
45	6.6 (1.17)	6.5 (0.97)	6.7 (0.77)	6.7 (1.09)
60	6.3 (1.21)	6.2 (1.15)	6.1 (0.75)	5.6 (0.7) *
90	5.7 (0.84)	5.5 (0.82)	5.5 (0.71)	5.8 (0.76)
120	5.4 (0.76)	5.2 (0.73)	5.3 (0.84)	5.4 (0.78)

* Significantly different from the sedentary concentration.

The blood glucose difference at the 60 min time point in the group who started activity at 45 min post-baseline was 0.44 mmol/L (95% CI 0.14 to 0.74). The mean (SD) iAUC in the sedentary and active conditions were 128.2 (65) and 128.8 (62) and were not different ($p = 0.842$). When comparing between the 15 and 45 min groups, there was no significant difference in iAUC in the sedentary ($p = 0.258$) or active conditions ($p = 0.483$).

4. Discussion

Our results suggest that the timing of physical activity undertaken after carbohydrate ingestion influences the postprandial blood glucose response. Our study has matched the intensity and duration of activity, suggesting that the timing of activity is responsible for the observed differences. Activity at the blood glucose peak occurred when insulin secretion had likely plateaued [19] and the majority of carbohydrate digestion had occurred [33]. In contrast, activity undertaken before peak glucose may have reduced the insulin response, as found by Aadland and colleagues [16], and consequentially slowed the rate of glucose disposal. This is speculative and a limitation of our work as we did not measure postprandial insulin or the rate of glucose disposal. An acute bout of exercise has been found to increase glucose disposal rate in obese people and in people with type 2 diabetes, but not in lean participants [34]. Assessing the effect of light activity on the rate of glucose disposal in relation to the timing of commencement of that activity after eating would be an interesting area for future research.

Previous studies of physical activity and blood glucose control in normal glucose tolerant adults [16,18–22,29,30,35–41] did not use the timing of activity as a variable. In studies that have considered timing, there has been no within-study comparison between different timings within the postprandial period [26–28]. Furthermore, in studies where change in postprandial blood glucose response was not observed, even with activity of higher intensities the timing of activity may have been an unacknowledged determinant [29,36,39,42].

A difference in blood glucose concentration was found at the 60 min timepoint and in the shape of the glucose response curve when activity commenced 45 min after baseline, but there was no difference in iAUC between the active and sedentary conditions. By inspection of Figure 2 in the 45 min condition, it is apparent that there is a decrease in iAUC during activity, which is offset by an increase in iAUC occurring over the 90–120 min timeframe after activity. A rebound phenomenon whereby blood glucose concentration increases has been found previously under conditions of longer (45 min) activity at greater intensity (55% VO_2 max), with those authors attributing it to ongoing carbohydrate absorption entering an environment of resting muscle [27]. However, in that study the blood glucose iAUC was less for the active condition compared with the sedentary condition. Our lack of difference is probably due to the short duration of the activity because blood glucose iAUC was lower after 20 min of slow walking compared with a sedentary control [26]. Therefore, it is clear that increasing the duration or intensity of the physical activity would have led to larger differences in postprandial blood glucose response. However, we specified very light intensity activity due to its low participant burden. Keeping the intensity of activity light is likely to be achievable for a wide range of individuals, including those with poor levels of fitness, with impairment, or people who are uncomfortable undertaking physical activity in public. It may be encouraging for some people to know that even small amounts of physical activity can make a difference. A limitation of our work is that it occurred for the duration of one meal only. Extending the current study to include several consecutive meals would have enabled us to test for a carry-over effect as previously reported [19,43–45]. Furthermore, consecutive bouts of activity throughout the day would serve to break up sedentary behaviours, an emerging independent factor in cardio metabolic risk [46].

Our results indicate the potential of physical activity to reduce blood glucose concentrations when they are high, including the postprandial period. Reduction of glycated haemoglobin in people with type 2 diabetes has been found both when targeting postprandial glycaemia with drugs [47] and with moderate physical activity undertaken for 40–50 min three times a week [48]. In a small study of two people, dampening of postprandial glycaemia and weight loss over one month was greater when walking for 30 min starting immediately after lunch and dinner compared with when an equivalent amount of exercise was started one hour after meals [49]. In another free-living crossover intervention, postprandial glycaemia was lower when 41 people with type 2 diabetes were advised to walk for 10 min after meals, starting 5 min after the finish of the meals, compared with when 30 min of activity was undertaken on a single daily occasion [50]. If people adopted just 10 min of post-meal activity after each of the three main meals of the day, this would make a contribution to fulfilling population-based activity recommendations with the added benefit of targeting postprandial glycaemia.

A limitation of the work is that two groups were studied. This design was adopted to suit the available resources and the demographics of the two groups were closely matched. Despite this limitation, a strength was that both groups had sample sizes larger than those of many other studies. Another limitation was the use of young, healthy adults. Activity could potentially be more beneficial for people with compromised glucose tolerance. However, it is encouraging to find an effect of very light activity on postprandial glucose dynamics even among healthy adults. A minimal intensity of activity was chosen on practical grounds, and we did not measure the effort. This is a limitation in the sense that we are unable to provide a numerical value for the power expended. Nevertheless, the study is reproducible if people use cycle ergometers set at zero resistance with a pedalling rate of 40 rotations per minute. Similarly, in another practically-oriented study, Lunde and colleagues did not measure power as the intervention simply required women to walk slowly [26]. Future research aimed at practically-achievable light activity interventions among people with conditions that could benefit from lowered glycaemia are warranted and urgently needed [51]. In our study, the potential for light activity to impact postprandial glycaemia was tested under controlled conditions after an overnight fast. Other factors that might impact the effect of activity on postprandial glycaemia could be time of day [52] and a second-meal effect, in which an earlier meal influences the glycaemic response to the following meal [53]. To explore effectiveness on a larger scale, the concept should be tested in the community to assess any effect on longer-term outcomes under usual living conditions, with options for people to choose a type and duration of activity to suit personal circumstances. In the meantime, physical activity is regarded as a cornerstone of diabetes management [54] and our results may have direct application for health care practitioners wanting to provide advice for control of postprandial blood glucose.

5. Conclusions

Our findings suggest that the timing of light physical activity shortly after eating affects the time-course of postprandial blood glucose. Activity initiated at the blood glucose peak may acutely lower blood glucose levels to a greater extent than the same amount of activity undertaken before the peak. These results support that activity, even for 10 min at very low intensity, may assist in the management of postprandial blood glucose if undertaken when blood glucose is high. Consumer acceptance might be high if the activity is easily achievable, while further work is necessary to consider these findings beyond the acute response and in people with impaired glucose tolerance.

Author Contributions: Conceptualization, B.J.V.; methodology, A.N.R., B.J.V.; resources, B.J.V.; data curation, A.N.R., B.J.V.; writing—original draft preparation, A.N.R., B.J.V.; writing—review and editing, A.N.R., B.J.V.; supervision, A.N.R., B.J.V.; project administration, A.N.R., B.J.V.; funding acquisition, A.N.R., B.J.V.

Funding: This research was funded by the University of Otago.

Acknowledgments: Associate Professor Sheila Williams is warmly acknowledged for her guidance of the statistical analysis.

Conflicts of Interest: The authors declare no conflicts of interest.

References

1. Danaei, G.; Finucane, M.M.; Lu, Y.; Singh, G.M.; Cowan, M.J.; Paciorek, C.J.; Lin, J.K.; Farzadfar, F.; Khang, Y.H.; Stevens, G.A.; et al. National, regional, and global trends in fasting plasma glucose and diabetes prevalence since 1980: Systematic analysis of health examination surveys and epidemiological studies with 370 country-years and 2.7 million participants. *Lancet* **2011**, *378*, 31–40. [CrossRef]
2. Bonora, E.; Muggeo, M. Postprandial blood glucose as a risk factor for cardiovascular disease in Type II diabetes: The epidemiological evidence. *Diabetologia* **2001**, *44*, 2107–2114. [CrossRef] [PubMed]
3. Bruno, A.; Biller, J.; Adams, H.P.; Clarke, W.R.; Woolson, R.F.; Williams, L.S.; Hansen, M.D. Acute blood glucose level and outcome from ischemic stroke. Trial of ORG 10172 in Acute Stroke Treatment (TOAST) Investigators. *Neurology* **1999**, *52*, 280–284. [CrossRef] [PubMed]
4. Control, G.; Turnbull, F.M.; Abraira, C.; Anderson, R.J.; Byington, R.P.; Chalmers, J.P.; Duckworth, W.C.; Evans, G.W.; Gerstein, H.C.; Holman, R.R.; et al. Intensive glucose control and macrovascular outcomes in type 2 diabetes. *Diabetologia* **2009**, *52*, 2288–2298.
5. Saydah, S.H.; Loria, C.M.; Eberhardt, M.S.; Brancati, F.L. Subclinical states of glucose intolerance and risk of death in the U.S. *Diabetes Care* **2001**, *24*, 447–453. [CrossRef] [PubMed]
6. Khaw, K.T.; Wareham, N.; Luben, R.; Bingham, S.; Oakes, S.; Welch, A.; Day, N. Glycated haemoglobin, diabetes, and mortality in men in Norfolk cohort of european prospective investigation of cancer and nutrition (EPIC-Norfolk). *BMJ* **2001**, *322*, 15–18. [CrossRef] [PubMed]
7. American Diabetes Association. Standards of Medical Care in Diabetes-2018 Abridged for Primary Care Providers. *Clin. Diabetes* **2018**, *36*, 14–37.
8. Wannamethee, S.G.; Shaper, A.G.; Alberti, K.G. Physical activity, metabolic factors, and the incidence of coronary heart disease and type 2 diabetes. *Arch. Intern. Med.* **2000**, *160*, 2108–2116. [CrossRef] [PubMed]
9. Sigal, R.J.; Kenny, G.P.; Wasserman, D.H.; Castaneda-Sceppa, C. Physical activity/exercise and type 2 diabetes. *Diabetes Care* **2004**, *27*, 2518–2539. [CrossRef] [PubMed]
10. Tremblay, M.S.; Warburton, D.E.; Janssen, I.; Paterson, D.H.; Latimer, A.E.; Rhodes, R.E.; Kho, M.E.; Hicks, A.; Leblanc, A.G.; Zehr, L.; et al. New Canadian physical activity guidelines. *Appl. Physiol. Nutr. Metab.* **2011**, *36*, 36–46. [CrossRef] [PubMed]
11. National Health Service England. A Practical Guide to Healthy Ageing. 2015. Available online: https://www.england.nhs.uk/wp-content/uploads/2015/09/hlthy-ageing-brochr.pdf (accessed on 17 October 2018).
12. Ceriello, A. Postprandial hyperglycemia and diabetes complications: Is it time to treat? *Diabetes* **2005**, *54*, 1–7. [CrossRef] [PubMed]

13. Woerle, H.J.; Neumann, C.; Zschau, S.; Tenner, S.; Irsigler, A.; Schirra, J.; Gerich, J.E.; Goke, B. Impact of fasting and postprandial glycemia on overall glycemic control in type 2 diabetes Importance of postprandial glycemia to achieve target HbA1c levels. *Diabetes Res. Clin. Pract.* **2007**, *77*, 280–285. [CrossRef] [PubMed]
14. Austin, G.E.; Mullins, R.H.; Morin, L.G. Non-enzymic glycation of individual plasma proteins in normoglycemic and hyperglycemic patients. *Clin. Chem.* **1987**, *33*, 2220–2224. [PubMed]
15. Englert, V.; Wells, K.; Long, W.; Hickey, M.S.; Melby, C.L. Effect of acute prior exercise on glycemic and insulinemic indices. *J. Am. Coll. Nutr.* **2006**, *25*, 195–202. [CrossRef] [PubMed]
16. Aadland, E.; Hostmark, A.T. Very light physical activity after a meal blunts the rise in blood glucose and insulin. *Open Nutr. J.* **2008**, *12*, 94–99. [CrossRef]
17. Short, K.R.; Pratt, L.V.; Teague, A.M. The acute and residual effect of a single exercise session on meal glucose tolerance in sedentary young adults. *J. Nutr. Metab.* **2012**, *2012*. [CrossRef] [PubMed]
18. Bailey, D.P.; Locke, C.D. Breaking up prolonged sitting with light-intensity walking improves postprandial glycemia, but breaking up sitting with standing does not. *J. Sci. Med. Sport* **2015**, *18*, 294–298. [CrossRef] [PubMed]
19. Charlot, K.; Pichon, A.; Chapelot, D. Exercise prior to a freely requested meal modifies pre and postprandial glucose profile, substrate oxidation and sympathovagal balance. *Nutr. Metab. (Lond.)* **2011**, *8*, 66. [CrossRef] [PubMed]
20. Hashimoto, S.; Hayashi, S.; Yoshida, A.; Naito, M. Acute effects of postprandial aerobic exercise on glucose and lipoprotein metabolism in healthy young women. *J. Atheroscler. Thromb.* **2013**, *20*, 204–213. [CrossRef] [PubMed]
21. Enevoldsen, L.H.; Simonsen, L.; Macdonald, I.A.; Bulow, J. The combined effects of exercise and food intake on adipose tissue and splanchnic metabolism. *J. Physiol.* **2004**, *561*, 871–882. [CrossRef] [PubMed]
22. Nygaard, H.; Tomten, S.E.; Hostmark, A.T. Slow postmeal walking reduces postprandial glycemia in middle-aged women. *Appl. Physiol. Nutr. Metab.* **2009**, *34*, 1087–1092. [CrossRef] [PubMed]
23. Haxhi, J.; Scotto di Palumbo, A.; Sacchetti, M. Exercising for metabolic control: Is timing important? *Ann. Nutr. Metab.* **2013**, *62*, 14–25. [CrossRef] [PubMed]
24. Chacko, E. Timing and intensity of exercise for glucose control. *Diabetologia* **2014**, *57*, 2425–2426. [CrossRef] [PubMed]
25. McConell, G.; Fabris, S.; Proietto, J.; Hargreaves, M. Effect of carbohydrate ingestion on glucose kinetics during exercise. *J. Appl. Physiol. (1985)* **1994**, *77*, 1537–1541. [CrossRef] [PubMed]
26. Lunde, M.S.; Hjellset, V.T.; Hostmark, A.T. Slow post meal walking reduces the blood glucose response: An exploratory study in female Pakistani immigrants. *J. Immigr. Minor Health* **2012**, *14*, 816–822. [CrossRef] [PubMed]
27. Nelson, J.D.; Poussier, P.; Marliss, E.B.; Albisser, A.M.; Zinman, B. Metabolic response of normal man and insulin-infused diabetics to postprandial exercise. *Am. J. Physiol.* **1982**, *242*, E309–E316. [CrossRef] [PubMed]
28. Borer, K.T.; Wuorinen, E.C.; Lukos, J.R.; Denver, J.W.; Porges, S.W.; Burant, C.F. Two bouts of exercise before meals, but not after meals, lower fasting blood glucose. *Med. Sci. Sports Exerc.* **2009**, *41*, 1606–1614. [CrossRef] [PubMed]
29. Altenburg, T.M.; Rotteveel, J.; Dunstan, D.W.; Salmon, J.; Chinapaw, M.J. The effect of interrupting prolonged sitting time with short, hourly, moderate-intensity cycling bouts on cardiometabolic risk factors in healthy, young adults. *J. Appl. Physiol. (1985)* **2013**, *115*, 1751–1756. [CrossRef] [PubMed]
30. Welle, S. Metabolic responses to a meal during rest and low-intensity exercise. *Am. J. Clin. Nutr.* **1984**, *40*, 990–994. [CrossRef] [PubMed]
31. Wolever, T.M.; Jenkins, D.J.; Jenkins, A.L.; Josse, R.G. The glycemic index: Methodology and clinical implications. *Am. J. Clin. Nutr.* **1991**, *54*, 846–854. [CrossRef] [PubMed]
32. Matthews, J.N.; Altman, D.G.; Campbell, M.J.; Royston, P. Analysis of serial measurements in medical research. *BMJ* **1990**, *300*, 230–235. [CrossRef] [PubMed]
33. Dickinson, S.; Colagiuri, S.; Faramus, E.; Petocz, P.; Brand-Miller, J.C. Postprandial hyperglycemia and insulin sensitivity differ among lean young adults of different ethnicities. *J. Nutr.* **2002**, *132*, 2574–2579. [CrossRef] [PubMed]
34. Burstein, R.; Epstein, Y.; Shapiro, Y.; Charuzi, I.; Karnieli, E. Effect of an acute bout of exercise on glucose disposal in human obesity. *J. Appl. Physiol. (1985)* **1990**, *69*, 299–304. [CrossRef] [PubMed]

35. Buckley, J.P.; Mellor, D.D.; Morris, M.; Joseph, F. Standing-based office work shows encouraging signs of attenuating post-prandial glycaemic excursion. *Occup. Environ. Med.* **2014**, *71*, 109–111. [CrossRef] [PubMed]

36. Hardman, A.E.; Aldred, H.E. Walking during the postprandial period decreases alimentary lipaemia. *J. Cardiovasc. Risk* **1995**, *2*, 71–78. [CrossRef] [PubMed]

37. Heiss, C.J.; Tollefson, M. Postprandial light exercise attenuates the glycemic effect of a candy bar. *Top. Clin. Nutr.* **2014**, *29*, 132–138. [CrossRef]

38. Hostmark, A.T.; Ekeland, G.S.; Beckstrom, A.C.; Meen, H.D. Postprandial light physical activity blunts the blood glucose increase. *Prev. Med.* **2006**, *42*, 369–371. [CrossRef] [PubMed]

39. Zhu, W.L.; Zhong, C.F.; Yu, Y.J.; Li, K.J. Acute effects of hyperglycaemia with and without exercise on endothelial function in healthy young men. *Eur. J. Appl. Physiol.* **2007**, *99*, 585–591. [CrossRef] [PubMed]

40. Peddie, M.C.; Bone, J.L.; Rehrer, N.J.; Skeaff, C.M.; Gray, A.R.; Perry, T.L. Breaking prolonged sitting reduces postprandial glycemia in healthy, normal-weight adults: A randomized crossover trial. *Am. J. Clin. Nutr.* **2013**, *98*, 358–366. [CrossRef] [PubMed]

41. Katsanos, C.S.; Moffatt, R.J. Acute effects of premeal versus postmeal exercise on postprandial hypertriglyceridemia. *Clin. J. Sport Med.* **2004**, *14*, 33–39. [CrossRef] [PubMed]

42. Farah, N.M.; Gill, J.M. Effects of exercise before or after meal ingestion on fat balance and postprandial metabolism in overweight men. *Br. J. Nutr.* **2013**, *109*, 2297–2307. [CrossRef] [PubMed]

43. Larsen, J.J.; Dela, F.; Kjaer, M.; Galbo, H. The effect of moderate exercise on postprandial glucose homeostasis in NIDDM patients. *Diabetologia* **1997**, *40*, 447–453. [CrossRef] [PubMed]

44. Pfeiffer, M.; Ludwig, T.; Wenk, C.; Colombani, P.C. The influence of walking performed immediately before meals with moderate fat content on postprandial lipemia. *Lipids Health Dis.* **2005**, *4*, 24. [CrossRef] [PubMed]

45. DiPietro, L.; Gribok, A.; Stevens, M.S.; Hamm, L.F.; Rumpler, W. Three 15-min bouts of moderate postmeal walking significantly improves 24-h glycemic control in older people at risk for impaired glucose tolerance. *Diabetes Care* **2013**, *36*, 3262–3268. [CrossRef] [PubMed]

46. Henson, J.; Yates, T.; Biddle, S.J.; Edwardson, C.L.; Khunti, K.; Wilmot, E.G.; Gray, L.J.; Gorely, T.; Nimmo, M.A.; Davies, M.J. Associations of objectively measured sedentary behaviour and physical activity with markers of cardiometabolic health. *Diabetologia* **2013**, *56*, 1012–1020. [CrossRef] [PubMed]

47. Bastyr, E.J.; Stuart, C.A.; Brodows, R.G.; Schwartz, S.; Graf, C.J.; Zagar, A.; Robertson, K.E. Therapy focused on lowering postprandial glucose, not fasting glucose, may be superior for lowering HbA1c. IOEZ Study Group. *Diabetes Care* **2000**, *23*, 1236–1241. [CrossRef] [PubMed]

48. Najafipour, F.; Mobasseri, M.; Yavari, A.; Nadrian, H.; Aliasgarzadeh, A.; Mashinchi Abbasi, N.; Niafar, M.; Houshyar Gharamaleki, J.; Sadra, V. Effect of regular exercise training on changes in HbA1c, BMI and VO2max among patients with type 2 diabetes mellitus: An 8-year trial. *BMJ Open Diabetes Res. Care* **2017**, *5*, e000414. [CrossRef] [PubMed]

49. Hijikata, Y.; Yamada, S. Walking just after a meal seems to be more effective for weight loss than waiting for one hour to walk after a meal. *Int. J. Gen. Med.* **2011**, *4*, 447–450. [CrossRef] [PubMed]

50. Reynolds, A.N.; Mann, J.I.; Williams, S.; Venn, B.J. Advice to walk after meals is more effective for lowering postprandial glycaemia in type 2 diabetes mellitus than advice that does not specify timing: A randomised crossover study. *Diabetologia* **2016**, *59*, 2572–2578. [CrossRef] [PubMed]

51. Solomon, T.P.J.; Eves, F.F.; Laye, M.J. Targeting postprandial hyperglycemia with physical activity may reduce cardiovascular disease risk. but what should we do, and when is the right time to move? *Front Cardiovasc. Med.* **2018**, *5*, 99. [CrossRef] [PubMed]

52. Leung, G.K.W.; Huggins, C.E.; Bonham, M.P. Effect of meal timing on postprandial glucose responses to a low glycemic index meal: A crossover trial in healthy volunteers. *Clin. Nutr.* **2017**. [CrossRef] [PubMed]

53. Jovanovic, A.; Gerrard, J.; Taylor, R. The second-meal phenomenon in type 2 diabetes. *Diabetes Care* **2009**, *32*, 1199–1201. [CrossRef] [PubMed]

54. International Diabetes Federation Guideline Development Group. Guideline for management of postmeal glucose in diabetes. *Diabetes Res. Clin. Pract.* **2014**, *103*, 256–268. [CrossRef] [PubMed]

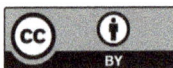

nutrients

MDPI

Review

Starchy Carbohydrates in a Healthy Diet: The Role of the Humble Potato

Tracey M. Robertson, Abdulrahman Z. Alzaabi, M. Denise Robertson and Barbara A. Fielding *

Department of Nutritional Sciences, University of Surrey, Guildford, GU2 7WG, UK;
t.m.robertson@surrey.ac.uk (T.M.R.); a.alzaabi@surrey.ac.uk (A.Z.A.); m.robertson@surrey.ac.uk (M.D.R.)
* Correspondence: b.fielding@surrey.ac.uk; Tel.: +44-(0)-1483-688649

Received: 4 October 2018; Accepted: 6 November 2018; Published: 14 November 2018

check for
updates

Abstract: Potatoes have been an affordable, staple part of the diet for many hundreds of years. Recently however, there has been a decline in consumption, perhaps influenced by erroneous reports of being an unhealthy food. This review provides an overview of the nutritional value of potatoes and examines the evidence for associations between potato consumption and non-communicable diseases. Potatoes are an important source of micronutrients, such as vitamin C, vitamin B6, potassium, folate, and iron and contribute a significant amount of fibre to the diet. However, nutrient content is affected by cooking method; boiling causes leaching of water-soluble nutrients, whereas frying can increase the resistant starch content of the cooked potato. Epidemiological studies have reported associations between potato intake and obesity, type 2 diabetes and cardiovascular disease. However, results are contradictory and confounded by lack of detail on cooking methods. Indeed, potatoes have been reported to be more satiating than other starchy carbohydrates, such as pasta and rice, which may aid weight maintenance. Future research should consider cooking methods in the study design in order to reduce confounding factors and further explore the health impact of this food.

Keywords: potato; obesity; satiety; T2DM; CVD; nutrition; resistant starch; fibre

1. Introduction

According to current UK government guidelines, carbohydrate (CHO) intake should be maintained at a population average of approximately 50% of total energy intake [1] and this is strongly supported by a recent meta-analysis indicating that a carbohydrate intake of 50–55% is optimal [2]. The intake of free sugars within the recommendation should not exceed 5% [1]. This is broadly in line with the WHO Scientific Update on carbohydrates in human nutrition (2007) which recommends a minimum of 50% of total energy intake from CHO, with free sugars restricted to <10% [3]. It is further recommended that carbohydrates consist mainly of starchy foods, such as potatoes, pasta, rice and bread, at about one-third of our total food intake [4].

The potato is historically a starch-rich staple food, originating over 7000 years ago in Peru as reviewed [5]. Potatoes have been an important, affordable food in our diet for hundreds of years and the economic and health consequences of the Irish potato famine between 1845 and 1849 are widely known. As a staple food, the potato still plays an important role in global food security, providing a sustainable food supply and lessening poverty and malnutrition in many parts of the world as highlighted in the Food and Agriculture Organization of the United Nations (FAO) review 'International Year of the Potato' [6]. Sustainability of a crop is partly determined by the area of land required, and the water and energy requirements. A ton of potato produced requires only 0.06 ha of land, while rice and wheat require 0.24 and 0.35 ha of land, respectively [7]. Moreover, potato and wheat need less water compared to rice [7] and despite the potato having the highest water content (80%), the energy produced per litre of water is greatest for the potato. In addition, the potato has the lowest carbon footprint of the three [7]. As a crop, potatoes require cool, but frost-free conditions, suiting many geographical areas. However, during storage, potatoes, require chilling and ventilation, which increases the demand for energy [5]. Most cultivated varieties are of the species *Solanum tuberosum* [8], and over the last 60 years, plant biotechnology has complemented conventional potato breeding resulting in specific genotypes or cultivars [9]. The potato is a globally important crop, with an estimated 377 million tonnes harvested in 2016, only falling short of the other starch staples, maize, wheat, and rice (Figure 1).

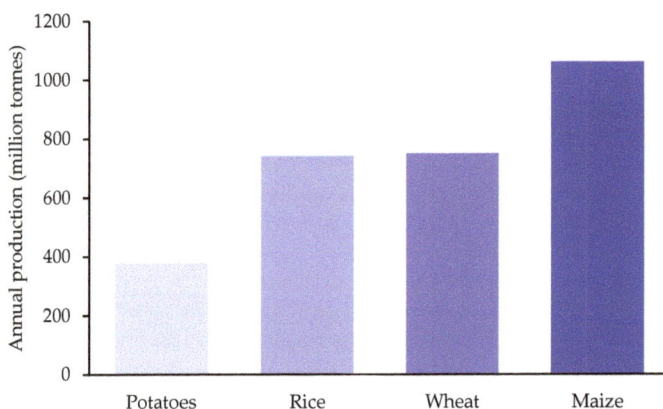

Figure 1. Global production of major starchy carbohydrate crops in 2016 [10].

China is estimated to produce the most potatoes in the world with many European countries in the top twelve (Figure 2).

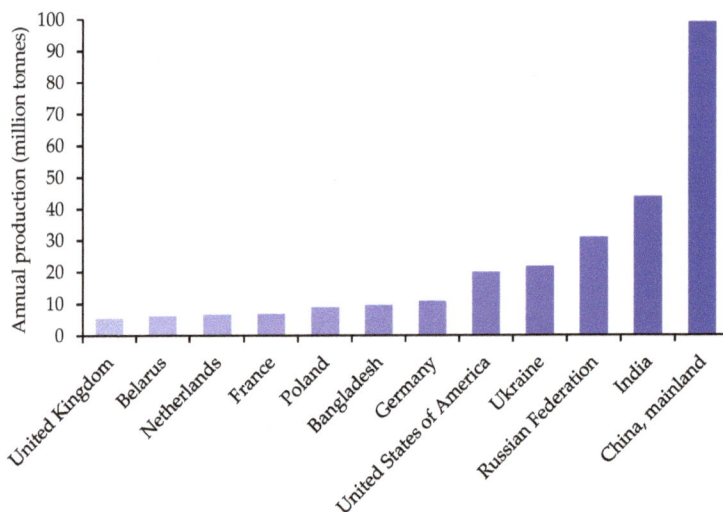

Figure 2. Top twelve producers of potato by country in 2016 [10].

Many European countries are also in the top ten worldwide potato consumers, when potato supply per capita is used as an estimate of consumption (Figure 3).

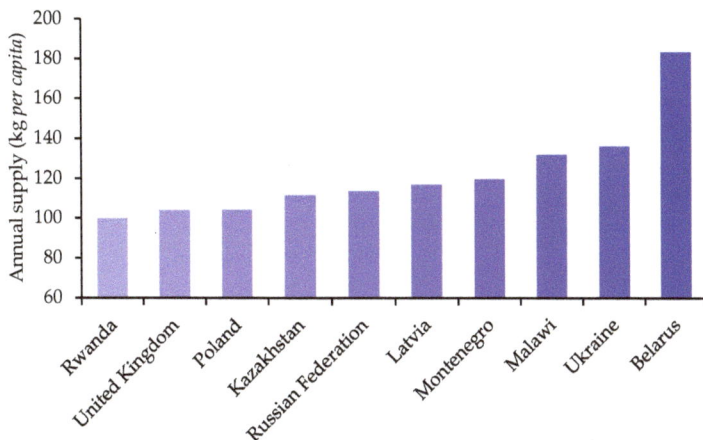

Figure 3. Annual per capita supply of potatoes, available for food, in 2013, as a marker of potential consumption [10]. Figures estimated based on the amounts produced, exported and imported, with deductions made for losses during storage and transport and amounts used for seed, animal feed, and non-food uses.

Annual per capita data from 2013 also shows that potatoes and potato products are the third most consumed in the diet, behind wheat and rice [10]. Although maize rates higher in terms of world production, it is used in large quantities as a raw material for the manufacture of glucose, fructose, and high glucose corn syrup, as animal feed, and is also increasingly used for industrial applications [11].

Despite the current recommendations for starch in the diet, the nutritional value of the potato could easily be overlooked, partly because it is not counted towards the 'five-a-day' fruit and vegetable intake recommendation [4] and because it is often prepared with fats or oils. Indeed, as far back as 1918, the popularity of the potato was attributed to the fact that 'the lack of flavour makes it possible to confer palatability upon it by the addition of milk, butter, and cream, salt and pepper, or by frying in fats' [12]. In a UK survey from 2008–2011, potatoes were found to contribute 7% of energy intake [13]. However, potatoes have recently lost favour with an 8.8% reduction in intake from 2013 to 2016/17 in the UK [14]. The reasons for the decline in potato consumption are varied and include changes in food preferences [7]. Potato consumption was recently examined in a Norwegian cohort of women who reported a 15% reduction in consumption from 1998 to 2005 [15]. Increase in income and a perceived association of potato consumption with weight gain and chronic diseases like type 2 diabetes mellitus (T2DM) have been identified as some of the factors responsible for the change, although low-carbohydrate, weight-reducing diets have given conflicting results [16]. Moreover, an increase in prevalence of T2DM has also been identified as a factor leading to a reduction in intake because of dietary advice [15]. However the nutritional benefits of the potato include a relatively high content of micronutrients such as potassium, vitamins such as the B vitamins, and fibre if the skin is eaten [13].

There have been many reviews on potatoes and health in the past; systematic reviews and meta-analyses have covered specific diseases, or focused on specific nutrients, or examined cooking methods [17–22]. In this Narrative Review, we have brought these aspects together under the remit of this special edition. In doing so, we have placed our emphasis on the associations between potato intake and non-communicable diseases, such as obesity, cardiovascular disease (CVD), and T2DM. The association between dietary potato intake and health is complex because of confounders such as cooking method, variety, and storage. We will evaluate the effect of such confounders on satiety and metabolic response, and to what extent these have been accounted for in the literature.

2. Nutrient Composition

2.1. Macronutrients

2.1.1. Carbohydrate

The starch content of a potato can be highly variable. In general terms fresh potatoes contain ~20% dry matter (DM) of which 60–80% is starch, with 70–80% of this starch as amylopectin [23]. This variability is primarily the result of genotype and growing environment.

2.1.2. Fibre

Dietary fibre (DF) is a mixed group of heterogeneous compounds, for the most part, as carbohydrate polymers and oligomers. All definitions identify DF as materials that escape digestion in the small intestine and pass into the large intestine, where they will be fermented by the resident microbiota to a variable extent. DF and their fermentation products, specifically the short-chain fatty acids may contribute many of the beneficial effects of DF consumption for the host. Although there is evidence for the metabolic benefit of DF ingestion from nutritional epidemiology, intervention studies, animal studies and in vitro work, it has mostly been assumed that all DF which share basic physiochemical features; such as solubility, monomeric unit or even botanical source will behave in an identical way, physiologically speaking. However, evidence suggests that different DF may also provide unique properties. The DF composition of potatoes is made up of resistant starch (RS) (major component, see Section 2.1.2.1), with smaller amounts of non-starch polysaccharides such as cellulose (0.45–0.7%) [24], hemi-cellulose (0.32–0.46%), lignin (0.15–0.22%), and pectin (0.32–0.38%) of raw potato mass [25].

The individual fraction responsible for most of the variability in DF content is the RS. Potato tubers are always cooked before consumption so DF values are not typically provided in databases as they are of potentially limited value, however DF values are known to be affected by cooking and serving temperature and typically multiple different values for DF for "potato" will be provided. A major limitation of many epidemiological studies is both the lack of detail on food preparation methods collected as part of the dataset and issues with the laboratory measurement of RS. Despite this obvious limitation, according to the most recent National Diet and Nutrition Survey (NDNS 2015–2016), it is estimated that "potatoes and potato products" contribute ~11% of the AOAC DF intake in adults (19–64 years) in the UK, contributing ~2 g/day [26]. In comparison with other starchy CHO, it contributes less DF than bread (total: ~20%), but more than "pasta, rice, pizza, and other miscellaneous cereals" (8%).

2.1.2.1. Resistant Starch

Resistant starches are the sum of both intact starch and starch degradation products that reach the large intestine for fermentation. The molar yield of butyrate produced by the gut microbiota differentiated RS from other DF fractions [27,28]. RS can be classified into five subtypes; namely, physically entrapped starch (RS1), raw starch granules (RS2), retrograded starch (RS3), chemically modified starch (RS4), and amylose-lipid complex (RS5). The starch in a raw potato tuber is ~75% RS2, with granules resistant to enzyme digestion [29,30]. Data on the exact RS2 content of raw potato tubers is sparse as potatoes would not normally be consumed raw, but estimates are in the region of 47–59% of DM, dependent on variety [29,30]. Thus, an "average" raw potato would contain 10 g RS/100 g wet weight. Potatoes are cooked before consumption and when the starch is heated in excess water gelatinization occurs and the starch becomes highly digestible. Both heat source and water have an impact on this process and following cooking the residual RS2 remaining in the cooked product is relatively low (2–4% DM) but consistently follows the following hierarchy: baked > microwaved > boiled. Cooking time and intensity also affect the amount of RS in the cooked potato, with lower temperature and longer cooking time resulting in greater RS retention for fried potato chips [31].

The practicalities of this should, however, be considered as both longer and shorter cooking times may result in an unpalatable product. If the gelatinized starch is allowed to cool, the amylose and amylopectin chains recrystalise by a process known as retrogradation. Recrystalised or retrograded amylose is resistant to the action of small intestinal α-amylase and this now forms RS3. Raatz et al. compared baking and boiling cooking methods for three different varieties of potato and measured the RS content at three service temperatures, hot, chilled and reheated [32]. Whilst they found no significant differences between varieties, they reported more RS in baked versus boiled across all varieties, and more RS in chilled potatoes than in hot or reheated. The greatest difference reported was in the Yukon Gold variety, where the baked/chilled combination (5.4 $\pm$ SD 0.05 g/100 g) had more than double the RS of the boiled/reheated combination (2.2 $\pm$ SD 0.05 g/100 g). When potatoes are deep-fried, the resulting RS [31] may be derived from the formation of complexes between the starch and other compounds in the potato or the food matrix, such as lipids [33]. This would now be termed RS5. In one study, potato that had been boiled and cooled was compared with potato that had been boiled then deep- or shallow-fried then cooled, the amount of total RS was as follows: boiled/cooled: 1.78 $\pm$ SD 0.24% > shallow fried/cooled: 1.11 $\pm$ SD 0.05% > deep fried/cooled: 1.04 $\pm$ SD 0.13% [34]. It was hypothesized that the frying process created RS5, which inhibited RS3 formation during retrogradation, such that the fried/cooled potato had more RS5 but less RS3, resulting in less total RS than the boiled/cooled potato. It is feasible that if the potato had been cooled before the addition of oil and deep-fried later, then both RS3 and RS5 formation would be maximized, however, to our knowledge, this has not yet been tested in the potato. It should be ensured, however, that any lipid consumed remains within current dietary guidelines for content and composition, until the metabolic fate of fat 'trapped' in RS5 is known. To summarise, any potato product eaten will contain variable amounts of RS2, RS3 and RS5, due to variation in cooking methods, length of cooking and both cooking and storage temperatures.

2.1.3. Protein and Fat

Quantitatively, potatoes are not a good source of protein, with an average content of 2–3 g/100 g (Table 1). To put this into context, the average potato intake in the UK is 85 g per capita per day [13] which we estimate would provide about 4% of the Reference Nutrient Intake (RNI) of protein for a 70 kg adult [35]. Interestingly, as recently reviewed, about 0.6 g/100 g of the protein is associated with the starch matrix in isolated potato starch, and proteomic analysis of potato starch revealed 36 different proteins [36], indicating possible targets for modifying starch biosynthesis and metabolism. The amount of fat in a potato is even less than protein. Without the addition of extra fat during preparation, the fat content in potato crop is ~0.1% of fresh weight.

Table 1. Nutrient composition per 100 g potato according to cooking method.

Nutrient	Raw (Flesh and Skin)	Boiled (Flesh Only) Cooked Without Skin	Boiled (Flesh Only) Cooked in Skin	Baked (Flesh and Skin)	Microwaved (Flesh and Skin)	Oven-Baked Chips[1]	Fried Chips[2]	Daily RNI; (M/F)
Water (g)	79.3	77.5	77.0	74.9	72.0	64.4	38.6	-
Energy (kcal)	77	86	87	93	105	158	312	-
Protein (g)	2.1	1.7	1.9	2.5	2.4	2.8	3.3	-
Fat (g)	0.1	0.1	0.1	0.1	0.1	5.5	14.7	-
Carbohydrate (g)	17.5	20.0	20.1	21.2	24.2	25.6	41.4	-
Fibre * (g)	2.1	1.8	1.8	2.2	2.3	2.0	3.8	-
Minerals								
Calcium (mg)	12	8	5	15	11	12	18	700
Iron (mg)	0.81	0.31	0.31	1.08	1.24	0.57	0.81	8.7/14.8
Magnesium (mg)	23	20	22	28	27	24	35	300/270
Phosphorus (mg)	57	40	44	70	105	87	125	550
Potassium (mg)	425	328	379	535	447	478	579	3500
Sodium (mg)	6	5	4	10	8	324 **	210 **	1600
Zinc (mg)	0.30	0.27	0.30	0.36	0.36	0.35	0.50	9.5/7.0
Vitamins								
Vitamin C (mg)	19.7	7.4	13.0	9.6	15.1	8.7	4.7	40
Thiamin (mg)	0.081	0.098	0.106	0.064	0.120	0.130	0.170	1.0/0.8
Riboflavin (mg)	0.032	0.019	0.020	0.048	0.032	0.032	0.039	1.3/1.1
Niacin (mg)	1.061	1.312	1.439	1.410	1.714	2.077	3.004	17/13
Vitamin B6 (mg)	0.298	0.269	0.299	0.311	0.344	0.261	0.372	1.4/1.2
Folate (µg)	15	9	10	28	12	23	30	200
Vitamin B12 (µg)	0.00	0.00	0.00	0.00	0.00	0.00	0.00	1.5
Vitamin A (µg)	0.00	0.00	0.00	0.00	0.00	0.00	0.00	700/600
Vitamin E (mg)	0.01	0.01	0.01	0.04	0.01	0.39	1.67	-
Vitamin D (µg)	0.00	0.00	0.00	0.00	0.00	0.00	0.00	10
Vitamin K (µg)	2.0	2.2	2.2	2.0	2.0	7.4	11.2	-

Data obtained from the USDA National Nutrient Database for Standard Reference, Release April 2018 [37]; Reference Nutrient Intake (RNI) values obtained from COMA Dietary Reference Values for Food Energy and Nutrients for the United Kingdom, 1991, and the UK Scientific Advisory Committee on Nutrition (SACN); M:male; F:female; * Total dietary fibre analysed by enzymatic gravimetric methods AOAC, does not include resistant starch; [1] Frozen, home-prepared, also known as French Fries; ** includes sodium added during product processing; [2] Fast foods, fried in vegetable oil, also known as French Fries.

2.2. Micronutrients

Potatoes are important sources of several micronutrients, including potassium, magnesium, vitamin C, vitamin B6, folate and thiamin. Various factors, such as variety, cooking method, and type/length of storage, affect how much of a given micronutrient is present; the effects of variety and storage will be discussed in detail in later sections. Boiling causes leaching of water-soluble vitamins and minerals. The scale of the losses are affected by duration of boiling and also surface area of the potato pieces. In one study [38], potassium losses of over 50% were observed when potatoes were cut into 1 cm cubes and boiled for 10 min, with even greater losses (70–75%) observed when the potatoes were shredded; substantial losses were also reported for iron, magnesium, manganese, phosphorus, sulphur, and zinc. These losses can be mitigated somewhat by boiling the potatoes in their skins, rather than after peeling (Table 1). Conversely, cooking methods that do not involve water preserve more of the water soluble vitamin and mineral content [39]. For example, vitamin C losses were lower when potatoes were microwaved (<33%), baked (<51%) and sautéed (<67%) than boiled (<88%) [40]. Interestingly, in the same study, addition of salt to the boiling water slightly reduced the vitamin C loss to 61–79%.

Table 1 shows the micronutrient composition of 100 g potato comparing various cooking methods with the content of raw potato. To put these figures in context, a medium-sized baked potato (200 g), for example, would contribute 24% of the UK daily reference nutrient intake (RNI) for iron for a man, 18% for magnesium, 30% for potassium, 48% for vitamin C, 44% for vitamin B6, 28% for folate and only 2% for sodium, with 14%, 10%, 30%, 48%, 52%, 28%, and 2% respectively for a woman. Furthermore, in an analysis of data from the NDNS (2008–2011), Gibson and Kurilich reported that potato consumption contributed 15% of potassium, 15% of B6, 14% of vitamin C, 10% of folate and 9% of magnesium in the UK diet [13].

2.3. Phytonutrients

Potatoes contain several types of phytonutrients including carotenoids, anthocyanins, and chlorogenic and caffeic acids [41] which are all antioxidants. Chu et al. analysed samples of ten different vegetables for total phenolic content, measured for antioxidant activity as gallic acid equivalents, measured by TOSC (total oxyradical scavenging capacity) assay, and anti-proliferative activity, measured in HepG$_2$ cells [42]. Potatoes were reported as having approximately <40 mg gallic acid equivalents/100 g, compared to the highest measured, broccoli, which had >100 mg gallic acid equivalents/100 g. They were in the lowest group for antioxidant activity, displaying 4.86 µmol of vitamin C equiv/g of sample, compared with the highest, red pepper, which displayed 46.95 µmol of vitamin C equiv/g of sample and also displayed minimal anti-proliferative activity. They did not, however, report which variety of potato they measured, but it is likely that it was a white potato variety as they stated that the vegetables were selected based on their per capita consumption in the US. Whilst these relative amounts are quite low, a different picture emerges when actual consumption patterns are considered. Kyoung Chun et al. measured total phenolic and antioxidant content of 14 fruits and 20 vegetables and estimated per capita consumption based on data from the United States Department of Agriculture [43]. They reported that although concentrations of total phenolics and antioxidants were relatively low in potatoes, they were the highest vegetable contributor and the third highest overall, behind oranges and apples, to the US diet, due to higher amounts being consumed. Whilst dietary antioxidants demonstrate strong antioxidant and anti-proliferative action in vitro, their bioavailability is highly variable [44]. It has been suggested that, in comparison with endogenous antioxidants, they play a minor role in direct antioxidant activity and rather that their main contribution is via indirect means, such as their effects on cell signalling and gene expression [45].

2.4. Effects of Potato Variety on Nutrient Composition

There is a fairly narrow range of nutrients in different potato varieties and cultivars as traditional breeding strategies are not possible [9]. Thus, a narrow range of amylose content in potatoes is usually reported e.g., 20–27% amylose (w/w) of total starch depending on variety and method of determination; 23% to 43% has also been cited [17]. However, genetic modification can increase this, with reports in excess of 80% [46]. Depending on the variety of potato, the protein content varies from 1 g to 4.2 g per 100 g of potato [8,20]. The colour of potato flesh can be an indicator of nutrient content, for example, yellow fleshed potatoes contain the carotenoids lutein and zeaxanthin [47]. The antioxidant content of potatoes, particularly coloured varieties and cultivars has been well reviewed [48]. For example, potatoes with purple and red skin/flesh contain high levels of anthocyanins and have been reported to contain the highest gallic acid equivalent total phenolic content, in comparison with both yellow and white varieties [49]. The 'golden potato' was developed by gene modification resulting in enrichment of β-carotene (>3000 fold over the wild type), lutein (30-fold), β-β-xanthophylls (nine-fold) and α-carotene [50]. The results from an in vitro study of bioaccessibility has led to the suggestion that the golden potato could be useful in boosting the dietary intake of retinol activity equivalents and vitamin E in children and women of reproductive age in developing countries [50]. This is important since Vitamin A deficiency is the major cause of blindness in children.

2.5. Effects of Storage on Nutrient Composition

Potatoes are usually planted in Spring and harvested in Autumn, yet consumers require potatoes throughout the year. This means that the fresh potato purchased by the consumer may have been stored for up to a year post harvest. In order to keep potatoes at their best for such a long period of time, their environment must be tightly regulated. Typically this means, for the fresh product, keeping them at 6–10 °C, in a well-ventilated, dark, humid environment [51]. Storing potatoes at lower temperatures further inhibits sprout production, but increases reducing sugar content, which is not desirable for potatoes destined for frying as the sugars take part in the Maillard reaction, which is responsible for the browning of potatoes when fried at high temperatures. Higher amounts of reducing sugars result in an overly-brown end-product, with increased amounts of acrylamide [52]. In one study carried out in Sweden, storage of potatoes for five months, resulted in a 60% decrease in vitamin C and a 20% increase in vitamin B6 content, with no difference in the amounts of potassium, thiamin or other vitamins and minerals [53]. Cold storage (4 °C) of a number of different cultivars for seven months, resulted in reduced vitamin C content in all cultivars (mean decrease, 52%) and slightly increased total polyphenol content in two pigmented varieties [51].

3. Relationship between Potato Consumption and Non-Communicable Diseases

3.1. Obesity

There is conflicting evidence from observational studies examining potato consumption and predictors of obesity, such as increases in weight, body mass index (BMI) and waist circumference (WC). Mozaffarian et al. reported a small weight gain of 0.71 lb (95% CI: 0.53–0.89) over a four year period for every 1 serving/day increase in boiled, baked, or mashed potato, and a larger weight gain (4.11 lb; 95% CI: 3.46–4.76) for every 1 serving/day increase in French fries [54]. French fries have also been associated with weight gain in women but not in men [55]. Consumption of French fries, but not other potato types, has been associated with increased BMI [56]. Some have observed an association between total potato intake and increased WC in women [57], whereas others have found no association between total potato intake and WC [58]. Details of these studies are reported in Table 2. A systematic review of these observational studies concluded that there was no evidence for an association between potato consumption and obesity, however, there may be some evidence for an association between French fries and obesity. Overall there were few studies and those that were included were of relatively poor quality [18].

Table 2. Summary of cohort studies investigating associations between potato consumption and weight change, BMI, and waist circumference.

Reference	Study Type; Follow-Up/Duration	n (%F); BMI; Age (years); Criteria	Exposure; Assessment Method	Results	Potato Categories	Comments
French et al., 1994 [55]	Cross-sectional and prospective cohort (two years)	3552 (53.9%) Normal weight to obese 37.3 ± 10.7 years (F) 39.1 ± 9.8 years (M)	Participating in a workplace weight loss intervention FFQ (18 items)	A trend for an association (p = 0.06) between consumption of French fries/fried potatoes and higher bodyweight in women at baseline Increased consumption of French fries associated with weight gain in women	French fries and fried potatoes in a single category; no other potatoes measured	Data from the Healthy Worker Project [59] Participants were fully clothed, including shoes, for weight measurement. Time of day was not standardised. FFQ contained only 15 highest contributors to energy and fat intake; fruit and vegetable intake was not assessed.
Halkjaer et al., 2004 [58]	Cohort (six years)	2300 (49.2%) Normal weight to obese 30–60 years Of Danish origin	Habitual diet FFQ (26 items)	A weak inverse association between potato consumption and waist circumference; insignificant after adjustment for changes in obesity	Potatoes (unspecified)	Data from the MONICA1 study Intake remained largely unchanged over the time period measured
Linde et al., 2006 [56]	Cross-sectional and prospective cohort (2 years)	1801 (71.8%) Overweight and obese (BMI > 27) >18 years	Participating in weight loss intervention Block Screening Questionnaires for Fat (15 Items) and Fruit/Vegetable/Fibre (nine items) Intake	Consumption of French fries associated with higher BMI in women, but not men at baseline Increased consumption of French fries associated with increased BMI over two years for men and women No association between potatoes and BMI at baseline or over the course of the intervention	Potatoes; French fries	
Halkjaer et al., 2009 [57]	Cohort (five years)	42,696 (52.9%) BMI 20–33.5 50–64 years	Habitual diet FFQ (192 items, 21 groups)	Energy intake from potatoes was associated with five year increase in waist circumference in women	Potatoes (not including French fries)	Data from the Danish Diet, Cancer and Health Study [60] French fries were incorporated into a Snack Foods group. potatoes were in a group of their own. All analysis by group, not individual food item.
Mozaffarian et al., 2011 [54]	Three cohorts (four year intervals)	120,877 (81.3%) Non-obese at baseline 18–64 years Energy intake 900–3500 kcal/day	Habitual diet FFQ (61/131 items)	Four year weight change was positively associated with potato intake (all categories)	Total potato intake; Boiled, baked or mashed; French fries; Potato chips	Data from the Nurses' Health Study I and II [61] and the Health Professionals Follow-up Study [62]

BMI: body mass index; FFQ: food frequency questionnaire; MONICA1: the Danish Monitoring Trends and Determinants of Cardiovascular Disease cohort.

Nutrients **2018**, *10*, 1764

Whilst these studies, and those discussed in later sections on T2DM and CVD, attempted to control for other dietary and lifestyle factors, utilising multivariate linear regression models, it is possible that other unidentified factors are confounding their results. For example, few studies included socioeconomic status (SES) in their analysis, although other factors associated with SES, such as activity levels, fruit and vegetable intake, smoking and alcohol intake were included in most analyses. Dietary intake was measured by food frequency questionnaires (FFQs), often containing a very restricted number of food items. The use of these questionnaires whilst practical for studies involving large numbers of participants, limits the amount of information that can be obtained. When considering potato consumption they appear to have been limited to very few options, sometimes only reporting on total potato consumption [63–65], or grouping baked, boiled and mashed potato as a single item [66]. Where more detail is provided, it is still insufficient with regard to cooking methods. For example, boiled potatoes will differ in nutrient content, particularly fibre, depending on whether or not they are cooked and consumed with their skins on. Additionally, French fries are often cited as producing a different effect from other preparation methods, however what is classed as a French fry varies from country to country. In the US any type of potato that has been sliced into batons and fried is classed as a French fry, regardless of size of the baton, whereas in the UK and parts of Europe the size of the baton determines the name; a very thin baton would be classed as a skinny chip, a wide-cut baton as a chip and only a medium sized baton referred to as a French fry. An additional point of confusion is that in the USA and other countries, 'chips' would be a thin, fried potato snack sold in bags, known as 'crisps' in the UK. When deep-frying, the surface area-to-volume ratio affects the amount of fat absorbed, with thinner-sliced batons absorbing more oil than their thicker counterparts. Furthermore, there is no distinction between oven-baked and deep-fried French fries, two preparation methods which could vary widely in fat content.

When food intake is assessed by dietary recall methods, answers may not be very accurate, particularly if a person's diet has changed in the intervening years. Reverse causality can also be a concern when interpreting results as it is common for people to make changes to their diet after learning they are at increased risk of a particular disease, for example reducing saturated fat intake after receiving a high cholesterol report. If these dietary changes are not made in time to affect their health, this could lead to people with apparently healthy diets being erroneously reported to be more likely to develop a particular disease.

As changes in weight, BMI and WC take place over a relatively long period of time, it would be difficult to design a well-controlled, longer-term intervention examining their effect on these markers, particularly as potatoes are not consumed alone, but within the context of a mixed diet. Instead of measuring weight gain directly, several acute studies have compared the effects of consuming different starchy carbohydrates, including potatoes, on satiety and subsequent energy intake [67–72]. A variety of methodologies have been implemented, such as matching for carbohydrate or energy content or allowing ad libitum intake; some served the carbohydrate on its own, whereas others served it within the context of a mixed meal. These studies are summarised in Table 3.

Table 3. Acute studies examining the effects of potato consumption on satiety measures and energy intake.

Reference	Participants	Study Type	Test Meals	Measures	Results
Holt et al., 1996 [67]	n = 11–13 per group BMI 22.7 ± 0.4 22.1 ± 2.9 years	Crossover	1000 kJ portions of 38 test foods split into food groups, carbohydrate-rich group included. Along with 220 mL water. White bread as reference food.	Seven-point scale for satiety ratings	Boiled potatoes had the highest satiety score of all foods. An inverse association between satiety score and subsequent ad libitum energy intake was observed.
Erdmann et al., 2007 [68]	11 M BMI 23.5 ± 0.5 24.4 ± 0.3 years	Crossover	150 g lean pork steak, served with ad libitum amount of boiled white pasta, boiled white rice or boiled white potatoes, all in tomato sauce. Participants asked to consume foods until comfortably satiated. Ad libitum sandwich meal provided 4 h later.	VAS scores for hunger and satiety every 15 min	Comparable amounts of potato, pasta and rice consumed at first meal (353–372 g), but energy intake significantly lower for potato meal (2177 kJ) than rice (2829 kJ) and pasta (3174 kJ). Greater satiety and less hunger following pasta and rice meals during hour 4. No difference in energy consumption at second ad libitum meal (+4 h) No differences in satiety and hunger following second meal.
Leeman et al., 2008 [69] Study 1	9 M, 4 F BMI 21.8 ± 3.1 19–27 years	Crossover	Isoenergetic 1000 kJ portions of boiled potatoes, French fries or instant mashed potatoes (reconstituted with 200 or 330 g water), providing 32.5–50.3 g available CHO, all served with 250 water or milk/water mix and 150 mL tea/coffee.	Nine-point scale (painfully hungry–full to nausea)	French fries produced a lower satiety AUC than boiled potatoes over 4 h and lower satiety AUC than the small portion of mashed potato over 0–70 min.
Leeman et al., 2008 [69] Study 2	6 M, 8 F BMI 21.9 ± 2.0 20–28 years	Crossover	50 g available CHO portions of French fries and boiled potatoes, with or without 15.4 g sunflower oil (963–534 kJ), white wheat bread reference, all served with 150 water and 150 mL tea/coffee.	Nine-point scale (painfully hungry–full to nausea)	No significant differences between meals.

Table 3. *Cont.*

Reference	Participants	Study Type	Test Meals	Measures	Results
Geliebter et al., 2013 [70]	6 M, 6 F BMI 22.4 ± 2.0 22–30 years	Crossover	240 kcal portions (50 g CHO) of peeled baked potato, instant mashed potato, steamed brown rice and boiled pasta. White bread as control (273 kcal, 50 g CHO). Variable amount of water (180–363 g) served on the side to bring total water content of each meal to 400 g.	Scales for hunger, fullness, desire to eat and prospective consumption	Both potato meals reduced appetite compared to pasta and rice. No differences between meals on subsequent (2 h) energy intake.
Akilen et al., 2016 [71]	Study 1: 12 M, 8 F Study 2: 6 M, 6 F 11–12 years (children) normal weight	Crossover	100 g meatballs, served with ad libitum boiled mashed potatoes (from frozen), served with milk and butter), pasta (with milk, butter and cheese powder), boiled white rice (with butter and rice seasoning), oven fries or French fries. All served 4 h after a standardised breakfast.	VAS for satiety ratings	A smaller amount of oven fries and French fries was consumed than pasta. Energy intake was lower for boiled mashed potato than all other meals. No difference between meals for mean appetite scores until adjusted for energy intake. Adjusted post-meal appetite scores were lower for boiled mashed potatoes than other test meals.
Diaz-Toledo et al., 2016 [72]	16 M, 17 F BMI 22.7 ± 0.3 34.1 ± 2.4 years	Crossover	858 kJ portions of French fries (deep-fried from frozen), baked potato (pre-prepared, microwaved from frozen), mashed potato (pre-prepared, microwaved from chilled), or potato wedges (microwaved and served chilled). Pasta (boiled) as control. All served with meatballs in tomato sauce, salad and Caesar dressing (total energy from meal, 1883 kJ). All served 3 h after a standardized, personalised breakfast. Ad libitum sandwich and yoghurt meal provided 4 h after test meal.	VAS for satiety ratings (hunger, fullness, desire to eat and prospective consumption)	Higher satiety ratings (4 h AUC) for French fries, compared to pasta. Each potato meal compared to pasta meal only; no comparisons performed between potato-based meals. No difference in energy consumption at second ad libitum meal (+4 h).

AUC: area under the curve; CHO: carbohydrate; VAS: visual analogue scale

When isoenergetic portions of starchy carbohydrates are consumed, potatoes have been reported to be more satiating than pasta, rice and bread [67,70]. Furthermore, when 38 different test foods were compared, boiled potatoes were reported to have the highest satiety index of all test foods, even when compared to protein and fat-rich foods [67]. When different preparation/serving methods were compared, Leeman et al. reported both boiled and mashed potatoes to be more satiating than French fries when meals were energy matched, but not when matched for carbohydrate content [69]. This is likely due to boiled potatoes being less energy dense and, therefore, having a larger portion size than French fries when energy matched, as feelings of fullness and satiety are affected by stomach distension and capacity [73]. Indeed, a 1000 kJ portion of boiled potatoes weighs 368 g in comparison to a matched portion of French fries which weighs only 93 g [74]. Geliebter et al. compared isoenergetic (~1000 kJ) amounts of instant mashed potato, peeled baked potato, pasta, and brown rice [70]. Each test meal was accompanied by a variable amount of water designed to bring the total meal water content to 400 g, which could potentially ameliorate some of the effects of meal volume. However, despite this, they found that both potato meals reduced appetite compared to pasta and rice. This may be because water served alongside a meal has been demonstrated to have no effect on satiety in contrast to water incorporated into a meal [75].

In contrast to these studies, Diaz-Toledo et al. reported higher satiety ratings for French fries compared to an energy-matched pasta control, with no differences between baked potato or mashed potato and the pasta control for any satiety measure [72]. There were several differences between their study and the other isoenergetic studies. Their participants were given a personalised breakfast 3 h prior to the test meal and so were not fasted when they consumed the test meal. Furthermore, their test meal was a mixed meal, containing meatballs in tomato sauce, salad and dressing; the starchy test food was not consumed in isolation. The mashed potato was a pre-prepared dish, which included a comparable amount of fat to the French fries, resulting in a smaller difference in portion weight and energy density between the two. Finally the overall energy content of the test meal was 1883 kJ, almost double that of other isoenergetic studies. These differences in energy density, macronutrient content and total energy may contribute to the contradictory results from this study.

When adult participants were given ad libitum amounts of boiled pasta, rice or potatoes, along with a fixed amount of meat, and instructed to eat until they were no longer hungry, equivalent amounts of the carbohydrate element were eaten (353–372 g), however, because of the lower energy density of the potatoes, less total energy was consumed in that meal [68]. After 4 h, satiety and hunger levels had returned to baseline for those consuming the potato meal, whereas they had not for the pasta and rice meals. Plasma insulin was lower after the potato meal, with no difference between meals for glucose, despite potatoes having a reported higher glycaemic index than pasta and rice [76]. This discrepancy is likely due to the smaller amount of carbohydrate in the potato meal.

Similarly, Akilen et al. served ad libitum amounts of potato (either boiled and mashed, oven fries or French fries), boiled pasta or rice with a fixed portion of meatballs to a group of normal-weight children [71]. Lower weights of oven fries and French fries were consumed compared to pasta, however when energy intake was compared, energy from the boiled mashed potato meal was lower than all other meals. In this study, there was no difference between meals for appetite scores until they were adjusted for energy intake, which resulted in a lower mean appetite rating/kcal for the boiled mashed potato meal in the 2 h following the meal.

Evidence for a relationship between satiety scores and energy intake at a subsequent ad libitum meal is mixed. When isoenergetic portions are compared, some have reported no difference in subsequent energy intake either between different potato preparation methods or in comparison to other starchy carbohydrates, despite higher satiety scores for boiled potatoes [70,72]. Holt et al., however, reported an inverse association between satiety score and energy intake at a second meal [67] across their 38 test foods, with a tendency for a lower total energy intake across the whole day from the most satiating foods. When participants were permitted ad libitum amounts of potato, pasta or rice at a first meal, the lower energy intake and lower 4 h satiety score from the potato meal did not translate into a greater energy intake at a subsequent ad libitum sandwich meal [68].

Of the studies that measured postprandial glucose and insulin responses [67,69], neither reported any direct correlation between glycaemic or insulinaemic response and satiety score, although an indirect relationship between insulin response and satiety was suggested by Holt et al., who reported inverse associations between both insulin score and satiety score with subsequent ad libitum energy intake.

In summary, isoenergetic portions of potatoes, in particular boiled potatoes, appear to be more satiating than other starchy carbohydrates when eaten in isolation. When ad libitum consumption is permitted, less energy is consumed in mixed meals containing potato, with no compensatory increase in energy intake at a subsequent meal, despite lower satiety ratings. It should be noted that the evidence is limited as there have been few studies of this type, particularly those examining the effects of ad libitum consumption of potatoes in the context of a mixed meal. Despite this, the results from studies so far do not support a link between potato consumption and risk of overweight and obesity.

3.2. Type 2 Diabetes Mellitus (T2DM)

An association between total potato consumption and risk of developing T2DM has been reported [66,77,78], with the highest risk associated with consumption of French fries. Muraki et al., in an analysis of data from three prospective cohort studies [66], reported that, for every three servings/week of boiled, mashed or baked potatoes there was an increased risk of T2DM (HR, 1.04; 95% CI 1.01–1.08), with a greater risk associated with French fries (HR, 1.19; 95% CI 1.13–1.25).

It has been suggested that the high glycaemic index (GI) of potatoes may be a contributory factor, as high GI diets have been associated with an increased risk of T2DM [79,80]. GI is a measure of how much a carbohydrate-containing food raises blood glucose in relation to a control (glucose):

$$GI = incremental\ area\ under\ the\ 2\ h\ glucose\ response\ curve\ (IAUC)\ for\ the\ test\ food\ \div\ IAUC\ for\ glucose\ \times 100$$

Foods with a GI > 70 are classed as high GI, whereas those with a GI < 55 are classed as low GI. Various factors affect the GI of the potato, such as variety, cooking method, and length of cooking. Shorter boiling times, in particular, may lead to incomplete gelatinization of the starch, with residual RS2 contributing to a lower GI. This is well demonstrated with the Carisma potato, which has been labelled low GI [81]. This is likely due to its higher onset of gelatinization temperature than other cultivars [82], as this would result in less extensive gelatinization, and therefore more resistant starch, when cooked for the same length of time as other varieties. Using GI as a predictor of a food's effect on blood glucose is also problematic. It is calculated based on consumption of a fixed amount of CHO, usually 50 g; it does not take portion size into account. Thus, a food may have a high GI but have little effect on blood glucose because the carbohydrate density is low, resulting in a small amount of carbohydrate being consumed in a standard portion. This has led to the suggestion that glycaemic load (GL) may give a better representation of the actual effect a food has on the glycaemic response as it considers portion size along with GI:

$$GL = GI \times amount\ of\ available\ CHO\ in\ a\ portion\ (g) \div 100$$

A GL less than 10 is considered low, with high GL categorized as a GL > 20. Typical GI and GL values, along with the amount of available CHO in a standard portion, for some common methods of preparing and serving potatoes are shown in Table 4. To put these values in context with other starchy CHO, boiled/steamed rice typically has a GI of 68–87 and a GL of 25–33 (150 g portion), depending on rice type and cooking time, whereas pasta has a GI of 51–61 and a GL of 24–29 (180 g portion) [83].

Table 4. Glycaemic index, glycaemic load, and available carbohydrate values for potatoes prepared according to domestic cooking methods.

Potato Variety and Cooking Method	Glycaemic Index	Glycaemic Load (150 g Portion)	Available CHO (g per 150 g Portion)
Charlotte (waxy), boiled 15 min	66	15	23
Nicola (waxy), boiled 15 min	58–59	9	16
Carisma (waxy), boiled 8–9 min	53	8	16
Desiree, boiled 35 min	101	17	17
Pontiac, boiled 35 min	88	16	18
Russet Burbank, unpeeled, microwaved for 18 min	77 ± 9	19	25
White with skin, baked	69	19	27
Instant mashed potato	79–97	16–19	20
Desiree, mashed	102	26	26
Pontiac, mashed	91	18	20
French fries, baked 15 min	64	21	32
Irish potato, peeled, fried in oil	70	21	30

Data taken from "International Tables of Glycemic Index and Glycemic Load Values: 2008" [83], except Carisma cultivar [81].

It appears from the reported GI values that GI alone cannot explain the association observed between French fries and T2DM risk, as French fries typically have a lower GI than other potato preparations. They do have a higher GL, which may partially explain the reported associations, however, other factors such as fat content and other unidentified, unhealthy lifestyle choices cannot be discounted. It should also be considered that potatoes are not usually eaten in isolation; other foods in the meal will affect the overall GI/GL of the meal. For example, serving a baked potato with cheese reduced the GI from 93 to 39 [84] and serving chicken breast, salad, and oil with mashed potato resulted in a reduction in GI from 108 to 54 compared to mashed potato served alone [85].

Furthermore, not all studies agree, with some reporting either no association [64,65,86] or an inverse association between potato consumption and development of T2DM [63,87]. Farhadnejad et al. reported a lower incidence of T2DM in those who consumed higher amounts of potatoes (55.5 g/day) compared to the lowest (7.3 g/day) consumption range [87]. A significant inverse association was observed for both total potato consumption and boiled potatoes with a trend observed for fried potatoes. These studies are summarized in Table 5.

A recent systematic review and meta-analysis [19] reported a slightly increased risk of T2DM (RR: 1.09, 95% CI 1.01, 1.18) for every 150 g/day increase in boiled, baked and mashed potatoes, with a stronger association reported for French fries (RR: 1.66, 95% CI 1.43, 1.94). The authors reported, however, that the quality of evidence was low for total potato consumption and moderate for French fries. The contradictory and limited evidence from the epidemiology does not support any recommendation to reduce total potato intake, with the possible exception of French fries, at this time.

Table 5. Summary of cohort studies investigating associations between potato consumption and T2DM risk.

Reference	Study Type; Follow-Up/Duration	n (%F); BMI (kg/m²); Age (years); Criteria	Exposure; Assessment Method	Results	Potato Categories	Comments
Salmerón et al., 1997 [88]	Cohort (six years)	42,759 (0%); normal weight to obese; 40–75 years; Energy intake 400–4200 kcal/day	Habitual diet FFQ (131 items)	Consumption of French fries, but not total potato intake, was associated with increased risk of T2DM	Cooked potato; French fries	Data from the Health Professionals Follow-up Study [62]
Salmerón et al., 1997 [78]	Cohort (six years)	65,173 (100%); normal weight to obese; 40–65 years; Energy intake 600–3502 kcal/day	Habitual diet FFQ (134 items)	Intake of both total potatoes and French fries was associated with increased risk of T2DM	Cooked potato; French fries	Data from the Nurses' Health Study [61]
Hodge et al., 2004 [64]	Cohort (four years)	31,641 (59%); normal weight to obese; 27–75 years	Habitual diet FFQ (121 items)	Total potato intake was not associated with risk of T2DM Total carbohydrate intake was inversely associated with T2DM incidence High dietary GI was associated with increased risk of T2DM	Total potato intake	Data from The Melbourne Collaborative Cohort Study [89]
Liu et al., 2004 [65]	Cohort (8 to 9 years)	38,018 (100%); normal weight to obese; ≥45 years	Habitual diet FFQ (131 items)	Total potato intake was not associated with risk of T2DM	Total potato intake	Data from the Women's Health Study [90]
Halton et al., 2006 [77]	Cohort (20 years)	84,555 (100%); normal weight to obese; 30–55 years at baseline; Energy intake 500–3500 kcal/day	Habitual diet FFQ (61 items at baseline, rising to 131 items), repeated assessment	Baked or mashed potato intake was associated with risk of T2DM in obese women only Intake of French fries was associated with increased risk of T2DM for all women	French fries; Baked or mashed	Data from the Nurses' Health Study [61] Potato and French fries consumption patterns did not change over time

Table 5. *Cont.*

Reference	Study Type; Follow-Up/Duration	n (%F); BMI (kg/m²); Age (years); Criteria	Exposure; Assessment Method	Results	Potato Categories	Comments
Villegas et al., 2007 [63]	Cohort (4.6 years)	64,227 (100%); normal weight to obese; 40–70 years	Habitual diet FFQ (77 food items/groups)	Potato consumption associated with lower risk of T2DM	Total potato intake	Data from the Shanghai Women's Health Study [91] Study population did not consume much potato (median intake 8.1 g/day); their main CHO was rice
Von Ruesten et al., 2013 [86]	Cohort (eight years)	23,531 (61%); normal weight to obese; 35–65 years Energy intake 800–6000 kcal/day	Habitual diet FFQ (148 food items)	No associations between potato or fried potato consumption and T2DM risk	Potatoes (potatoes, mashed, potato dumpling, potato salad); Fried potatoes (French fries, croquettes, fried potatoes, potato pancake)	Data from the EPIC Potsdam Study [92]
Muraki et al., 2016 [66]	Three cohorts (four years)	199,181 (80%) Normal weight to obese; 40–75 years;	Habitual diet FFQ (61/131 items)	Consumption of potatoes, especially French fries was associated with increased risk of T2DM	Total potato intake; Boiled, baked or mashed; French fries	Data from the Nurses' Health Study I and II [61] and the Health Professionals Follow-up Study [62]
Farhadnejad et al., 2018 [87]	Cohort (six years)	1981 (53.8%) normal weight to obese 38.9 ± 13.4 years		Total potato and boiled potato consumption both associated with lower risk of T2DM	Total potato intake; Boiled potatoes;Fried potatoes	Data from the Tehran Lipid and Glucose Study [93] Median intake 22.4 g/day

3.3. Cardiovascular Disease (CVD) and CVD Risk Factors

Several cohort studies have examined associations between potato consumption and CVD and its risk factors; a summary of these studies is presented in Table 6. Larsson et al., investigated associations between potato consumption and risk of myocardial infarction, heart failure, stroke or mortality from CVD in Swedish men and women [94]. They found no significant association between total potato intake and risk of major CVD event or mortality from CVD. Nor did they report any associations between boiled, fried, or French-fried potato consumption and any CVD outcome. In a large cohort study investigating the relationship between fruit and vegetable consumption and risk of ischemic stroke, total potato consumption was not associated with ischemic stroke risk, although individual preparation methods were not explored [95].

Studies examining the relationship between hypertension (HT) and potato intake have reported mixed results. In a Chinese cohort, total potato consumption, stir-fried and non-stir-fried potato consumption were all associated with increased risk of developing HT [96]. However, when non-potato-consumers were excluded from the analysis, higher intakes of total potato and stir-fried potato were associated with lower risk of HT. Borgi et al. also reported an association between total potato consumption and HT for those consuming ≥ 1 serving/day and an increased risk of HT for those consuming ≥ 4 servings/week of French fries. Consuming ≥ 4 servings/week of boiled, baked and mashed potatoes was associated with increased HT risk in women but not men [97]. In contrast to these two studies, Hu et al. reported no association between total potato consumption and change in blood pressure (BP) or HT risk in either the PREDIMED or SUN cohort over four years [98].

In their systematic review and dose-response meta-analysis, Schwingshackl et al. examined associations between potato consumption and risk of chronic disease [19]. They reported no association between total potato consumption and risk of coronary heart disease or stroke, even for the highest total potato intake (150 g/day). However, high consumption of French fries (150 g/day), but not other preparation methods (boiled, mashed or baked) was associated with increased risk of HT. Again, the authors noted that quality of evidence was low for boiled, mashed, and baked potatoes and moderate for French fries. They also stated that the studies' results were confounded by only reporting total potato consumption in the majority of cases.

There have been few interventional-type studies examining the effect of potato consumption on CVD risk factors. One explanation may be that any intervention examining these measures, would have to be carried out over a longer period of time, unlike, for example, those investigating effects on postprandial glucose metabolism. Furthermore, in order to maintain energy balance, an intervention would have to remove some other component of the diet in order to incorporate potatoes. This in itself would confound the results, because any effect may be the result of what has been removed, rather than what has been added. If potatoes were added to the diet, without removing anything then overall energy intake could increase, potentially resulting in weight gain, although this was not observed in one of the studies discussed here [99].

Arterial stiffness is an independent risk factor for the development of CVD [100]. Tsang et al. explored the effects of an anthocyanin-rich potato, Purple Majesty (PM), on pulse wave velocity (PWV), a clinical measure of arterial stiffness [101]. They found that consumption of 200 g/day of PM potatoes, for 14 days, significantly reduced carotid-femoral PWV, in healthy individuals, whereas consumption of an equivalent amount of white potato had no effect. They reported no change in blood pressure, fasted glucose, insulin, triacylglycerol or HDL-, LDL-, and total cholesterol for either potato variety. They hypothesized that anthocyanins in the PM potatoes contributed to the observed results as anthocyanin intake has been associated with reduced arterial stiffness [102].

Vinson et al. also investigated the effects of the PM potato in two separate trials [99]. In an acute study, they investigated the effects of the PM potato on plasma antioxidant activity and urinary polyphenols compared to a control biscuit containing an equivalent amount of potato starch. Plasma antioxidant capacity, measured by ferric reducing antioxidant power, was non-significantly higher following the PM potato meal and urinary polyphenols were increased by 92% ($p = 0.09$ for trend) following PM consumption, compared to controls. Urinary polyphenols are a marker for polyphenol intake, with higher concentrations associated with reduced risk of HT [103]. In a second study, they investigated the effect of PM potatoes on BP in 18 individuals, 14 of whom were hypertensive, of which 13 were taking antihypertensive medication. In this crossover trial they compared the effects of four weeks consumption of PM potatoes at lunch and dinner with no potatoes for the same time period. They reported a significant (4 mmHg) reduction in diastolic blood pressure (DBP) following PM consumption, with no significant effects on systolic blood pressure (SBP), body weight, glucose, HDL- or total cholesterol and triacylglycerol. These interventional studies are reported in Table 7.

In summary, the epidemiology generally reports no associations between potato consumption and the risk of CVD, with the possible exception of HT, where some, but not all, have reported increased risk from both total potato consumption and French fries. Potatoes are a rich source of potassium, which has been associated with reduced risk of CVD [104], however, French fries are often consumed with salt which could attenuate any beneficial effect of potassium as high salt intake is associated with HT and could increase the risk of CVD [105]. In contrast, interventional studies have demonstrated some beneficial effects from an anthocyanin-rich pigmented potato variety on PWV and DBP. Whilst these results are interesting, it should be noted that these results are confined to a single pigmented potato cultivar and no effect on PWV was observed following consumption of white potatoes. Clearly, further research is required, utilizing different, commonly consumed potato cultivars, before conclusions can be drawn.

Table 6. Summary of cohort studies investigating associations between potato consumption and cardiovascular disease.

Reference	Study Type; Follow-Up/Duration	n (%F); BMI; Age (years); Criteria	Exposure; Assessment Method	Results	Cooking Methods	Comments
Joshipura et al., 1999 [95]	Two cohorts (NHS: eight years; HPFS: 14 years)	114,276 (66%); mean BMI 24.3–25.45 kg/m²; M: 40–75 years; F: 34–59 years; CVD-, cancer- and T2DM-free at baseline	Habitual diet FFQ (61/131 items)	No association between potato consumption and ischemic stroke risk	Not Specified	Data from the Nurses' Health Study I and II [61] and the Health Professionals Follow-up Study [62]
Larsson et al., 2016 [94]	Two cohorts (13 years)	69,313 (47.3%); M: 45–79 years; F: 49–83 years; CVD-, cancer- and T2DM-free at baseline	Habitual diet FFQ (96 items)	Neither total potato consumption nor any individual cooking method was associated with risk of major CVD events (myocardial infarction, heart failure, stroke) or mortality from CVD	Total potatoes; Boiled potatoes; Fried potatoes; French fries	Data from the Cohort of Swedish Men and the Swedish Mammography Cohort Median total potato consumption 4.5–5.5 times/week, mainly from boiled potatoes (3.5 times/week)
Borgi et al., 2016 [97]	Three cohorts (max 24–34 years) Health questionnaires every two years	187,453 (80.4%) Non-hypertensive at baseline BMI 20.9–31.8 kg/m² F: 25–55 years M: 40–75 years	Habitual diet FFQ (61/131 items)	≥1 serving/day of potato (all types) associated with increased risk of hypertension, compared to <1 serving/month ≥4 servings/week of boiled, baked or mashed potatoes associated with increased risk of hypertension in women but not men, compared to <1 serving/month ≥4 servings/week French fries associated with increased risk of hypertension, compared to <1 serving/month	Total potato intake; Boiled, baked or mashed; French fries; Potato chips	Data from the Nurses' Health Study I and II [61] and the Health Professionals Follow-up Study [62]

Table 6. *Cont.*

Reference	Study Type; Follow-Up/Duration	n (%F); BMI; Age (years); Criteria	Exposure; Assessment Method	Results	Cooking Methods	Comments
Hu et al., 2017 [98]	2 cohorts 4 and 6–7 years follow-ups)	PREDIMED: 6940 55–80 years CVD free, but at high risk (T2DM or ≥3 of: smoking, hypertension, high LDL, low HDL, overweight, family history of CVD) SUN project: 13,837 M: 42.7 ± 13.3 years F: 35.1 ± 10.7 years	PREDIMED: Mediterranean diet FFQ (137 items) SUN: Habitual diet FFQ (136 items)	Total potato intake not associated with change in BP or incidence of hypertension over 4 years	PREDIMED: Potato chips (crisps), homemade fries, cooked or boiled potatoes SUN: Fried potatoes, cooked or roasted potatoes	Data from the PREDIMED [106] and SUN [107] cohorts
Huang et al., 2018 [96]	Cohort Mean 11.3 years	11,763 (54.6%) 20–93 years No hypertension, infarction or diabetes at baseline	Habitual diet, three day dietary recall	Sweet potato associated with HT in urban residents Potatoes (p = 0.1225), stir-fried potatoes (p = 0.2168) and non-stir-fried potatoes (p = 0.0456) all associated with HT When non-potato consumers were excluded, higher consumption of total potatoes and stir-fried potatoes associated with lower risk of HT	Total potatoes; Sweet potatoes; Stir-fried potatoes; Non stir-fried potatoes	Data from the China Health and Nutrition Survey [108] Urban residents more likely to consume sweet potato in snack form (fried chips, sugar-cured fries) Rice was the main starchy CHO in the diet, potato consumption was much lower than Western countries; potatoes were more often consumed as a side dish

HDL: high density lipoprotein cholesterol; HPFS: Health Professionals' Follow-up Study; HT: hypertension; LDL: low density lipoprotein cholesterol; NHS: Nurses' Health Study; PREDIMED: PREvención con DIeta MEDiterránea; SUN: Seguimiento University of Navarra.

Table 7. Summary of intervention studies investigating effects of potato consumption on cardiovascular disease risk factors.

Reference	Study Type; Follow-up/Duration	n (F); BMI; age (years); Criteria	Exposure; Assessment Method	Results	Cooking Methods	Potato Type	Comments
Vinson et al., 2012 [99]	1. RCT: Single meal 2. Supplementation: Crossover (four weeks)	8 (1); 5 normal weight, 2 overweight, 1 obese; 23 ± 9 years; Healthy 18 (11); 5 normal weight, 6 overweight, 7 obese; 54 ± 10 years; 14/18 hypertensive; 13/18 taking BP lowering medication	6–8 small potatoes (~138 g), microwaved; Biscuit containing equivalent amount of potato starch served as control; Plasma samples (0, 0.5, 1, 2, 4, and 8 h) 24 h urine collection (urine polyphenols), pre- and post-study 6–8 small potatoes, microwaved, twice a day (lunch and dinner); No potatoes consumed on alternate arm; (BP, body weight, glucose, HDL, TAG, TC) pre/post trial	Non-significantly lower plasma antioxidant capacity following control meal, compared to potatoes ($p = 0.11$) Urine polyphenols increased by 92% following potato consumption and decreased by 3.5% following control biscuit ($p = 0.09$ for trend) 4 mmHg reduction in DBP following potato supplementation ($p < 0.01$); No effect on plasma glucose, HbA1c or lipids No effect on SBP or body weight	Microwaved, consumed with skins	Purple majesty (pigmented potato)	Participants followed a low polyphenol diet for three days prior to the acute study
Tsang et al., 2018 [101]	RCT (14 days, with seven days washout between treatments)	14 (8F); BMI: 19.4–31.2 kg/m² (11 normal weight, 2 overweight, 1 obese) 20–55 years; Healthy; Normotensive	200 g/day of PM potato versus white potato control; PWV, BP, bodyweight Plasma samples (TAG, HDL, LDL, TC, CRP, insulin, glucose)	Consumption of PM potatoes, but not white potatoes, significantly reduced PWV; No changes in any other measure for either PM or white potato	Boiled with skin	Purple Majesty (PM)	PM potatoes contain significantly higher amounts of anthocyanins than white potatoes (control); Participants were forbidden certain high-polyphenol foods and drinks and advised to limit fruit, vegetable and potato intake during the study

CRP: C-reactive protein; TAG: triacylglycerol; TC: total cholesterol.

Nutrients **2018**, *10*, 1764

4. Conclusions

We have reviewed substantive literature that has investigated the health consequences of consuming potatoes. We have found that authors have not been able to sufficiently take into account the cooking method, which is a major determinant of nutrient content of the potato as eaten. In addition, no studies measured the RS content. However, evidence did suggest a positive association between obesity, risk of T2DM, and CVD and the consumption of French fries/'chips' in the UK. A limited number of studies investigated satiety/energy intake after the consumption of potatoes, and made specific comparisons with other starchy CHO foods. Isoenergetic portions of potatoes, particularly boiled potatoes, appeared to be more satiating when eaten in isolation. Furthermore, studies suggest that less energy is consumed if potato rather than pasta or rice is eaten as part of a mixed meal. Potatoes are a valuable source of several key nutrients and the evidence reviewed here supports their inclusion in a healthy balanced diet, in line with current dietary guidelines.

There are always limitations and caveats for determining the diet of free-living individuals but assessing the nutritional impact of potatoes consumed by their quantity alone is particularly misleading. We should, therefore, be aware of the limitations of epidemiological studies in this respect and indeed, further research, particularly randomized controlled trials, is required to understand the role of food preparation on the nutrient content of potatoes, particularly in regard to resistant starch content.

Summary points:

- The nutritional content of a medium-sized baked potato weighing 200 g can provide a significant contribution to vitamin and micronutrient needs, containing almost half of the UK daily RNI for a man for vitamin C and vitamin B6, 30% for potassium, 28% for folate, 24% for iron, and 18% for magnesium.
- The total fibre content of 4.4 g is 15% of the 30 g per day recommended for an adult. However, these figures are markedly altered by the cooking method, for example, the vitamin C content would be 50% higher in a microwaved potato, and the iron content would be reduced by over 70%.
- A major limitation when assessing the nutrient quality of the potato is that the RS content of potatoes is not included in the gold standard AOAC method for total fibre. Therefore, the total fibre content of potatoes listed in food databases underestimates actual total fibre content, and consequently the nutritional value.
- The interaction between meal components, such as starch and lipid, is a somewhat under-explored but particularly exciting and important area, as there is the potential to change the RS starch content of a meal by making simple changes to cooking methods. Considering other meal components and portion size is also important with respect to the overall GL of a meal.

Author Contributions: All authors contributed to the writing of the manuscript.

Funding: This research was funded by the Biotechnology and Biological Sciences Research Council Diet and Health Research Industry Club (BBSRC DRINC) grant number BB/N021274/1.

Conflicts of Interest: The authors declare no conflict of interest.

References

1. Scientific Advisory Committee on Nutrition. *SACN Carbohydrates and Health Report*; Public Health England: London, UK, 2015.
2. Seidelmann, S.B.; Claggett, B.; Cheng, S.; Henglin, M.; Shah, A.; Steffen, L.M.; Folsom, A.R.; Rimm, E.B.; Willett, W.C.; Solomon, S.D. Dietary carbohydrate intake and mortality: A prospective cohort study and meta-analysis. *Lancet Public Health* **2018**. [CrossRef]

3. Mann, J.; Cummings, J.H.; Englyst, H.N.; Key, T.; Liu, S.; Riccardi, G.; Summerbell, C.; Uauy, R.; van Dam, R.M.; Venn, B.; et al. FAO/WHO Scientific Update on carbohydrates in human nutrition: Conclusions. *Eur. J. Clin. Nutr.* **2007**, *61*, S132–S137. [CrossRef] [PubMed]
4. Eat Well—NHS.UK. Available online: https://www.nhs.uk/live-well/eat-well/ (accessed on 6 August 2018).
5. Haverkort, A.J.; de Ruijter, F.J.; van Evert, F.K.; Conijn, J.G.; Rutgers, B. Worldwide Sustainability Hotspots in Potato Cultivation. 1. Identification and Mapping. *Potato Res.* **2013**, *56*, 343–353. [CrossRef]
6. Thomas, G.; Sansonetti, G. *Food and Agriculture Organization of the United Nations. New Light on a Hidden Treasure: International Year of the Potato 2008, an End-of-Year Review*; Food and Agriculture Organization of the United Nations: Rome, Italy, 2009.
7. Riley, H. Potato consumption in the UK—Why is "meat and two veg" no longer the traditional British meal? *Nutr. Bull.* **2010**, *35*, 320–331. [CrossRef]
8. Burlingame, B.; Mouillé, B.; Charrondière, R. Nutrients, bioactive non-nutrients and anti-nutrients in potatoes. *J. Food Compos. Anal.* **2009**, *22*, 494–502. [CrossRef]
9. Barrell, P.J.; Meiyalaghan, S.; Jacobs, J.M.E.; Conner, A.J. Applications of biotechnology and genomics in potato improvement. *Plant Biotechnol. J.* **2013**, *11*, 907–920. [CrossRef] [PubMed]
10. Food and Agriculture Organization of the United Nations. FAOSTAT. Available online: http://www.fao.org/faostat/en/#home (accessed on 23 August 2018).
11. Ranum, P.; Peña-Rosas, J.P.; Garcia-Casal, M.N. Global maize production, utilization, and consumption. *Ann. N. Y. Acad. Sci.* **2014**, *1312*, 105–112. [CrossRef] [PubMed]
12. McCollum, E.V.; Simmonds, N.; Parsons, H.T. The dietary properties of the potato. *J. Biol. Chem.* **1918**, *36*, 197–210.
13. Gibson, S.; Kurilich, A.C. The nutritional value of potatoes and potato products in the UK diet. *Nutr. Bull.* **2013**, *38*, 389–399. [CrossRef]
14. Family Food 2016/17: Purchases—GOV.UK. Available online: https://www.gov.uk/government/publications/family-food-201617/purchases (accessed on 1 October 2018).
15. Attah, A.O.; Braaten, T.; Skeie, G. Change in potato consumption among Norwegian women 1998–2005-The Norwegian Women and Cancer study (NOWAC). *PLoS ONE* **2017**, *12*, e0179441. [CrossRef] [PubMed]
16. Churuangsuk, C.; Kherouf, M.; Combet, E.; Lean, M. Low-carbohydrate diets for overweight and obesity: A systematic review of the systematic reviews. *Obes. Rev.* **2018**. [CrossRef] [PubMed]
17. Camire, M.E.; Kubow, S.; Donnelly, D.J. Potatoes and Human Health. *Crit. Rev. Food Sci. Nutr.* **2009**, *49*, 823–840. [CrossRef] [PubMed]
18. Borch, D.; Juul-Hindsgaul, N.; Veller, M.; Astrup, A.; Jaskolowski, J.; Raben, A. Potatoes and risk of obesity, type 2 diabetes, and cardiovascular disease in apparently healthy adults: A systematic review of clinical intervention and observational studies. *Am. J. Clin. Nutr.* **2016**, *104*, 489–498. [CrossRef] [PubMed]
19. Schwingshackl, L.; Schwedhelm, C.; Hoffmann, G.; Boeing, H. Potatoes and risk of chronic disease: A systematic review and dose–response meta-analysis. *Eur. J. Nutr.* **2018**. [CrossRef] [PubMed]
20. McGill, C.R.; Kurilich, A.C.; Davignon, J. The role of potatoes and potato components in cardiometabolic health: A review. *Ann. Med.* **2013**, *45*, 467–473. [CrossRef] [PubMed]
21. King, J.C.; Slavin, J.L. White potatoes, human health, and dietary guidance. *Adv. Nutr.* **2013**, *4*, 393S–401S. [CrossRef] [PubMed]
22. Tian, J.; Chen, J.; Ye, X.; Chen, S. Health benefits of the potato affected by domestic cooking: A review. *Food Chem.* **2016**, *202*, 165–175. [CrossRef] [PubMed]
23. Zeeman, S.C.; Kossmann, J.; Smith, A.M. Starch: Its Metabolism, Evolution, and Biotechnological Modification in Plants. *Annu. Rev. Plant Biol.* **2010**, *61*, 209–234. [CrossRef] [PubMed]
24. Lewosz, J.; Reda, S.; Ryś, D.; Jastrzębski, K.; Piątek, I. Chemical composition of potato tubers and their resistance on mechanical damage. *Biul. Inst. Ziemn.* **1976**, *18*, 31–46.
25. Kita, A. The influence of potato chemical composition on crisp texture. *Food Chem.* **2002**, *76*, 173–179. [CrossRef]
26. Public Health England. *National Diet and Nutrition Survey: Results from Years 7 and 8 (Combined) of the Rolling Programme (2014/2015 to 2015/2016)*; Public Health England: London, UK, 2018.
27. Slavin, J.L. Carbohydrates, Dietary Fiber, and Resistant Starch in White Vegetables: Links to Health Outcomes. *Adv. Nutr.* **2013**, *4*, 351S–355S. [CrossRef] [PubMed]

28. Li, Y.-D.; Xu, T.-C.; Xiao, J.-X.; Zong, A.-Z.; Qiu, B.; Jia, M.; Liu, L.-N.; Liu, W. Efficacy of potato resistant starch prepared by microwave–toughening treatment. *Carbohydr. Polym.* **2018**, *192*, 299–307. [CrossRef] [PubMed]

29. Zhao, X.; Andersson, M.; Andersson, R. Resistant starch and other dietary fiber components in tubers from a high-amylose potato. *Food Chem.* **2018**, *251*, 58–63. [CrossRef] [PubMed]

30. Yang, Y.; Achaerandio, I.; Pujolà, M. Effect of the intensity of cooking methods on the nutritional and physical properties of potato tubers. *Food Chem.* **2016**, *197*, 1301–1310. [CrossRef] [PubMed]

31. Goñi, I.; Bravo, L.; Larrauri, J.A.; Calixto, F.S. Resistant starch in potatoes deep-fried in olive oil. *Food Chem.* **1997**, *59*, 269–272. [CrossRef]

32. Raatz, S.K.; Idso, L.; Johnson, L.K.; Jackson, M.I.; Combs, G.F. Resistant starch analysis of commonly consumed potatoes: Content varies by cooking method and service temperature but not by variety. *Food Chem.* **2016**, *208*, 297–300. [CrossRef] [PubMed]

33. Kawai, K.; Takato, S.; Ueda, M.; Ohnishi, N.; Viriyarattanasak, C.; Kajiwara, K. Effects of fatty acid and emulsifier on the complex formation and in vitro digestibility of gelatinized potato starch. *Int. J. Food Prop.* **2017**, *20*, 1500–1510. [CrossRef]

34. Singh Yadav, B. Effect of frying, baking and storage conditions on resistant starch content of foods. *Br. Food J.* **2011**, *113*, 710–719. [CrossRef]

35. British Nutrition Foundation. Protein. Available online: https://www.nutrition.org.uk/nutritionscience/nutrients-food-and-ingredients/protein.html (accessed on 2 October 2018).

36. Helle, S.; Bray, F.; Verbeke, J.; Devassine, S.; Courseaux, A.; Facon, M.; Tokarski, C.; Rolando, C.; Szydlowski, N. Proteome Analysis of Potato Starch Reveals the Presence of New Starch Metabolic Proteins as Well as Multiple Protease Inhibitors. *Front. Plant Sci.* **2018**, *9*, 746. [CrossRef] [PubMed]

37. USDA Food Composition Databases. Available online: https://ndb.nal.usda.gov/ndb/ (accessed on 6 August 2018).

38. Bethke, P.C.; Jansky, S.H. The Effects of Boiling and Leaching on the Content of Potassium and Other Minerals in Potatoes. *J. Food Sci.* **2008**, *73*, H80–H85. [CrossRef] [PubMed]

39. Finglas, P.M.; Faulks, R.M. Nutritional composition of UK retail potatoes, both raw and cooked. *J. Sci. Food Agric.* **1984**, *35*, 1347–1356. [CrossRef]

40. Han, J.-S.; Kozukue, N.; Young, K.-S.; Lee, K.-R.; Friedman, M. Distribution of Ascorbic Acid in Potato Tubers and in Home-Processed and Commercial Potato Foods. *J. Agric. Food Chem.* **2004**, *52*, 6516–6521. [CrossRef] [PubMed]

41. Lachman, J.; Hamouz, K. Red and purple coloured potatoes as a significant antioxidant source in human nutrition—A review. *Plant Soil Environ.* **2005**, *51*, 477–482. [CrossRef]

42. Chu, Y.-F.; Sun, J.; Wu, X.; Liu, R.H. Antioxidant and Antiproliferative Activities of Common Vegetables. *J. Agric. Food Chem.* **2002**, *50*, 6910–6916. [CrossRef] [PubMed]

43. Kyoung Chun, O.; Kim, D.-O.; Smith, N.; Schroeder, D.; Taek Han, J.; Yong Lee, C. Daily consumption of phenolics and total antioxidant capacity from fruit and vegetables in the American diet. *J. Sci. Food Agric.* **2005**, *85*, 1715–1724. [CrossRef]

44. Manach, C.; Scalbert, A.; Morand, C.; Rémésy, C.; Jiménez, L. Polyphenols: Food sources and bioavailability. *Am. J. Clin. Nutr.* **2004**, *79*, 727–747. [CrossRef] [PubMed]

45. Gordon, M.H. Significance of Dietary Antioxidants for Health. *Int. J. Mol. Sci.* **2011**, *13*, 173–179. [CrossRef] [PubMed]

46. Andersson, M.; Melander, M.; Pojmark, P.; Larsson, H.; Bülow, L.; Hofvander, P. Targeted gene suppression by RNA interference: An efficient method for production of high-amylose potato lines. *J. Biotechnol.* **2006**, *123*, 137–148. [CrossRef] [PubMed]

47. Burgos, G.; Muñoa, L.; Sosa, P.; Bonierbale, M.; zum Felde, T.; Díaz, C. In vitro Bioaccessibility of Lutein and Zeaxanthin of Yellow Fleshed Boiled Potatoes. *Plant Foods Hum. Nutr.* **2013**, *68*, 385–390. [CrossRef] [PubMed]

48. Brown, C.R. Antioxidants in potato. *Am. J. Potato Res.* **2005**, *82*, 163–172. [CrossRef]

49. Stushnoff, C.; Holm, D.; Thompson, M.D.; Jiang, W.; Thompson, H.J.; Joyce, N.I.; Wilson, P. Antioxidant Properties of Cultivars and Selections from the Colorado Potato Breeding Program. *Am. J. Potato Res.* **2008**, *85*, 267–276. [CrossRef]

50. Chitchumroonchokchai, C.; Diretto, G.; Parisi, B.; Giuliano, G.; Failla, M.L. Potential of golden potatoes to improve vitamin A and vitamin E status in developing countries. *PLoS ONE* **2017**, *12*, e0187102. [CrossRef] [PubMed]

51. Külen, O.; Stushnoff, C.; Holm, D.G. Effect of cold storage on total phenolics content, antioxidant activity and vitamin C level of selected potato clones. *J. Sci. Food Agric.* **2013**, *93*, 2437–2444. [CrossRef] [PubMed]

52. Alamar, M.C.; Tosetti, R.; Landahl, S.; Bermejo, A.; Terry, L.A. Assuring Potato Tuber Quality during Storage: A Future Perspective. *Front. Plant Sci.* **2017**, *8*, 2034. [CrossRef] [PubMed]

53. Öhrvik, V.; Mattisson, I.; Wretling, S.; Åstrand, C. *Potato—Analysis of Nutrients*; National Food Administration: Uppsala, Sweden, 2010.

54. Mozaffarian, D.; Hao, T.; Rimm, E.B.; Willett, W.C.; Hu, F.B. Changes in Diet and Lifestyle and Long-Term Weight Gain in Women and Men. *N. Engl. J. Med.* **2011**, *364*, 2392–2404. [CrossRef] [PubMed]

55. French, S.A.; Jeffery, R.W.; Forster, J.L.; McGovern, P.G.; Kelder, S.H.; Baxter, J.E. Predictors of weight change over two years among a population of working adults: The Healthy Worker Project. *Int. J. Obes. Relat. Metab. Disord.* **1994**, *18*, 145–154. [PubMed]

56. Linde, J.A.; Utter, J.; Jeffery, R.W.; Sherwood, N.E.; Pronk, N.P.; Boyle, R.G. Specific food intake, fat and fiber intake, and behavioral correlates of BMI among overweight and obese members of a managed care organization. *Int. J. Behav. Nutr. Phys. Act.* **2006**, *3*, 42. [CrossRef] [PubMed]

57. Halkjær, J.; Tjønneland, A.; Overvad, K.; Sørensen, T.I.A. Dietary Predictors of 5-Year Changes in Waist Circumference. *J. Am. Diet. Assoc.* **2009**, *109*, 1356–1366. [CrossRef] [PubMed]

58. Halkjaer, J.; Sørensen, T.I.A.; Tjønneland, A.; Togo, P.; Holst, C.; Heitmann, B.L. Food and drinking patterns as predictors of 6-year BMI-adjusted changes in waist circumference. *Br. J. Nutr.* **2004**, *92*, 735–748. [CrossRef] [PubMed]

59. Jeffery, R.W.; Forster, J.L.; French, S.A.; Kelder, S.H.; Lando, H.A.; McGovern, P.G.; Jacobs, D.R., Jr.; Baxter, J.E. The Healthy Worker Project: A work-site intervention for weight control and smoking cessation. *Am. J. Public Health* **1993**, *83*, 395–401. [CrossRef] [PubMed]

60. Tjønneland, A.; Olsen, A.; Boll, K.; Stripp, C.; Christensen, J.; Engholm, G.; Overvad, K. Study design, exposure variables, and socioeconomic determinants of participation in Diet, Cancer and Health: A population-based prospective cohort study of 57,053 men and women in Denmark. *Scand. J. Public Health* **2007**, *5*, 432–441. [CrossRef] [PubMed]

61. Nurses' Health Study. Available online: http://www.nurseshealthstudy.org/ (accessed on 1 August 2018).

62. Health Professionals Follow-Up Study. Available online: https://sites.sph.harvard.edu/hpfs/ (accessed on 1 August 2018).

63. Villegas, R.; Liu, S.; Gao, Y.-T.; Yang, G.; Li, H.; Zheng, W.; Shu, X.O. Prospective Study of Dietary Carbohydrates, Glycemic Index, Glycemic Load, and Incidence of Type 2 Diabetes Mellitus in Middle-aged Chinese Women. *Arch. Intern. Med.* **2007**, *167*, 2310–2316. [CrossRef] [PubMed]

64. Hodge, A.M.; English, D.R.; O'Dea, K.; Giles, G.G. Glycemic index and dietary fiber and the risk of type 2 diabetes. *Diabetes Care* **2004**, *27*, 2701–2706. [CrossRef] [PubMed]

65. Liu, S.; Serdula, M.; Janket, S.-J.; Cook, N.R.; Sesso, H.D.; Willett, W.C.; Manson, J.E.; Buring, J.E. A prospective study of fruit and vegetable intake and the risk of type 2 diabetes in women. *Diabetes Care* **2004**, *27*, 2993–2996. [CrossRef] [PubMed]

66. Muraki, I.; Rimm, E.B.; Willett, W.C.; Manson, J.E.; Hu, F.B.; Sun, Q. Potato Consumption and Risk of Type 2 Diabetes: Results from Three Prospective Cohort Studies. *Diabetes Care* **2016**, *39*, 376–384. [CrossRef] [PubMed]

67. Holt, S.H.; Brand Miller, J.C.; Petocz, P. Interrelationships among postprandial satiety, glucose and insulin responses and changes in subsequent food intake. *Eur. J. Clin. Nutr.* **1996**, *50*, 788–797. [PubMed]

68. Erdmann, J.; Hebeisen, Y.; Lippl, F.; Wagenpfeil, S.; Schusdziarra, V. Food intake and plasma ghrelin response during potato-, rice- and pasta-rich test meals. *Eur. J. Nutr.* **2007**, *46*, 196–203. [CrossRef] [PubMed]

69. Leeman, M.; Östman, E.; Björck, I. Glycaemic and satiating properties of potato products. *Eur. J. Clin. Nutr.* **2008**, *62*, 87–95. [CrossRef] [PubMed]

70. Geliebter, A.; Lee, M.I.-C.; Abdillahi, M.; Jones, J. Satiety following Intake of Potatoes and Other Carbohydrate Test Meals. *Ann. Nutr. Metab.* **2013**, *62*, 37–43. [CrossRef] [PubMed]

71. Akilen, R.; Deljoomanesh, N.; Hunschede, S.; Smith, C.E.; Arshad, M.U.; Kubant, R.; Anderson, G.H. The effects of potatoes and other carbohydrate side dishes consumed with meat on food intake, glycemia and satiety response in children. *Nutr. Diabetes* **2016**, *6*, e195. [CrossRef] [PubMed]

72. Diaz-Toledo, C.; Kurilich, A.C.; Re, R.; Wickham, M.S.J.; Chambers, L.C. Satiety Impact of Different Potato Products Compared to Pasta Control. *J. Am. Coll. Nutr.* **2016**, *35*, 537–543. [CrossRef] [PubMed]

73. Geliebter, A. Gastric distension and gastric capacity in relation to food intake in humans. *Physiol. Behav.* **1988**, *44*, 665–668. [CrossRef]

74. Holt, S.H.; Miller, J.C.; Petocz, P.; Farmakalidis, E. A satiety index of common foods. *Eur. J. Clin. Nutr.* **1995**, *49*, 675–690. [PubMed]

75. Rolls, B.J.; Bell, E.A.; Thorwart, M.L. Water incorporated into a food but not served with a food decreases energy intake in lean women. *Am. J. Clin. Nutr.* **1999**, *70*, 448–455. [CrossRef] [PubMed]

76. Foster-Powell, K.; Miller, J.B. International tables of glycemic index. *Am. J. Clin. Nutr.* **1995**, *62*, 871S–890S. [CrossRef] [PubMed]

77. Halton, T.L.; Willett, W.C.; Liu, S.; Manson, J.E.; Stampfer, M.J.; Hu, F.B. Potato and French fry consumption and risk of type 2 diabetes in women. *Am. J. Clin. Nutr.* **2006**, *83*, 284–290. [CrossRef] [PubMed]

78. Salmerón, J.; Manson, J.E.; Stampfer, M.J.; Colditz, G.A.; Wing, A.L.; Willett, W.C. Dietary fiber, glycemic load, and risk of non-insulin-dependent diabetes mellitus in women. *JAMA* **1997**, *277*, 472–477. [CrossRef] [PubMed]

79. Barclay, A.W.; Petocz, P.; McMillan-Price, J.; Flood, V.M.; Prvan, T.; Mitchell, P.; Mitchell, P.; Brand-Miller, J.C. Glycemic index, glycemic load, and chronic disease risk—A meta-analysis of observational studies. *Am. J. Clin Nutr.* **2008**, *87*, 627–637. [CrossRef] [PubMed]

80. Oba, S.; Nanri, A.; Kurotani, K.; Goto, A.; Kato, M.; Mizoue, T.; Noda, M.; Inoue, M.; Tsugane, S.; Japan Public Health Center-Based Prospective Study Group. Dietary glycemic index, glycemic load and incidence of type 2 diabetes in Japanese men and women: The Japan public health center-based prospective study. *Nutr. J.* **2013**, *12*, 165. [CrossRef] [PubMed]

81. Ek, K.L.; Wang, S.; Copeland, L.; Brand-Miller, J.C. Discovery of a low-glycaemic index potato and relationship with starch digestion in vitro. *Br. J. Nutr.* **2014**, *111*, 699–705. [CrossRef] [PubMed]

82. Lin Ek, K.; Wang, S.; Brand-Miller, J.; Copeland, L. Properties of starch from potatoes differing in glycemic index. *Food Funct.* **2014**, *5*, 2509–2515. [CrossRef] [PubMed]

83. Atkinson, F.S.; Foster-Powell, K.; Brand-Miller, J.C. International Tables of Glycemic Index and Glycemic Load Values: 2008. *Diabetes Care* **2008**, *31*, 2281–2283. [CrossRef] [PubMed]

84. Henry, C.J.; Lightowler, H.J.; Kendall, F.L.; Storey, M. The impact of the addition of toppings/fillings on the glycaemic response to commonly consumed carbohydrate foods. *Eur. J. Clin. Nutr.* **2006**, *60*, 763–769. [CrossRef] [PubMed]

85. Hätönen, K.A.; Virtamo, J.; Eriksson, J.G.; Sinkko, H.K. Protein and fat modify the glycaemic and insulinaemic responses to a mashed potato-based meal. *Br. J. Nutr.* **2011**, *2011 106*, 248–253. [CrossRef]

86. von Ruesten, A.; Feller, S.; Bergmann, M.M.; Boeing, H. Diet and risk of chronic diseases: Results from the first 8 years of follow-up in the EPIC-Potsdam study. *Eur. J. Clin. Nutr.* **2013**, *67*, 412–419. [CrossRef] [PubMed]

87. Farhadnejad, H.; Teymoori, F.; Asghari, G.; Mirmiran, P.; Azizi, F. The Association of Potato Intake with Risk for Incident Type 2 Diabetes in Adults. *Can. J. Diabetes* **2018**. [CrossRef] [PubMed]

88. Salmerón, J.; Ascherio, A.; Rimm, E.B.; Colditz, G.A.; Spiegelman, D.; Jenkins, D.J.; Stampfer, M.J.; Wing, A.L.; Willett, W.C. Dietary fiber, glycemic load, and risk of NIDDM in men. *Diabetes Care* **1997**, *20*, 545–550. [CrossRef] [PubMed]

89. Melbourne Collaborative Cohort Study. Available online: https://www.cancervic.org.au/research/epidemiology/health_2020/health2020-overview (accessed on 1 August 2018).

90. Women's Health Study. Available online: http://whs.bwh.harvard.edu/ (accessed on 1 August 2018).

91. Zheng, W.; Chow, W.-H.; Yang, G.; Jin, F.; Rothman, N.; Blair, A.; Li, H.L.; Wen, W.; Ji, B.T.; Li, Q.; et al. The Shanghai Women's Health Study: Rationale, Study Design, and Baseline Characteristics. *Am. J. Epidemiol.* **2005**, *162*, 1123–1131. [CrossRef] [PubMed]

92. EPIC Centres—GERMANY. Available online: http://epic.iarc.fr/centers/germany.php (accessed on 2 August 2018).

93. Hosseinpanah, F.; Rambod, M.; Reza Ghaffari, H.R.; Azizi, F. Predicting isolated postchallenge hyperglycaemia: A new approach; Tehran Lipid and Glucose Study (TLGS). *Diabet. Med.* **2006**, *23*, 982–989. [CrossRef] [PubMed]

94. Larsson, S.C.; Wolk, A. Potato consumption and risk of cardiovascular disease: 2 prospective cohort studies. *Am. J. Clin. Nutr.* **2016**, *104*, 1245–1252. [CrossRef] [PubMed]

95. Joshipura, K.J.; Ascherio, A.; Manson, J.E.; Stampfer, M.J.; Rimm, E.B.; Speizer, F.E.; Hennekens, C.H.; Spiegelman, D.; Willett, W.C. Fruit and vegetable intake in relation to risk of ischemic stroke. *JAMA* **1999**, *282*, 1233–1239. [CrossRef] [PubMed]

96. Huang, M.; Zhuang, P.; Jiao, J.; Wang, J.; Chen, X.; Zhang, Y. Potato consumption is prospectively associated with risk of hypertension: An 11.3-year longitudinal cohort study. *Clin Nutr.* **2018**. [CrossRef] [PubMed]

97. Borgi, L.; Rimm, E.B.; Willett, W.C.; Forman, J.P. Potato intake and incidence of hypertension: Results from three prospective US cohort studies. *BMJ* **2016**, *353*, i2351. [CrossRef] [PubMed]

98. Hu, E.A.; Martínez-González, M.A.; Salas-Salvadó, J.; Corella, D.; Ros, E.; Fitó, M.; Garcia-Rodriguez, A.; Estruch, R.; Arós, F.; Fiol, M.; et al. Potato Consumption Does Not Increase Blood Pressure or Incident Hypertension in 2 Cohorts of Spanish Adults. *J. Nutr.* **2017**, *147*, 2272–2281. [CrossRef] [PubMed]

99. Vinson, J.A.; Demkosky, C.A.; Navarre, D.A.; Smyda, M.A. High-Antioxidant Potatoes: Acute in Vivo Antioxidant Source and Hypotensive Agent in Humans after Supplementation to Hypertensive Subjects. *J. Agric. Food Chem.* **2012**, *60*, 6749–6754. [CrossRef] [PubMed]

100. Safar, M.E. Systolic blood pressure, pulse pressure and arterial stiffness as cardiovascular risk factors. *Curr. Opin. Nephrol. Hypertens.* **2001**, *10*, 257–261. [CrossRef] [PubMed]

101. Tsang, C.; Smail, N.F.; Almoosawi, S.; McDougall, G.J.M.; Al-Dujaili, E.A.S. Antioxidant Rich Potato Improves Arterial Stiffness in Healthy Adults. *Plant Foods Hum. Nutr.* **2018**, *73*, 203–208. [CrossRef] [PubMed]

102. Jennings, A.; Welch, A.A.; Fairweather-Tait, S.J.; Kay, C.; Minihane, A.-M.; Chowienczyk, P.; Jiang, B.; Cecelja, M.; Spector, T.; Macgregor, A.; et al. Higher anthocyanin intake is associated with lower arterial stiffness and central blood pressure in women. *Am. J. Clin. Nutr.* **2012**, *96*, 781–788. [CrossRef] [PubMed]

103. Medina-Remón, A.; Zamora-Ros, R.; Rotchés-Ribalta, M.; Andres-Lacueva, C.; Martínez-González, M.A.; Covas, M.I.; Corella, D.; Salas-Salvadó, J.; Gómez-Gracia, E.; Ruiz-Gutiérrez, V.; et al. Total polyphenol excretion and blood pressure in subjects at high cardiovascular risk. *Nutr. Metab. Cardiovasc. Dis.* **2011**, *21*, 323–331. [CrossRef] [PubMed]

104. Aburto, N.J.; Hanson, S.; Gutierrez, H.; Hooper, L.; Elliott, P.; Cappuccio, F.P. Effect of increased potassium intake on cardiovascular risk factors and disease: Systematic review and meta-analyses. *BMJ* **2013**, *346*, f1378. [CrossRef] [PubMed]

105. Baldo, M.P.; Rodrigues, S.L.; Mill, J.G. High salt intake as a multifaceted cardiovascular disease: New support from cellular and molecular evidence. *Heart Fail. Rev.* **2015**, *20*, 461–474. [CrossRef] [PubMed]

106. PREDIMED Trial. Available online: http://www.predimed.es/introduction.html (accessed on 16 August 2018).

107. Martínez-González, M.A. The SUN cohort study (Seguimiento University of Navarra). *Public Health Nutr.* **2006**, *9*, 127–131. [CrossRef] [PubMed]

108. China Health and Nutrition Survey (CHNS). Available online: http://www.cpc.unc.edu/projects/china (accessed on 16 August 2018).

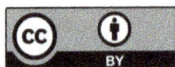

MDPI

St. Alban-Anlage 66

4052 Basel

Switzerland

Tel. +41 61 683 77 34

Fax +41 61 302 89 18

www.mdpi.com

Nutrients Editorial Office

E-mail: nutrients@mdpi.com

www.mdpi.com/journal/nutrients